UNDERSTANDING MENTAL DISORDERS

Your Guide to DSM-5-TR®

American Psychiatric Association

With Forewords by Abraham M. Nussbaum, M.D.
and Patrick J. Kennedy

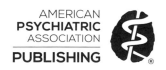

AMERICAN
PSYCHIATRIC
ASSOCIATION
PUBLISHING

Note: The publisher has tried to ensure that all information in this book is accurate at the time of publication and consistent with general psychiatric and medical standards, and that information concerning drugs is accurate at the time of publication and consistent with standards set by the U.S. Food and Drug Administration and the general medical community. As medical research and practice continue to advance, however, therapeutic standards may change. Moreover, specific situations may require a specific therapeutic response not included in this book. Readers should not use this guide for self-diagnosis or as a substitute for seeking and following the advice of a mental health care provider. Diagnosis and treatment of mental illness are individualized endeavors that require personal attention from a mental health care provider. Readers should seek the advice of physicians directly involved in their care or the care of a member of their family.

DSM, DSM-5, and DSM-5-TR are registered trademarks of the American Psychiatric Association (APA). Use of these terms is prohibited without permission of the APA.

Copyright © 2024 American Psychiatric Association
ALL RIGHTS RESERVED. Unless authorized in writing by the APA, no part of this book may be reproduced or used in a manner inconsistent with the APA's copyright. This prohibition applies to unauthorized uses or reproductions in any form, including electronic applications.

Manufactured in the United States of America on acid-free paper
27 26 25 24 23   5 4 3 2 1
Second Edition
Typeset in Adobe's Palatino LT Std and Helvetica Lt Std
American Psychiatric Association Publishing
800 Maine Avenue SW, Suite 900
Washington, DC 20024-2812
www.appi.org

Library of Congress Cataloging-in-Publication Data
Names: American Psychiatric Association, issuing body.
Title: Understanding mental disorders : your guide to DSM-5-TR / American
    Psychiatric Association ; with forewords by Abraham Nussbaum, and Patrick
    J. Kennedy.
Other titles: Understanding mental disorders (American Psychiatric Association)
Description: Second edition. | Washington, DC : American Psychiatric Association,
    [2024] | Includes bibliographical references and index.
Identifiers: LCCN 2023006319 (print) | LCCN 2023006320 (ebook) |
    ISBN 9781615375219 (paperback ; alk. paper) | ISBN 9781615375226 (ebook)
Subjects: MESH: Diagnostic and statistical manual of mental disorders. (Fifth
    edition, text revision) | Mental Disorders | Popular Work
Classification: LCC RC454 (print) | LCC RC454 (ebook) | NLM WM 75 |
    DDC 616.89—dc23/eng/20230511
LC record available at https://lccn.loc.gov/2023006319/
LC ebook record available at https://lccn.loc.gov/2023006320

British Library Cataloguing in Publication Data
A CIP record is available from the British Library.
Cover and Text Design—Tammy J. Cordova

Contents

Foreword vii

Foreword to the Prior Edition xi

Introduction xv

1 Disorders That Start in Childhood 3

2 Schizophrenia and Other Psychotic Disorders . . .29

3 Bipolar Disorders 45

4 Depressive Disorders 59

5 Anxiety Disorders 75

6 Obsessive-Compulsive Disorders 93

7 Trauma and Stress Disorders 107

8 Dissociative Disorders .131

9 Somatic (Physical) Symptom Disorders 139

10 Eating Disorders 149

11 Elimination Disorders 161

12 Sleep-Wake Disorders 169

13 Sexual Dysfunctions 191

14 Gender Dysphoria 205

15 Disruptive and Conduct Disorders 213

16 Addictive Disorders 225

17 Dementia and Other Memory Problems 243

18 Personality Disorders 267

19 Paraphilic Disorders 285

20 Treatment Essentials 295

Appendixes

   A.   Complete List of Mental Disorders
        in DSM-5-TR 317

   B.   Medications 323

   C.   Helpful Resources 333

   Index 355

Foreword

When I introduce myself to someone as their psychiatrist, I am offering to skillfully guide them through the confusing experience of mental distress. After an introduction, I listen as they describe their experience. Listening well is the beginning of my efforts to care for them medically.

People facing mental health concerns of their own or loved ones often have fears and shame about what they are going through and questions about seeking treatment. *Understanding Mental Disorders: Your Guide to DSM-5-TR* aims to dispel the fears and shame about mental illness and seeking treatment. It describes the symptoms of mental disorders and what to expect from treatment, offering knowledge and hope for those suffering from mental illness and the people who love and care for them.

◆

Psychiatry is a medical way to understand and help care for people experiencing behaviors, emotions, and thoughts in ways that other fields of medicine cannot. Psychiatric treatments are some of the most effective in all of medicine. I have seen patients whose minds and bodies were racing at the pace of mania settle into a normal rhythm after a few days of lithium. I've felt the joints of patients stiffened into immobility by catatonia relax into mobility after a week of electroconvulsive treatment. I've listened to patients whose disorganized and delusional thoughts became orderly and logical with a few weeks of clozapine. For the patients who respond, treatment can be life changing.

◆

When I meet a person as a patient, I want them to know what they can expect from mental health treatment. I begin by saying that I will be their psychiatrist. Then I pause. Experience has taught me to prepare for a range of responses. Based on what they say, I help them to understand what I do. I may say any of the following based on their concerns:

> *"Psychiatrists listen instead of reading minds."*
>
> *"Psychiatrists help people make changes they cannot make on their own."*
>
> *"Psychiatrists are people who can help a person seeking mental health."*

I share my hope that, together, we can explain and learn a little of what seemed before unknown to them.

There are three important things that a psychiatrist or other mental health care professional can offer to a person experiencing mental distress. These may occur in a different order or overlap one another: a name for the person's symptoms, a sense of what the symptoms mean, and care that treats the person's symptoms as part of a compassionate response to their experience.

A psychiatrist or other mental health care professional can offer a person experiencing mental distress a *name* for their symptoms.

With this kind of naming, I give a patient a category for understanding their experiences. Sometimes it takes time to find a name. Sometimes patients receive this kind of name as a label. I remind them that no patient is a "schizophrenic" or a "depressive," but a *person* receiving treatment for schizophrenia or major depressive disorder. A person is not their mental disorder, and a diagnosis is not an identity but a way to tame a confusing experience with a name.

It's often a relief to those seeking care (and their loved ones) that they are not alone in an isolating experience. *Understanding Mental Disorders* explains more about how psychiatrists like me reach a diagnosis. We use a diagnostic manual called DSM-5-TR, which this book explains and introduces, so you can understand more about the diagnosis you, or someone you care for, receives. For now, know that with a diagnosis, you have the company of others whose experience was enough like yours that it has a name, and you have a mental health care professional who can make some sense of those experiences.

> **A psychiatrist or other mental health care professional can offer *sense* to the experience of mental distress.**

We all engage the world through our senses. We know what smells attract us, what sights we cannot look away from, what tastes pucker our lips, and what feels rough to our touch. The experience of mental distress is harder to sense.

Are my worries normal or symptoms of an encompassing anxiety?

Is my sadness an expected response to life events or a sign of a devastating depression?

Am I thinking just a little slower than I used to or has my ability to think thinned to the point of disability?

No one knows you as well as yourself, but very few of us can make sense of ongoing, troubled behaviors, emotions, and thoughts without the help of other people. Our internal senses are simply harder to sort out than our external senses. A psychiatrist or other mental health care professional is trained to help distinguish worry from anxiety, sadness from depression, age-appropriate memory loss from dementia, and more. *Understanding Mental Disorders* will explain to you how a mental health care professional makes those distinctions.

> **When a psychiatrist like me gives a name and makes some sense of someone's mental distress, we open a door to treatment, to professional care. A psychiatrist or other mental health care professional can offer skillful *care*.**

A psychiatrist or other mental health care professional can offer care through listening with compassion to your experience and asking helpful questions to better understand your experience and point of view. We also offer care through treatment of symptoms. One of the treatments that psychiatrists and other mental health care professionals offer is psychotherapy (or "talk therapy"). Psychotherapy, in all its forms, is one of the most valued treatments offered by a mental health care professional, because it helps people solve problems they find too difficult to solve on their own.

When needed, medications support a person with mental illness as they make changes to reach their goals. A psychiatrist has a specialty in treating patients with medication for mental health care concerns or illnesses. Psychiatrists commit to a lifetime of learning about the range of medications that treat mental disorders. Medications can help a patient make changes in their behaviors, emotions, and thoughts that they could not make on their own.

Understanding Mental Disorders offers a wealth of helpful treatment information in Chapter 20, "Treatment Essentials." It provides must-read guidance on treatment, finding treatment, and staying healthy. Each chapter in this book also offers treatment information for the specific disorders featured.

◆

I encourage anyone with a mental health care concern for themselves or a loved one to seek help. You can find a skilled mental health care professional who can give a name to a seemingly nameless experience, make sense of a seemingly senseless suffering, and provide care beyond what you might try through your own efforts. You can also find support groups and other organizations that offer help and information in Appendix C, "Helpful Resources." Today is a good day to start, and *Understanding Mental Disorders* is a good companion to begin your journey toward understanding mental disorders and achieving mental health.

Abraham M. Nussbaum, M.D.
Professor of Psychiatry
University of Colorado School of Medicine

Foreword to the Prior Edition

Mental illness touches everyone. Nearly half of all Americans have a risk of mental disorder in the course of their lifetimes. We all know someone—parent, partner, child, friend, coworker, neighbor—who has suffered or is suffering from a psychiatric condition. Mental illness costs our nation and our world trillions of dollars every year. Yet as devastating as the financial toll clearly is, the cost in lives lost or severely compromised by mental illness is incalculably greater.

Across the globe, depression robs more people of more years lost to disease than any other condition. Suicide is the third leading cause of death among young people ages 10–24 in the United States. Our veterans, who have given so much for their country, are among the most vulnerable: every day 22 American veterans take their own lives. Just as tragic are the stories of the many Americans living in pain who are never diagnosed or treated. Too frequently, our society's response to mental disorders is to assign blame, leaving millions of Americans marginalized, neglected, vilified, or incarcerated because of their illness.

But mental illnesses are not a question of character; they are illnesses that can be treated. And like most illnesses, mental illnesses respond best to treatments that are timely and effective. Yet often we ignore or dismiss these illnesses in their earliest, most treatable stages—and respond only when they have escalated to critical and potentially life-threatening conditions. Simply put, too few of us know the signs and symptoms of mental illnesses, and countless people suffer as a result.

This is why *Understanding Mental Disorders: Your Guide to DSM-5* makes such an important contribution. By translating the psychiatric profession's most recent *Diagnostic and Statistical Manual of Mental Disorders* (DSM) into clear, accessible language, it empowers family members and friends to help identify individuals who might be at risk or who are already suffering from a mental disorder and need treatment. This book gives those of us with these conditions the keys to better understand our own situations.

Understanding Mental Disorders also helps us address the great challenge of stigma. People with mental disorders often experience fear, shame, and a terrible sense of being alone because their condition is not discussed. This invaluable guide will equip patients and families with the tools they need to break through stigma, seek professional diagnosis and care, and stick with their treatment. Mental health is the right of every citizen, and this guide will help us better understand how to claim that right.

When I was in Congress, I worked for years with my father, Senator Edward M. Kennedy, and many others on both sides of the aisle to pass the Mental Health Parity and Addiction Equity Act because so many Americans were being denied access to the treatments that could help them lead happier, more productive lives. This parity law—the first ever to ensure equal care for people with mental illnesses and substance use disorders—requires insurance providers to cover mental health treatments the same way they cover treatments for all other medical illnesses. The mental health parity act is a tremendously important milestone, but its true value will only be realized if all of us are informed and know what services to seek and expect. Researchers must continue to search for new and effective treatments, and patients and payers must make sure doctors are held accountable for providing such treatments—and then make sure insurers pay for them. We must ensure compliance with the law and demand enforcement.

When we talk about "parity" for mental illnesses, we should think not only about insurance coverage but also about how our society approaches these common disorders. If it's unacceptable to withhold treatment until a cancer hits Stage IV or diabetes is claiming a patient's vision or limbs, surely it must be wrong to wait until a mental illness has become life threatening before making treatment available. Early intervention is as appropriate for mental illnesses as it is for all other conditions, and we should all expect our health care providers to monitor our mental health as carefully as they do our blood pressure or cholesterol levels.

Every routine physical exam should include a "check-up from the neck up." This guide gives us the language to use in sometimes critical discussions about mental health with all of the medical professionals we encounter.

Back in 1963, in the months before his assassination, my uncle, President John F. Kennedy, described the national lack of attention to mental health as a "situation that has been tolerated for too long" because too many Americans viewed mental illness "only as a problem, unpleasant to mention…and despairing of solution."

My belief is that Americans today are more ready than ever to step up and address mental health issues. As this guide shows, we have solutions to the problems caused by mental illness. Do we use these solutions effectively and get them to the people who need them most? Not yet, but this guide helps to point the way.

The struggle to change this perspective is gaining ground, but we need to accelerate the campaign to enhance mental health awareness. This guide is a valuable addition to a growing list of transformative approaches—recovery and wellness self-management strategies, family education, and mental health first-aid among them—that will empower us as individuals and, ultimately, change our society's understanding of mental illness. All of us can do our part. It is time to stop marginalizing people with mental disorders and to show greater compassion and love. You can't eradicate bigotry just by passing a law, but you can help create a new culture that embraces the need for treating those with mental illness in the same manner as those with physical illness. Remember: If you help just one person, you help the world.

Understanding Mental Disorders gives individuals with mental disorders and their loved ones something they have too long been denied: the power that comes from knowledge and understanding.

Patrick J. Kennedy
Member, U.S. House of Representatives
Rhode Island, 1st District, 1995–2011

Introduction

Mental illness affects people of all ages. Most everyone has had a friend, a coworker, or a loved one with a mental illness. About 1 in 4 adults suffers from mental illness at some point in their lives, and nearly 1 in 5 children are also affected.

In the past, the subject of mental illness was surrounded by mystery, shame, and fear. Today, there has been major progress in the understanding of and ability to treat mental illness. This book was written to help people better understand mental disorders and how to manage them.

◆

Understanding Mental Disorders: Your Guide to DSM-5-TR explains mental disorders, their diagnosis, and their treatment in basic terms for those seeking mental health care and for their loved ones. This book is a practical guide to the disorders described in the current edition of the *Diagnostic and Statistical Manual of Mental Disorders* (DSM). The most recent edition of DSM is the *Diagnostic and Statistical Manual of Mental Disorders, Fifth Edition, Text Revision* (DSM-5-TR).

DSM describes all recognized mental disorders in the United States and is used worldwide. It also provides a common language for health care providers who diagnose mental illnesses. The American Psychiatric Association (APA) is the official organization that represents more than 38,000 psychiatrists (medical doctors who treat mental disorders) and supports the delivery of high-quality mental health care. The APA publishes DSM and developed *Understanding Mental Disorders* to help people whose lives have been touched by mental illness.

Understanding Mental Disorders was first written after the publication of the fifth edition of DSM (DSM-5). This new edition of *Understanding Mental Disorders* reflects changes made to DSM-5-TR and has been fully updated.

About Mental Illness

Mental illness has a major impact on quality of life for both individuals and their families, yet it is a treatable health problem. Common warning signs of mental illness include a change in sleep (more or less than usually needed), changes in weight (gain or loss), changes in mood or attention, and feeling "not normal." Of note, an expected response to a source of stress or loss, such as the death of a loved one, is not a mental disorder. Likewise, it is normal at times to have feelings of being down, anxious, fearful, or angry.

A *mental disorder* is a major disturbance in an individual's thinking, feelings, or behavior that reflects a problem in mental function. Mental disorders cause distress or reduced function in work or school tasks, as well as in social or family relationships.

There may be challenges in recognizing that someone may need to seek care for a mental illness:

- Children may be too young to clearly relay in words what is wrong.
- An older person with dementia may be confused and not understand what is occurring.
- People may express or describe mental disorders in different ways based on their culture or background.
- Some mental illnesses can have an intense effect on the mind, clouding judgment and leading to harmful behaviors, such as use of alcohol or other drugs. The person may be unable to think clearly enough to help themselves, and others must intervene on their behalf and for their good.

Living with a mental illness, whether it affects you or a loved one, can be very hard—but help is available. People can learn how to maintain a healthy mind and body, connect with others for support, and make positive changes that can improve quality of life and outlook. Being alert to warning signs and knowing when to seek help and what to expect from treatment can be vital. *Understanding Mental Disorders* can help increase knowledge and awareness about signs and symptoms of mental illness.

Diagnosis

Key to overcoming a mental illness is to recognize its symptoms, to know when to seek help, and to get the right treatment. This may be hard for someone who is struggling with mental illness. *Understanding Mental Disorders* is designed to help.

Each person and their symptoms are unique. There is no single approach to diagnosing something as complex as a mental illness. The same diagnosis does not look alike in all people.

A mental health care professional is best equipped to address these challenges and to evaluate the many behaviors, symptoms, and in some cases biological causes to determine the correct diagnosis, and thus, best treatment. In some cases, those caring for an individual with a mental illness—whether it is a spouse, sibling, or parent—can have more insight about the effects of the illness than the person with the disorder. These caregivers often serve as the "eyes and ears" of those who may not recognize symptoms in themselves. They can help answer questions that a mental health care professional may have about the person's symptoms.

Specific symptoms define mental disorders and help lead to a correct diagnosis. These symptoms, as well as other factors that could determine the diagnosis, are described in each chapter of *Understanding Mental Disorders*. These symptoms can be used to help explain thoughts and feelings to a mental health care professional. All the symptoms listed need not be present for a diagnosis. The degree of distress and effect on daily living also are important factors.

Although self-diagnosis based on the symptoms in this book is tempting, seeking a mental health care professional is needed for an accurate diagnosis and treatment. Some of the same symptoms occur in many different disorders. For example, anxiety is a symptom that occurs in people with depression, schizophrenia, and posttraumatic stress disorder. Some mental disorders can be related to a medical problem, such as heart disease or diabetes.

Communicating clearly and honestly with the mental health care professional about symptoms, including when they first arose and the problems they cause, will help in getting the most appropriate diagnosis and the very best care. Lab tests and other assessments are often used to help gather information about symptoms and progress. Some measures that assess symptoms can be found at www.psychiatry.org/psychiatrists/practice/dsm/educational-resources/assessment-measures.

Understanding Mental Disorders is designed to help those who are facing a possible diagnosis, as well as their loved ones. It helps people know more about their mental illness once there is a diagnosis and provides information about the major forms of treatment.

Treatment

Good treatment is tailored by a healtn care provider for each person and their unique needs and symptoms. Often more than one type of treatment is needed. Unfortunately, the early signs of mental illness often go unnoticed, and those who would most benefit from treatment do not receive it. They may be reluctant to admit to having a problem, or they may not be aware of the signs and symptoms that signal the presence of a mental illness. For this reason, it is important to have a guide such as *Understanding Mental Disorders* to know when to seek care early, when treatment is most effective.

As with any medical illness, early recognition and treatment improve the chances of a better outcome. Treatment can relieve symptoms and reduce suffering. *Understanding Mental Disorders* can help caregivers to notice signs of an illness that may need attention and can help patients to receive the care they need. Treatment options for specific disorders or groups of disorders are discussed briefly in each chapter, along with information on what to expect—and when to look at other options.

This book cannot replace individual diagnosis and care with a mental health care professional and does not provide in-depth details on treatment of specific disorders. Rather, it gives an overview of the treatments for these conditions—both talking therapies and psychiatric medications. In addition to treatment options in each chapter, other helpful information is included:

- A healthy lifestyle can promote optimal mental health. This involves getting sufficient exercise and adequate sleep, having a healthy diet, and learning to confide in friends and trusted family members. It also means learning how to better cope with life's stresses. Even small steps toward these goals help improve health and well-being. Tips for maintaining good mental health are found throughout *Understanding Mental Disorders*.
- Chapter 20, "Treatment Essentials," presents an overview of mental health treatments and how they work. It also reviews types of mental health care professionals, what to expect from a first session, types of therapies and medications, and ways to support general mental health.
- Appendix B provides a list of medications often prescribed for mental disorders.

- One way of dealing with mental illness is by seeking support from people who care. In addition to a helpful doctor or mental health care professional, support groups and other organizations can provide sound knowledge for coping with the disorder for individuals and their loved ones. Appendix C includes a listing of these additional resources.

About DSM

The *Diagnostic and Statistical Manual of Mental Disorders* (DSM) specifies symptoms that must be present for a given diagnosis and organizes these diagnoses together into a classification system. The drive to organize such a system began during World War II, when it became clear that psychiatrists needed to communicate clearly with one another in describing mental disorders. First published in 1952, DSM has evolved to serve as the foundation for defining and diagnosing mental disorders in a variety of settings. Psychiatrists, psychologists, other mental health care professionals, other physicians, nurses, lawyers, and social workers use DSM as a clinical guide and textbook. It is used in schools, hospitals, courtrooms, and the insurance industry to define mental disorders.

Published in 2013, DSM-5 reflects more than a decade of research and the expertise of hundreds of mental health care doctors and professionals who focus on the mental disorders that are their specialty. Published in 2022, DSM-5-TR includes fully revised text and updates to diagnostic criteria since DSM-5 was printed. Text updates are based on current scientific literature. DSM-5-TR features a new disorder, prolonged grief disorder. Mentions of all other DSM-5-TR disorders, guidelines, and criteria in this book also refer to those that were included in DSM-5.

More than 200 subject matter experts helped to develop DSM-5 and DSM-5-TR, crossing medical and mental health disciplines such as psychiatry, psychology, pediatrics, nursing, social work, neuroscience, biology, genetics, statistics, and public health.

More About This Book

Understanding Mental Disorders: Your Guide to DSM-5-TR is a version of DSM-5-TR for the general public—although it is not meant for use in self-diagnosis (just as any version of DSM is not meant for self-diagnosis). Rather, this book describes most of the disorders contained in DSM-5-TR. This book can be a helpful resource when talking with a health care provider before or after a diagnosis is received. The content of this book mirrors that of DSM-5-TR—it describes symptoms, risk factors, and related disorders. It defines mental disorders based on their symptoms and explores special needs or concerns.

In *Understanding Mental Disorders*, as in DSM-5-TR, similar disorders are grouped on the basis of their symptoms and when they first appear in life. Thus, disorders that begin in childhood are found in the first chapter, while disorders that begin in adulthood appear later in the book. For ease of use, each chapter explains the major and most common DSM-5-TR disorders that occur within these groups. Disorder names are in *italics* to aid notice within chapters, and terms are defined within the text. A complete listing of all DSM-5-TR mental disorders is found in Appendix A.

Chapters include personal stories that show how mental illness may have affected individuals, and their families and friends. Names, ages, and other information have been changed to disguise each real-life person in these stories. (If a real person matches any of these stories, it is by chance and is not the intent of the authors.)

Understanding Mental Disorders is designed to help combat mental illness through education about the disorders and their symptoms, about when to seek help, and what to expect from treatment. Overcoming mental illness will take work and effort, but there is always hope—and help.

◆

Acknowledgments

The American Psychiatric Association wishes to acknowledge the invaluable help of the following individuals in the creation of this book:

The American Psychiatric Association (APA) is a national medical specialty society representing more than 38,000 physician members specializing in diagnosis, treatment, prevention, and research of mental illnesses, including substance use disorders. Visit the APA at www.psychiatry.org.

Note: *The publisher has tried to ensure that all information in this book is accurate at the time of publication and consistent with general psychiatric and medical standards, and that information concerning drugs is accurate at the time of publication and consistent with standards set by the U.S. Food and Drug Administration and the general medical community. As medical research and practice continue to advance, however, therapeutic standards may change. Moreover, specific situations may require a specific therapeutic response not included in this book. Readers should not use this guide for self-diagnosis or as a substitute for seeking and following the advice of a mental health care professional. Diagnosis and treatment of mental illness are individualized endeavors that require personal attention from a mental health care professional. Readers should seek the advice of physicians directly involved in their care or the care of a member of their family.*

Donald W. Black, M.D., for his helpful review and edits of text across the book; Holly G. Prigerson, Ph.D., for reviewing, editing, and writing text sections on prolonged grief disorder, including the case vignette in Chapter 7, "Trauma and Stress Disorders"; William Byne, M.D., Ph.D., and Annelou L.C. de Vries, M.D., Ph.D., for their careful review and edits to Chapter 14, "Gender Dysphoria"; Abraham M. Nussbaum, M.D., for his helpful contributions to Chapter 20, "Treatment Essentials"; Robert B. MacArthur, Pharm.D., M.S., for his expertise in thoroughly updating Appendix B, "Medications."

We also acknowledge the contributions of the following staff of the American Psychiatric Association for their thoughtful review and suggestions for Appendix C, "Helpful Resources": Amy Porfiri, Managing Director, American Psychiatric Association Foundation; Ginnie Titterton, Director, Corporate Communications and Public Affairs; Deborah Cohen, Associate Director, Public Education; Madonna Delfish, M.P.H., Senior Program Manager, Division of Diversity and Health Equity; and Veronica Handunge, M.P.H., Senior Program Manager, Division of Diversity and Health Equity.

The following staff of American Psychiatric Association Publishing made valuable and essential contributions to this work: John McDuffie, former Publisher, for recognizing the need for this new edition and initiating its publication; Ann M. Eng, DSM Managing Editor, for revising the text and shepherding it through to completion; Tammy J. Cordova, Graphics Design Manager, for designing the book cover, interior, and graphics, and for selection of chapter images; and Erika Parker, Acquisitions Editor, and Annie Earl-Birge, Acquisitions Coordinator, for their help in researching and writing draft descriptions for the organizations listed in Appendix C, "Helpful Resources."

Most of all, we are grateful for the mental health care professionals who work with compassion and dedication on behalf of individuals suffering with mental illness. With them, we recognize and acknowledge the spoken and unspoken stories, the seen and unseen hard work, and the ongoing courage of all who have a mental illness and their loved ones who witness and walk with them on their journey.

Illustration Credits

Unless otherwise noted, all interior images are used under license from Shutterstock.com.

chapter graphics: notebook with pen, Copyright © Kae Deezign; *chapter images:* Chapter 1, "Disorders That Start in Childhood": Copyright © Natty_Blissful; Chapter 2, "Schizophrenia and Other Psychotic Disor-

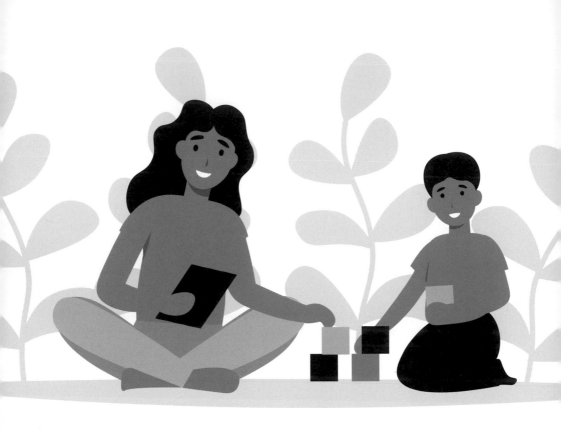

Autism Spectrum Disorder

Attention-Deficit/Hyperactivity Disorder (ADHD)

Intellectual Disability (Intellectual Developmental Disorder)

Other Disorders That Start in Childhood

    Communication Disorders

    Specific Learning Disorder

    Motor Disorders

For a complete list of DSM-5-TR disorders, see Appendix A.

CHAPTER 1

Disorders That Start in Childhood

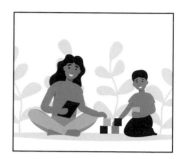

The disorders that begin during childhood featured in this chapter are also known as *neurodevelopmental disorders*. This means they affect the development and function of the brain. They often begin before a child enters grade school and can impair personal, social, school, or work function. Some of these disorders may last only during childhood. They may get better on their own or with treatment. Others can last longer or may not be noticed or diagnosed until the teen or adult years. For all these disorders, symptoms begin at an early age, even if they are mild.

These disorders include *autism spectrum disorder, attention-deficit/ hyperactivity disorder, intellectual disability, communication disorders* (such as problems with speech), *specific learning disorder* (such as reading, math, or writing problems), and *motor disorders* (such as tic disorders). A child can have more than one of these disorders—for instance, both autism spectrum disorder and intellectual disability.

These disorders can cause great distress and concern to parents and children, and the impact of the child's symptoms can affect the whole family. Seeking help from a doctor or mental health care professional will provide a diagnosis if a disorder is present (versus just normal childhood struggles). Treatment can lead to learning new skills and ways to manage symptoms, resources for support and coping, and in some cases, medications to relieve symptoms. It also can offer hope. Many children with these disorders can go on to lead full and rewarding lives. Undiagnosed and untreated disorders increase the risk for more severe problems and hardships as the child grows.

Autism spectrum disorder is a single diagnosis that combines disorders that used to be separate conditions before DSM-5 was published. These other conditions that are now within autism spectrum disorder are autistic disorder (autism), Asperger's disorder, childhood disintegrative disorder, Rett's disorder, and pervasive developmental disorder not otherwise specified.

Intellectual disability (also called *intellectual developmental disorder*) describes problems with mental abilities that occur at an early age. These abilities include reasoning, problem solving, and academic learning. These problems also may involve other types of thinking and behavior beyond just pencil-and-paper types of tests (sometimes called "formal intelligence testing" or IQ test scores).

Autism Spectrum Disorder

Autism spectrum disorder is marked by two main symptoms: problems with the child's ability to relate to others, and having a fixed set of interests or repetitive behaviors. The disorder name reflects a range, or spectrum, of symptoms that vary greatly by age and person.

Many people with the disorder may not be able to handle changes in their daily routines. They may show a lack of eye contact, social response to others, and shared play. Signs of autism spectrum disorder begin during early childhood and often last through a person's lifetime. Some people with the disorder need a lot of help in their daily lives, and others need less. Symptoms can improve with treatment.

Autism spectrum disorder has been reported in about 1%–2% of children and adults in the general public in the United States and non-U.S. countries. Rates may be rising, but it remains unclear whether this is due to increased awareness or different ways of diagnosing the disorder across studies.

Symptoms are often seen in the first 2 years of life and can be seen before 12 months—or after 24 months if symptoms are milder. Babies who are less likely to smile and coo or babble back and forth with parents may be showing early autism spectrum disorder symptoms. First symptoms also involve delayed speaking in toddlers and a low interest in social contact. Some children show a slow or sudden loss of speaking or social skills during the first 2 years of life. Such a loss of skills is rare for other disorders and may be a sign (or a "red flag") for autism spectrum disorder.

In other children with the disorder, symptoms may not appear until there is a change in their routine. This may include going to preschool or a new setting where they must try out new social skills. Sometimes children may learn ways to avoid social contacts that are challenging for them, and their symptoms are not fully known. But over time, their symptoms are seen more clearly as social contact becomes a bigger part of daily life as they mature. Studies have found that the diagnosis is often delayed in children of color, which can delay treatment.

Symptoms of autism spectrum disorder can be more pronounced during childhood and early school years. Interest in social contact may increase in later childhood. Adults with the disorder may learn coping methods for their problems with social cues (such as when or how to join a conversation, or what not to say). This requires great effort on their part to think through how to engage with others. People with autism spectrum disorder may struggle to know how other people find such social contact to be natural or easy. The need to learn coping methods and build new skills to improve function can persist through life. People with autism spectrum disorder are able to keep learning over time and often have a sense of purpose about learning new social skills.

Because a diagnosis of autism spectrum disorder can be made in those with good levels of language and thinking skills, people with this disorder are often able to find work that matches their special interests and skills. Those with higher skills may have different or more challenges with relationships. Features of treatment for autism spectrum disorder should be designed with the goals and strengths in mind of those with the disorder. Access to *vocational rehabilitation services* greatly improves the prospect of stable work for youth with the disorder. These services help them prepare for and stay employed.

People with autism spectrum disorder may also have *intellectual disability, language disorder, attention-deficit/hyperactivity disorder, developmental coordination disorder, anxiety disorders,* and *depressive disorders.* Other medical conditions, such as epilepsy, sleep problems, and constipation, also may occur. *Avoidant/restrictive food intake disorder* is somewhat common, in which only a narrow range of foods is eaten.

Autism Spectrum Disorder

There is a great range of abilities and traits in people with autism spectrum disorder, and no two people reflect the disorder in the same way.

The following symptoms must be present in the child's early developmental stage for a diagnosis of autism spectrum disorder:

- Frequent and sustained problems in social communication and interaction in many settings:
    - Limited back-and-forth exchange of sounds, expressions, or talking. For instance, there may be reduced sharing of feelings, thoughts, or interests; or failure to start or respond to social contact.
    - Problems with nonverbal communication used in social contact, such as lack of eye contact, gestures like pointing or waving, or facial expressions like smiling or frowning. For instance, there may be a failure to look where someone is pointing.
    - Problems with building, keeping, and understanding relationships. For instance, the child may have problems changing behavior to suit the setting, making friends, or sharing pretend play; or may have a lack of interest in peers.
- Fixed and repeating patterns of behaviors, interests, or tasks in at least two of the following:
    - Repeating body movements, use of objects, or speech. For instance, the child may often flap their hands, repeat sounds or phrases, spin coins, or line up toys again and again.
    - Insisting on the same routines and behaviors. For instance, there may be extreme distress with small changes, problems with shifting to another task, rigid routines in greeting, or a firm need to eat the same foods each day.
    - Having strongly fixed interests with extreme or intense focus beyond what is normal. For instance, the child may be attached to unusual objects (such as vacuum cleaners or fans).
    - Showing great response or no response to certain sights, sounds, smells, textures, and tastes. For instance, there may be no or dulled response to pain, heat, or cold; great dislike for certain sounds or textures; or high pleasure for lights or movement.

These symptoms can cause problems in social, school, and work function. They can range from mild to severe and can change over time or by setting (see Table 1 for levels of support needed).

Diagnosing and treating autism spectrum disorder early are important aims to reduce symptoms and improve quality of life for children and their families. Under federal law, any child suspected of having a developmental disorder can get a free evaluation. The Centers for Disease Control and Prevention (CDC) recommends that all children be screened for autism spectrum disorder at well-child visits with their pediatrician at 18 and 24 months of age.

There is no medical test for autism spectrum disorder. Doctors often diagnose autism spectrum disorder by talking with the child, watching how the child talks and acts compared with others the same age (keeping in mind stages of child development), asking questions of parents and other caregivers, and using screening questionnaires. They assess the type of behavior, how often it occurs, and how intense it is.

Table 1. Levels of support needed for autism spectrum disorder		
Severity level	Social communication	Restricted, repetitive behavior
Level 3 "Requiring very substantial support"	Severe lack of verbal and nonverbal communication that causes severe problems in social interactions. Speaks few understandable words and rarely starts social contact.	Preoccupations, fixed rituals, and/or repetitive behaviors that disrupt all areas of function. Very distressed when rituals or routines are interrupted.
Level 2 "Requiring substantial support"	Marked lack of verbal and nonverbal communication. Speaks in simple sentences and has very odd nonverbal communication.	Restricted and repetitive behaviors occur often enough to be noticed by the casual observer. Distress or frustration is clear when behaviors are changed or interrupted.
Level 1 "Requiring support"	Without support in place, impaired social communication causes clear problems. Can speak in full sentences and engage in communication but fail in back-and-forth communication with others.	Repetitive behavior causes great interference with daily function. Trouble switching between tasks. Problems organizing and planning that hamper independence.

In some cases, the primary care doctor may refer the child and family to a specialist to better assess any symptoms. These include developmental pediatricians (doctors with special training in child development and children with special needs), child neurologists (doctors who work on the brain, spine, and nerves), child psychologists (specialists with a Ph.D. or Psy.D. degree; they treat mental disorders with psychotherapy and may specialize in psychological testing and evaluation), or child psychiatrists (doctors who know about the human mind, emotions, thinking, and behavior; they can prescribe medicine and conduct psychotherapy).

Risk Factors

There are no known causes of autism spectrum disorder. Risk factors include the following:

- **Environment.** Children born to older parents, born very early, or whose mothers used valproate (a medication used to treat seizures, migraines, and *bipolar disorder*) during pregnancy are more likely to have autism spectrum disorder.
- **Genetics.** The risk of autism spectrum disorder is much greater if there is a family member with the disorder. Genes play a major role in autism spectrum disorder, but they are not the only elements. A combination of several genes and many other factors seem to affect whether the disorder occurs. About 15% of children with autism spectrum disorder have a genetic basis for the disorder.

Much debate has occurred over the belief that childhood vaccines cause autism spectrum disorder. One reason people believe that autism spectrum disorder is linked to vaccines is that the signs of the disorder sometimes do not appear until around the same age as vaccines are given. If a child is diagnosed shortly after getting a vaccine, this may seem like the vaccine caused the disorder. Many studies have been conducted over many years, and there is no proof of a link between vaccines and autism spectrum disorder. Parents are strongly urged to have their child immunized to protect against serious childhood diseases.

Adam's Story

Adam, a 12-year-old boy, was brought in by his mother for psychiatric evaluation. He had temper tantrums that were causing problems for him at school. She said that school had always been stressful for Adam and that it had become worse after he entered middle school.

Adam's sixth-grade teachers reported that he could do classroom work, but that he had a hard time making friends. He seemed to mistrust the motives of classmates who were sincere and nice to him. Instead, he believed others who laughed and faked interest in the toy cars and trucks that he brought to school. The teachers noted that he often cried and rarely spoke in class.

When interviewed, Adam mumbled when asked questions about school, classmates, and his family. When asked if he liked toy cars, however, Adam lit up. He pulled out several cars and trucks from his backpack. He did not make good eye contact but talked at length about the vehicles, using their correct names, such as front-end loader, B-52, and Jaguar.

Adam spoke his first word at age 11 months and began to use short sentences by age 3. He had always been very focused on cars and trucks. His mother said that he had always been "very shy" and had never had a best friend. He struggled with childhood jokes and banter because "he takes things so literally." Adam's mother had always seen this behavior as "a little odd." She added that this behavior was like that of Adam's father, a successful lawyer, who had the same focus in his interests. Both of them were "sticklers for routine" who "lacked a sense of humor."

During the exam, Adam was shy and made below-average eye contact. The doctor diagnosed him with *autism spectrum disorder without intellectual impairment*. Adam has trouble interacting with classmates and holding a conversation—both symptoms of social communication problems. Adam also has fixed interests—he is interested in cars and trucks and little else. Perhaps because his autism spectrum symptoms were like his father's behavior, his mother viewed Adam as "a little odd" but did not seek an evaluation and diagnosis.

Treatment

In most cases, autism spectrum disorder is a lifelong disorder. Although there is no cure, children who are diagnosed and treated early can get better. There is no single treatment, but rather different approaches suited to each child to improve behavior and communication. These include intensive skill-building and education sessions. They provide structure, direction, and organization for the child and family.

Methods of *applied behavior analysis* often are used. This approach involves types of rewards to support desired behavior and lessen those that can cause harm or block learning. These methods can improve skills such as listening, looking, reading, and relating with others. A child also may receive speech and language therapy, occupational therapy (to help with tasks of daily living), and social skills training. The child's family plays a key role in treatment.

There are no medications to treat the core symptoms (problems with social communication and repetitive behavior) of autism spectrum disorder. Some children and adults with autism spectrum disorder also have other disorders, such as an *anxiety* or *depressive disorder* or *attention-deficit/hyperactivity disorder* (ADHD). These disorders may improve with psychotherapy or medication. Improved or reduced symptoms of these disorders may help in the treatment of autism spectrum disorder.

Many types of special diets have been discussed and explored by those seeking to find better ways to help autism spectrum disorder. These diets often try to avoid foods or substances that might cause problems or allergies. These include excess sugar, gluten, casein, food additives (used to improve taste or flavor), and colorings. Nutrient supplements, such as antioxidants and flavonoids (luteolin), have also become popular with many parents who believe that they help improve autism spectrum disorder symptoms. There is little scientific proof that special diets or supplements work. Parents should check with a doctor before adding a supplement or changing the child's diet, to ensure the child receives the proper vitamins and nutrients for healthy growth.

Ways to Cope

- Having a child with autism spectrum disorder affects the whole family. It can be stressful and require much time to manage the disorder. Paying attention to the physical and emotional health of the entire family is important. The following steps can help:

  - **Learn as much as possible.** Get trusted, reliable information about the diagnosis from organizations such as the Autism Society (www.autismsociety.org) and the Autism Science Foundation (http://autismsciencefoundation.org).

  - **Provide structure and routine.** Many who have autism spectrum disorder function better if the day is consistent and predictable. Stick to a schedule for daily activities, including mealtimes, schoolwork, and play.

  - **Connect with other parents.** Talking to parents who share your experiences can help you cope with your child's challenges. The Autism Society offers online support groups for parents and families, as well as help finding resources around the country.

  - **Know your child's rights.** A federal law known as the Individuals with Disabilities Education Act (IDEA) requires that special services be available for children with a disability. The services can include early treatment and support for birth through age 2, and "free and appropriate" special education funded by the government for ages 3–21. Read more about IDEA at http://idea.ed.gov.

Attention-Deficit/Hyperactivity Disorder

Attention-deficit/hyperactivity disorder (ADHD) is one of the most common mental disorders in children. Although this disorder begins in childhood, it also can affect adults. Main features include *inattention* (not being able to keep focus), *hyperactivity* (excess movement that is not fitting to the setting), and *impulsivity* (hasty acts that occur in the moment without thought). It can disrupt school, social, and work tasks or function and cause problems in development.

About 7% of children and 2.5% of adults have ADHD. It occurs twice as often in boys than in girls. Parents may notice symptoms in their toddlers, but usually ADHD is diagnosed during elementary school, when problems paying attention become clear. During the teen years, hyperactivity may be expressed as being fidgety, restless, or impatient. In adults, inattention, poor planning, restless feelings, and impulsivity may cause problems in all aspects of life, including relationships.

People with ADHD also may have *oppositional defiant disorder* or *disruptive mood dysregulation disorder*. *Specific learning disorder* is also common.

 ADHD

Symptoms must be noticed before age 12 and last for at least 6 months. In children, at least six symptoms must be present. In older teens and adults (age 17 and older), at least five symptoms must be present. The symptoms are *not* due only to disobedience or rebellion, defiance, hostility, or failure to understand tasks or instructions. The symptoms clearly disrupt or reduce the quality of social, school, or work function.

ADHD occurs when there is a lasting and frequent pattern of inattention and/or hyperactivity or impulsivity that disrupts function or development, as shown in the following types of symptoms.

Inattention: Six (or five, for those 17 and older) of the following symptoms occur *often*:

- Doesn't pay close attention to details or makes careless mistakes in school or job tasks.

- Has problems staying focused in tasks or leisure, such as during lectures, conversations, or long reading.

- Does not seem to listen when spoken to (mind seems to be elsewhere).

- Does not follow through on instructions and doesn't finish schoolwork, chores, or job duties (may start tasks but quickly loses focus).

- Has problems bringing order to tasks and work (for instance, does not manage time well; has messy, disorganized work; misses deadlines).
- Avoids or dislikes tasks that require sustained mental effort, such as schoolwork or homework. Older teens and adults may avoid preparing reports and completing forms.
- Often loses things needed for tasks or daily life, such as school papers, books, keys, wallet, cell phone, and eyeglasses.
- Is easily distracted.
- Forgets daily tasks, such as doing chores and running errands. Older teens and adults may forget to return phone calls, pay bills, and keep appointments.

Hyperactivity and impulsivity: Six (or five, for those 17 and older) of the following symptoms occur *often*:

- Fidgets with or taps hands or feet or squirms in seat.
- Not able to stay seated (in the classroom, workplace).
- Runs about or climbs where it is inappropriate.
- Unable to play or do leisure activities quietly.
- Always "on the go," as if driven by a motor.
- Talks too much.
- Blurts out an answer before a question has been finished (for instance, may finish people's sentences, can't wait to speak in conversations).
- Has difficulty waiting their turn, such as while waiting in line.
- Interrupts or intrudes on others (for instance, cuts into conversations, games, or activities; or starts using other people's things without permission). Older teens and adults may take over what others are doing.

The symptoms must occur in two or more settings, such as school, home, or work, and with family and friends. They are not due to other disorders such as *schizophrenia, anxiety disorder,* or *substance intoxication.* The disorder can be mild, moderate, or severe based on the symptoms and how much there are problems in social, school, or work function.

ADHD is diagnosed based on the types of symptoms that occur over the past 6 months: *Combined type* is diagnosed when the required number of symptoms occurs for both inattention and hyperactivity or impulsivity. *Inattentive type* is diagnosed when the required number of inattentive symptoms is present, but not all required symptoms of hyperactivity or impulsivity occur. *Hyperactive/impulsive type* is diagnosed when the required number of hyperactivity or impulsivity symptoms is present, but not all required symptoms of inattention occur.

Risk Factors

Some factors that may increase the risk of the disorder are as follows:

- **Environment.** Babies born early and with very low birth rate have an increased risk of ADHD; the lower the baby's weight at birth, the greater the risk. Exposure to cigarette smoke while in the womb is linked to the disorder. A mother who drinks alcohol while pregnant may increase a child's risk. A history of infections and exposure to toxins, such as lead, also might play a role. A very small number of cases may be linked with the child's diet.
- **Genetics and biology.** People with ADHD are much more likely to have a first-degree blood relative (parent or sibling) with ADHD.

Treatment

Behavior therapy and medication can improve the symptoms of ADHD. Both methods combined often work best.

- *Behavior therapy* focuses on helping parents and the child to better control the symptoms of ADHD. This may involve teaching parents how to give positive feedback for desired behaviors and negative results for undesirable ones.
- *Medication* helps children improve their attention span, perform tasks better, and control impulsive behavior. *Stimulants* increase the action of certain brain chemicals and have been safely used for decades when taken as the doctor prescribes. They include methylphenidate and amphetamines. *Nonstimulant medications* are an alternative to stimulants and include atomoxetine and guanfacine. Most children will improve with medication.

It is key for children who have ADHD to receive a correct diagnosis and proper treatment for their symptoms. Children who are not treated are at greater risk for problems with learning, failing school, behavior and discipline problems, and problems relating with others. As they grow older, added problems can include alcohol and drug use, depression, suicide, and job-related problems. Adults with the disorder can benefit from psychotherapy, cognitive-behavior therapy, medication, and learning how to use tools such as electronic reminders.

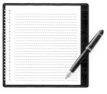

Charlie's Story

Charlie, a 6-year-old boy, was brought to a psychiatrist by his mother after a recent school meeting, in which it was pointed out that Charlie was having problems getting used to first grade.

Charlie's mother reported that he had always been a difficult child. As an infant, he was cranky and antsy. He learned to crawl at 7 months and was soon exploring the entire house, leaving a trail of emptied wastebaskets and cupboards behind him. As he learned to talk, he seemed to talk all the time and often needed attention from his parents.

He began to attend preschool at age 4 years. His teachers complained that he was rowdy and impulsive, seeming to have little thought for the other children. He would not sit in his seat like the other children and would often get up and run around the room. He could not work on a task for more than 5 minutes without losing focus. He would also distract his classmates by talking to them when they were supposed to be working quietly.

When meeting with the psychiatrist, Charlie was quite active. He entered the doctor's office with a firm, bold step. He jumped on his chair rather than sitting down, finally squirming into a sitting position, which he held for only 2 or 3 minutes. He then jumped up and began pulling books off the bookshelves. When told that they belonged to the doctor and should be placed back on the shelf, he threw one or two on the floor and went to the doctor's desk to handle the pens, pencils, and paperweights. Charlie's mother looked embarrassed and upset and tried to get him to sit back down.

The psychiatrist decided to prescribe methylphenidate. Within a week Charlie's mother said that the effects were "amazing." Charlie's behavior had improved. He showed a clear increase in his ability to stay focused, and his rowdy, hyper behavior had decreased. His teacher also noticed a big change. Charlie was able to complete the first grade with only minor problems and was found to have reached progress for his age in learning to read and to do very simple math.

Ways to Cope

- Being a parent of a child with ADHD can be a challenge. Along with regular treatment, these tips can help:
  - **Keep routines.** Structure helps keep a child from becoming too disorganized and distracted. Set a consistent time for homework, meals, playtime, bedtime, and wake time.

- **Stay organized.** Put schoolbags, clothing, and toys in the same place every day so your child will be less likely to lose them.
- **Make sure instructions are understood.** Give brief, clear directions and set limits. Children who have ADHD need to know exactly what others expect from them.
- **Avoid distractions.** Turn off the TV, music, and computer when your child is doing homework or needs to focus.
- **Limit choices.** Offer a choice between two things (this outfit, meal, toy, etc., or that one) so that your child isn't overwhelmed and overstimulated.
- **Have a plan for discipline.** Reward good behavior and respond to misbehavior with alternatives such as a time-out or loss of privileges.
- **Maintain communication with the child's teacher.** Being aware of how a child is doing each day with behavior and schoolwork is important to help track their progress.
- **Find support.** The group Children and Adults with Attention-Deficit/Hyperactivity Disorder (CHADD) provides online community discussions, resources, and a directory of local support groups in the United States (www.chadd.org).
- **Help your child find a talent.** All children need to have some success to feel good about themselves. Finding out what your child does well—and giving them support in these pursuits—can boost your child's social skills and self-esteem.
- **Know your child's rights.** The Individuals with Disabilities Education Act ensures children with ADHD receive care.

Intellectual Disability

Children with *intellectual disability* (also called *intellectual developmental disorder* and called "mental retardation" in the past) have problems both with their intellectual ability and with learning and doing the skills needed for day-to-day living. About 11 out of every 1,000 persons in the U.S. population has intellectual disability. By age 2, delayed motor skills (such as walking) and language (or speech) skills and social milestones may point to severe intellectual disability, which is found in about 6 of every 1,000 children. Mild intellectual disability may not be noticed until a child starts school and learning problems become clearer. See Table 2 for the levels of intellectual disability across types of function.

People with intellectual disability may struggle with communication and may not be able to express themselves clearly. Others may misunderstand what they mean, which can cause people with intellectual disability to lash out in an attempt to be understood. This may include yelling or trying too hard to communicate. They may become forceful toward others who don't know what they are trying to say. People with intellectual disability may also notice and feel awkward or ashamed that they are behind others their own age. As a result, they can act out, feel worried, or try to be alone and away from others. They may have symptoms of depression and problems with eating and sleeping because of the distress they feel. They may also be easily misled by others. This leaves them at risk for being victims of abuse and fraud, or being involved in crime without their knowledge or true consent.

Table 2. Levels of intellectual disability for each type of function (examples)		
Mild		
Conceptual	**Social**	**Practical**
For preschool children, there may be no clear problems. For school-age children and adults, learning reading, writing, math, time, or money is hard. Help is needed in one or more of these areas to meet standards for their age. In adults, planning, setting priorities, short-term memory, and use of academic skills in daily life (such as reading or dealing with money) are impaired.	Talking with others, knowing words, and picking up on social cues lag behind age standards. There may be trouble keeping feelings and behavior under control in ways that match their peers. These problems are noticed by peers in social settings.	May function in self-care and hygiene like others of the same age. In adults, help may be needed for grocery shopping, transportation, home and child care tasks, health care and legal choices, and banking and money management. Adults may hold jobs and can learn skills for work.

Table 2. Levels of intellectual disability for each type of function (examples) *(continued)*		
Moderate		
Conceptual	**Social**	**Practical**
For preschool children, delays in speech may occur. For school-age children, progress in reading, writing, math, and understanding of time and money lags behind peers. For adults, school skills (such as reading and math) remain at a grade school level. They need daily help for use of these skills in work and personal life.	They can form ties with family and friends, and they may have romantic bonds as adults. Caregivers must assist with life decisions. Help is needed to learn and apply social norms (such as manners and greetings).	By adult age, self-care and household tasks may be done with teaching and reminders. Adults may hold jobs with ongoing help from others on the job, as well as from caregivers. Help is needed to manage job duties, schedules, transportation, health benefits, and money.
Severe		
Conceptual	**Social**	**Practical**
There is little understanding of written language or of concepts that involve numbers, amounts, time, or money. Caregivers provide much support for problem solving throughout life.	Speech may be single words or phrases. Simple speech and gestures are understood. Ties with family members and familiar others are a source of pleasure and help.	Help is required for all functions of daily living, such as meals, dressing, bathing, and using the bathroom. Care is needed at all times to ensure safety and well-being. In adults, taking part in tasks at home, leisure, and work requires ongoing support and help. Learning skills involves long-term teaching and ongoing support.

Table 2. Levels of intellectual disability for each type of function (examples) *(continued)*		
Profound*		
Conceptual	**Social**	**Practical**
They may learn skills, such as matching and sorting based on size, shape, or color.	Simple instructions or gestures may be understood. They express desires and feelings mostly through nonverbal communication. They enjoy ties with well-known family members, caregivers, and familiar others, and start and respond to social contact through gestures and emotions.	Help from others is needed for all aspects of daily physical care, health, and safety, although they may take part in some of these activities as well. Those without severe physical impairments may assist with some daily work tasks at home, like carrying dishes to the table. Leisure activities may involve listening to music, watching movies, going out for walks, or water activities, all with the support of others.

*If present, motor and sensory (such as hearing or vision) problems may prevent taking part in activities in any area of function.

The disorder tends to be lifelong, although how severe it is may change over time. Early and ongoing treatment and support may improve daily function through childhood and adult years. In some cases, these services result in major improvement of intellectual function, such that the diagnosis of intellectual disability no longer applies. For this reason, when doctors assess infants and young children, they often delay diagnosis of intellectual disability until proper support services are given for a certain amount of time. For older children and adults, support services may allow them to take full part in all daily living skills and greatly improve their function.

People with intellectual disability often have other mental, neurodevelopmental, and physical conditions. For instance, other disorders such as cerebral palsy and epilepsy may occur three to four times more often in people with intellectual disability than in the general public. People with intellectual disability may not be able to explain their health problems. These can go untreated because the person may not mention or know how to talk about their physical symptoms. The most common mental and neurodevelopmental disorders that occur with intellectual disability include *ADHD*, *depressive* and *bipolar disorder, anxiety disorders, autism spectrum disorder,* and *impulse-control disorders.*

 ## Intellectual Disability

Intellectual disability begins during child development and involves problems in thinking, social, and real-world functions. All of the following must occur for a diagnosis:

- Impaired *intellectual function* that may be seen in problems with reasoning, problem solving, planning, academic learning, and learning from experience (for instance, problems with memory, knowing word meanings, solving problems, math concepts).

- Impaired *adaptive function* that results in failure to meet standards for age in being independent and socially responsible (such as being able to master real-life tasks). Ongoing support is needed to function in at least one setting of school, work, home, or community.

- Both of the above types of problems begin in the *developmental period* (before age 18).

Intellectual disability is measured in part through a standardized intelligence test given by a psychologist. The average score on such tests, often termed an IQ, is 100. Scores between 65 and 75 (based on the test) fall within the range for intellectual disability. Test scores alone cannot be used for the diagnosis, which must take into account adaptive function. *Adaptive function* means how well the child handles common skills needed for life on their own as compared with other children of the same age. It includes three skill types: conceptual (academic learning), social, and practical (daily life skills). Problems in these areas must be present for a diagnosis. Intellectual disability occurs across a range of levels: mild, moderate, severe, and profound. Table 2 provides examples for each skill type across levels.

Children are diagnosed based on an exam by a doctor (such as a pediatrician or a child psychiatrist), a standardized intelligence test, and assessment of their behavior or adaptive function. Many health care providers may be involved in making a diagnosis. These providers may be in the fields of neurology (the brain and nervous system), special education, hearing, speech, and vision.

Risk Factors

Anything that affects a baby's normal brain development before or after birth can cause or increase risk for intellectual disability:

- **Genetics.** Chromosomal (genetic) disorders, such as Down syndrome.
- **Environment.** A mother who has consumed or was exposed to alcohol, drugs, toxins, and certain infections or diseases.
- **Childbirth complications.** A baby deprived of oxygen or born before full term.
- **Illness or injury.** Brain injury, infections, seizure disorders, severe neglect or abuse, or exposure to toxins such as lead.

Treatment

After intellectual disability has been diagnosed, parents work with a team of professionals to develop a treatment plan. Goals include keeping the child at home whenever possible and helping them have a fulfilling life. This may involve speech therapy, occupational therapy, physical therapy, and family counseling. If the child's disability is mild, as in most cases, care is often given in the home by parents, along with outside support and special education. For children with more severe disabilities, health care providers may suggest a group home or a specialized institution to provide more needed care. Group homes and supported housing may help adults with intellectual disabilities reach their highest level of independence.

Children with intellectual disability qualify for special education services according to the Individuals with Disabilities Education Act (IDEA). The services can include early treatment and support for birth through age 2, and "free and appropriate" special education funded by the government for ages 3–21.

Parents of children with intellectual disability can benefit from learning as much as they can about the disorder and their child's rights under the law (such as IDEA). Talking with other parents who have children with intellectual disability can provide ideas and support, as well as help to maintain hope, build the child's skills at home, enjoy and learn from the child, and improve coping.

Other Disorders That Start in Childhood

These disorders are diagnosed when they cause distress, prevent progress, or create other problems with the child's self-care, home, social, or school tasks. They include *communication disorders, specific learning disorder,* and *motor disorders.* These disorders are not due to the effects of a drug or medication, brain condition, or any other mental disorder, although other conditions or mental disorders may also occur with these disorders. Without treatment or care, these disorders can cause greater problems for the child. Treatment for some disorders can allow complete recovery. Treatment also can relieve symptoms and lead to better coping to aid the child's present and future.

Communication Disorders

Communication disorders are problems in language, speech, or communication (any verbal or nonverbal behavior) that begin early in a child's development. They include *language disorder, speech sound disorder, stuttering,* and *social (pragmatic) communication disorder.* Differences in the way young boys and girls develop early communication abilities may explain the higher rate of these disorders in boys as compared with girls.

Language Disorder

Children with *language disorder* have chronic problems with learning and using language. They have trouble knowing what others' words mean (*receptive language*) and using words or gestures to express themselves (*expressive language*). Their language skills are well below what is normal for their age. Their first words and phrases are often delayed. Problems following instructions may result from struggles to recall new words and phrases. A family history of language disorders is often present. The disorder is lifelong, but speech therapy can improve skills. Psychotherapy can help relieve any problems with emotions or behavior that might result from the disorder. Key symptoms are as follows:

- Reduced vocabulary (for instance, trouble learning new words or often using the same words and phrases).
- Limited sentence structure (uses words and word endings incorrectly when forming sentences).
- Problems using vocabulary to have a conversation with someone or to explain a topic.

Speech Sound Disorder

With *speech sound disorder,* the child has not learned enough about sounds or is unable to make correct speech sounds with the jaw, tongue, or lips. These problems result in speech that cannot be understood well by others or problems in verbal communication of messages. The disorder is diagnosed when the child's speech is at lower than normal standards for their age. For instance, by age 4, most children's speech can be understood—and by age 7 or 8, most children speak clearly. The sounds *l, r, s, z, th,* and *ch* are often the latest for children to learn. A family history of speech or language disorders is often present, and boys more often than girls have the disorder. Most children with the disorder respond well to treatment with speech therapy, and problems with speech can improve over time. These are the key symptoms:

- Frequent problems with making speech sounds that cause speech to be unclear or that prevent verbal communication.
- The problem limits how well the person can express themselves and hinders social, school, or work function.

Stuttering

People with *stuttering* have frequent problems with the flow and timing of speech. The problem does not go away quickly, but it may end on its own in children. Stuttering that starts in childhood often occurs by age 6. The problem can start slowly or have a sudden onset. Once the problem starts, it becomes more frequent. Stress and anxiety can worsen the symptoms (such as for a school report or job interview). The risk of stuttering among first-degree blood relatives (parents, siblings) is three times higher than in the general public. Treatment includes speech therapy or cognitive-behavior therapy to address thoughts about speaking. The patience and support of parents to remind the child to take more time to speak greatly helps. The disorder is diagnosed when at least one of the following occurs:

- Repeated sounds and syllables ("W-W-W-Where did you go?").
- Lengthened consonant and vowel sounds ("SSSave me a seat").
- Broken words (pauses within a word).
- Pauses in speech that may be silent or filled with sound.
- Replaced words to avoid those that cause problems ("um um").
- Great physical tension with produced words.
- Repeated single-syllable whole words ("I-I-I-I see him").

Social (Pragmatic) Communication Disorder

Social (pragmatic) communication disorder involves problems in the social use of verbal and nonverbal communication. Problems can be seen by age 4 or 5 years. Milder forms of the disorder may not be known until the early teens, when social communication becomes more complex.

Some children greatly improve with speech, language, and behavior therapies that involve the family, special education teachers, and mental health care professionals. Other children may still have some struggles in social relationships that persist into adult years.

Because of the problems in social communication, this disorder might look like *autism spectrum disorder*, but those with this disorder do not have fixed interests or repeating behaviors. Those who in the past had a diagnosis of *Asperger's disorder* or *pervasive developmental disorder not otherwise specified* based on their problems in social communication might better fit this new diagnosis of social communication disorder. A family history of *autism spectrum disorder,* other *communication disorders,* or *specific learning disorder* increases risk for the disorder. All of the following must be shown for a diagnosis:

- Problems communicating for social reasons, such as greeting or chatting with someone just met.
- Problems changing communication to match the setting (such as a playground or classroom) or the needs of the listener (such as a child or adult).
- Problems with keeping the rules of conversation and storytelling, such as taking turns to speak or listen, and knowing how to use verbal and nonverbal signals to guide contact.
- Trouble understanding humor, figures of speech, what is not stated, and words that might have different meanings in other settings.

Specific Learning Disorder

Children with a *specific learning disorder* have frequent problems learning one or more key academic skills. The diagnosis includes problems with reading, writing, or math that result in school performance well below grade level. These problems can impair school or job function and success. If the disorder remains undiagnosed and untreated, a child may begin to dislike or feel upset by schoolwork, which can lead to low self-esteem, sadness, loneliness, and other problems. The learning problems are not due to *intellectual disability*, sight or hearing problems, low income, adverse home life, chronic absence from school, lack of education, brain or mental disorders, or lack of knowledge of the English language.

The diagnosis is made through standardized tests and an evaluation by a team that may include a psychologist, special education expert, and reading and speech-language specialists. Risk factors for a learning disorder include premature birth, low birth weight, and being exposed to air pollution or nicotine (such as cigarette smoke) while in the womb or during early childhood. Having a first-degree blood relative (parent or sibling) with a learning disorder increases risk four to eight times. The disorder occurs more often in boys, whose risk is at least two times higher than in girls. The disorder can be mild, moderate, or severe based on how hard it is for the child to learn the needed skills. Treatment includes learning new strategies and tools to grasp concepts and build on the child's strengths. About 4% of adults may have specific learning disorder.

Specific learning disorder is diagnosed when one or more of the following symptoms has lasted for at least 6 months:

- Incorrect or slow reading that requires great effort (for instance, reads words aloud incorrectly, often guesses at words, has problems sounding out words).
- Problems understanding the meaning of what is read.
- Problems with spelling (such as adding letters or leaving them out).
- Problems with writing (for instance, problems putting ideas in order, many grammar and punctuation mistakes).
- Poor understanding of numbers (counts on fingers, gets confused with math problems).
- Problems with mathematical reasoning (applying math facts or concepts).

Motor Disorders

Motor disorders begin early in the developmental years and involve problems with movement. They include *developmental coordination disorder, stereotypic movement disorder,* and *tic disorders.*

Developmental Coordination Disorder

Children with *developmental coordination disorder* sit, crawl, walk, climb stairs, button shirts, use zippers, or ride a bike later than others their age. Even when the skill is achieved, the movements may appear awkward, slow, or less precise than those of peers. Older children and adults may display slow speed or mistakes with tasks such as self-care skills or playing ball games, writing, typing, and driving.

The disorder is often not diagnosed until after age 5. Boys are twice as likely to have the disorder as girls. In children ages 5–11 years, 5%–8% may have the disorder. Low birth weight, premature birth, or mothers who drink alcohol while pregnant can also increase the risk. In 50%–70% of children affected, problems persist into the teenage years. There may be poor self-esteem, poor physical fitness, reduced physical activity, and behavior problems along with the disorder. Although the disorder is lifelong, treatment can include physical education (exercise), perceptual motor training (helps train the brain and body to improve coordination), and occupational therapy (helps adapt skills for daily life and self-care). Key symptoms for the disorder include the following:

- Learning and doing motor skills lags greatly behind that of peers and standards for age. The person may appear clumsy, drop or bump into things, and seem slow or make mistakes, such as when riding a bike or writing by hand.
- Symptoms often hinder or impair normal daily tasks at home, school, and play. For instance, there are challenges in getting dressed, eating meals, and using scissors, pencils, or rulers during class.
- Symptoms are not due to *intellectual disability*, vision problems, or brain disorders that affect movement (such as cerebral palsy).

Stereotypic Movement Disorder

Stereotypic movement disorder begins in the first 3 years of life. The child repeats movements such as hand shaking or waving. Some types of movement may cause self-injury, such as self-biting or head banging. Symptoms before age 3 may be a sign of another neurodevelopmental problem. In children with normal development (that is, meeting age standards for growth and skills), the movements resolve over time or can be stopped when the child is given attention, is asked to stop, or changes focus to another task. Being left alone for a long time or other stress in the child's home may increase risk for the behavior. In children with *intellectual disability*, 4%–16% may have symptoms. In these children, the behavior can last for years.

Treatment should focus on the cause, symptoms, and child's age. Settings around the child can be made safer to prevent harm. Behavior therapy and psychotherapy often help. Some medications, such as antidepressants or naltrexone, may help reduce symptoms.

The disorder may be mild, moderate, or severe. When the disorder is mild, the child can stop the behavior. When the disorder is moderate, measures are needed to protect the child and change the behavior. When the disorder is severe, constant watching and safety measures are needed to prevent great harm. Key symptoms include the following:

- Frequent movements that repeat over and over, such as hand shaking or waving, body rocking, head banging, self-biting, eye poking, face slapping, or hitting their own body.

- Movement that disrupts social, school, or other tasks and may result in self-harm (such as bruises, cuts, loss of fingers).

Tic Disorders

Tics are sudden, brief movements or vocal outbursts that the child may repeat over and over. They are not done on purpose. Often the person cannot control them but may be able to stop them for a certain amount of time before they occur. Tics get worse with worry, excitement, fatigue, and stressful events (such as taking a test). They may stop or lessen during times of calm or relaxing, or during focused tasks that require muscle control.

Tic disorders occur two to four times as much in boys as in girls. They often begin between ages 4–6 years and reach their peak at ages 10–12. Symptoms lessen during the teen years, but a small number of people may have tics worsen or last into adult years.

Risk factors include older age of the father, early birth, and smoking by the mother while pregnant. Those with a tic disorder may have anxiety or depression, withdraw from others, and be at risk for substance use. Treatment includes behavior therapy, parent training, and sometimes, medications.

Although few or many tics may occur, tic disorders are diagnosed when the tic has been present for at least 1 year. The different types of tic disorders all begin before age 18. (If Tourette's disorder is present, none of the other tic disorders can be diagnosed.)

- *Tourette's disorder*—a person has both multiple motor tics (such as blinking eyes, turning head, shrugging shoulders) and at least one vocal tic (such as grunting, clearing throat, repeating words, or unintentionally blurting out offensive words).
- *Persistent (chronic) motor or vocal tic disorder*—a person has one or more motor tics or one or more vocal tics, but not both.
- *Provisional tic disorder*—motor and/or vocal tics have been present for less than 1 year.

Key Points

- *Neurodevelopmental disorders* affect the growth and development of the brain and begin during childhood. Once these disorders are diagnosed, they can be treated. A range of support services may be available. With treatment and support, many children with these disorders can go on to lead full and rewarding lives. Untreated disorders increase the risk for more severe problems and hardships as the child grows.

- Many of these disorders (such as *autism spectrum disorder, attention-deficit/hyperactivity disorder, intellectual disability,* and *specific learning disorder*) will qualify a child for special services. A federal law known as the Individuals with Disabilities Education Act (IDEA) requires that special services be available for children with a disability. The services can include early treatment and support for birth through age 2, and "free and appropriate" special education funded by the government for ages 3–21. Read more about IDEA at http://idea.ed.gov.

- Treatment goals should focus on helping the child take part in life as fully as possible. Treatments should help find and build the child's strengths, as well as improve skills that lag behind those of peers or age standards. In most cases, the child will be able to reach these goals while staying with their family.

- Some of these disorders may last only during childhood. Others may be lifelong. The need to learn coping methods and build new skills can last through life—and lead to lasting gains.

- The treatment plan for the child's disorder should also include helping parents and families to learn new skills to adapt to the child's disorder. The physical and emotional health of the entire family is important. Learn as much as possible about the disorder and connect with other parents whose children also have these disorders. See Appendix C, "Helpful Resources," for support groups and organizations.

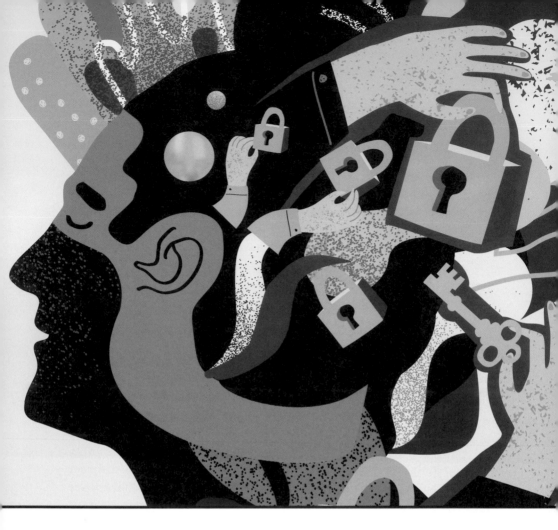

Schizophrenia

Schizoaffective Disorder

Delusional Disorder

Other Psychotic Disorders

    Brief Psychotic Disorder

    Schizophreniform Disorder

    Catatonia

For a complete list of DSM-5-TR disorders, see Appendix A.

CHAPTER 2

Schizophrenia and Other Psychotic Disorders

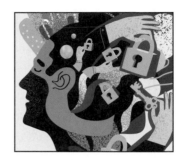

S*chizophrenia and other psychotic disorders* are illnesses that disrupt a person's sense of reality, and can affect their understanding of what they see, hear, and experience. These disorders involve psychotic symptoms that can make it very hard or impossible for a person to know what is real, to think clearly, or to communicate and relate with others. Their emotions and responses to others may appear greatly reduced, and they may have little interest in their work or social activities. When these symptoms occur, it can be hard to get through to the person or sometimes even to understand what they are trying to say. With treatment, many people with these disorders improve and can work and live on their own.

Schizophrenia is the most common psychotic disorder. Less common disorders are *schizoaffective disorder*, *delusional disorder*, *brief psychotic disorder*, *schizophreniform disorder*, and *catatonia*.

The psychotic symptoms of these disorders differ from person to person, yet one or more of these five key features must be present:

1. *Delusions* are false beliefs that do not change even with proof that the beliefs are not true, no matter what others may say. Delusions are called *bizarre* if they are clearly far-fetched, cannot occur in real life, or are not based on beliefs of the person's culture. There are several types of delusions:

    - *Persecutory delusions* are the most common. People believe that they are being harmed or harassed by another person or group (such as the government). They may believe that others are stealing from them or mocking them in some way. When people have persecutory delusions, they may be described by friends and family as "paranoid" (that is, suspicious of others).
    - *Referential delusions* are also common. People think that certain gestures and words from others are directed at them. Believing that people on television are sending special messages to them is a common referential delusion.
    - *Grandiose delusions* involve the person's belief in having exceptional abilities, wealth, or fame.
    - *Erotomanic delusions* center on the person's belief that another person is in love with them.
    - *Nihilistic delusions* lead a person to believe that a major crisis will happen or that they are doomed, dying, or already dead.
    - *Somatic delusions* involve the person's beliefs about their health or bodily functions, such as a belief that their organs are rotting away.

2. *Hallucinations* refer to hearing, seeing, smelling, or feeling things that are not there. They appear real to the person having them. The most common type of hallucination is "hearing voices." There may be one or more voices speaking to the person or speaking about the person. When people have these *auditory hallucinations*, they may appear to be talking to themselves when they are actually responding to what they are hearing. These voices may say bad things, such as "kill yourself," or they may give constant comments on what the person is doing, such as "John is brushing his teeth....John is going out to the street now."

3. *Disorganized thinking and speech* are scattered or jumbled thoughts and speech. The person is not thinking clearly and does not sound logical when talking (is not "making sense"). People with disorganized speech may appear alert and engaged in a conversation, but their words and sentences may not connect in a way that a listener can follow.

4. *Disorganized or abnormal motor behavior* are movements that seem nervous, restless, or frantic, or that repeat without a clear purpose.

Sometimes the person may be *catatonic* (in a daze, not moving or speaking for hours, even when asked questions). For persons with schizophrenia, the term *grossly disorganized* conveys severe problems in being able to complete routine daily tasks or behave in a normal way, beyond disorganized (scattered, inefficient, extra) movement.

5. *Negative symptoms* are observed when the person has little energy, may not speak as much as usual, has little interest in past pursuits that were once enjoyed, and has no desire to meet daily goals, express feelings, or have social contact. The person may appear to have no interest in the outside world and is not bothered at all by this lack of interest.

Schizophrenia and other psychotic disorders almost always begin during the late teen years or early 20s, but may start later. They may occur rarely in children and the elderly. When the main symptoms of the disorders appear, getting help quickly is key.

In diagnosing schizophrenia and other psychotic disorders, mental health care professionals look at factors such as culture, religion, ethnic background, and socioeconomic status. These factors can play a big role in what a person may consider a delusion or hallucination. For example, a belief in witchcraft might appear to be a delusion, but some cultures believe in witchcraft, and for that reason, this belief would not be a sign of a psychotic disorder for someone who belongs to that culture. "Hearing God's voice" is also a normal part of some religions, and this is not considered a psychotic symptom in those who belong to these religious groups.

Although there is no cure for these disorders, treatment can improve and relieve symptoms. Most people who receive treatment can live full and meaningful lives.

Schizophrenia

Schizophrenia is a brain disorder that can disturb a person's thoughts, speech, and behavior. It tends to remain for life once it begins and to cause problems with day-to-day living. Schizophrenia occurs in about 0.3%–0.7% of people in their lifetime, and rates differ across countries. It affects men and women equally.

Schizophrenia can have a sudden or slow start. For most people with the disorder, it begins slowly. A person might have a normal childhood and function very well until symptoms start. Most men have their first psychotic episode (that is, delusions or hallucinations) in their early to mid-20s. For most women, the first episode is in their late 20s.

People with schizophrenia are at high risk to abuse alcohol or other drugs. Over half of people with schizophrenia are regular cigarette smokers. A person with schizophrenia may use alcohol, marijuana, or other drugs to help cope with some of the symptoms of schizophrenia. These can make the illness worse and treatment more difficult. The rates of *obsessive-compulsive disorder* and *panic disorder* are high in people with schizophrenia as well.

Suicide is another major risk for those with schizophrenia. The person may hear voices telling them to take their own life, and drug use and symptoms of depression also can increase risk. About 5%–6% of people with the disorder take their own lives, and about 20% attempt suicide. Suicide risk is reduced with treatment, close support, and supervision. For this reason, finding a skilled mental health care professional for treatment is vital.

Schizophrenia often requires treatment with medications throughout life, and most people find relief from their symptoms with treatment, along with mental health care based on the recovery model. A recovery-based approach focuses on what the person can control; their strengths, abilities, and interests; and ways to maintain hope (see Chapter 20, "Treatment Essentials," for more information). Psychotic symptoms tend to lessen with age.

 ## Schizophrenia

Schizophrenia occurs when a person has at least two of the following symptoms for 1 month:

- Delusions
- Hallucinations
- Disorganized speech
- Grossly disorganized or catatonic behavior
- Negative symptoms

A person must have at least one of the first three symptoms. For most of the time since the symptoms began, the person's day-to-day function has worsened in one or more major areas, such as work, relationships, or personal hygiene. The signs of troubled behavior also have lasted for at least 6 months; they have not been temporary. A mental health care professional should rule out other disorders, such as *schizoaffective disorder, depressive disorders,* and *bipolar disorders.* If the symptoms are caused by a drug, medication, or other medical condition, schizophrenia cannot be diagnosed. If there is a history of *autism spectrum disorder* or a *communication disorder* that began in childhood, schizophrenia is only diagnosed if a person has had delusions or hallucinations and the other symptoms of the disorder for at least 1 month.

Risk Factors

Genes play a strong role in risk for schizophrenia. However, many with the disorder do not have a family history of the disease.

Myles's Story

Myles was a 20-year-old man who was brought to the emergency room by the campus police of the college from which he had been suspended several months ago. A professor had called and reported that Myles had walked into his classroom, accused him of taking his tuition money, and refused to leave.

Although Myles had much academic success as a teenager, his behavior had become increasingly odd during the past year. He quit seeing his friends and no longer seemed to care about his appearance or social pursuits. He began wearing the same clothes each day and seldom bathed. He lived with several family members but rarely spoke to any of them. When he did talk to them, he said he had found clues that his college was just a front for an organized crime operation. He had been suspended from college because of missing many classes. His sister said that she had often seen him mumbling quietly to himself and at times he seemed to be talking to people who were not there. He would emerge from his room and ask his family to be quiet even when they were not making any noise.

Myles began talking about organized crime so often that his father and sister brought him to the emergency room. On exam there, Myles was found to be a poorly groomed young man who seemed inattentive and preoccupied. His family said that they had never known him to use drugs or alcohol, and his drug screening results were negative. He did not want to eat the meal offered by the hospital staff and voiced concern that they might be trying to hide drugs in his food.

His father and sister told the staff that Myles's maternal grandmother had had a serious illness and had lived for 30 years in a state hospital. Myles's mother left the family when Myles was very young. She has been out of touch with them, and they thought she might have been treated for mental health problems.

Myles agreed to sign himself into the psychiatric unit for treatment.

Myles's story reflects a common case, in which a high-functioning young adult goes through a major decline in day-to-day skills. Although family and friends may feel this is a loss of the person they know, the illness can be treated and a good outcome is possible. In the case of Myles, he was having persecutory delusions, auditory hallucinations, and negative symptoms that had lasted for at least 1 year. All of these symptoms fit with a diagnosis of schizophrenia. It is key for the treating doctor to quickly rule out other causes of the problem, such as substance use, a head injury, or a medical illness. Treatment for these conditions differ from that for schizophrenia and may be lifesaving.

Treatment

Treatments can be effective in relieving the symptoms of schizophrenia. Medication and psychotherapy can help people with schizophrenia lead productive and rewarding lives. Some people with the illness may have more lasting problems in daily living despite treatment and family support. For most people with schizophrenia, recovery may mean that although some symptoms are still present, there is no major disability.

Treatment often begins with medications to reduce delusions and hallucinations. When symptoms are better controlled, other types of therapy and services can help those with schizophrenia (see "Key Support Options" later in this section). Taking care of general health and wellness (such as eating a healthy diet, quitting smoking, and getting exercise) is a key part of caring for the illness.

Family members and loved ones can play a key role in helping someone with schizophrenia get and stay better. Along with the person with schizophrenia, they should learn as much as possible about the disorder. With the help of a mental health care professional, family members can learn coping strategies and problem-solving skills. Family members can also help make sure their loved one sticks with treatment and takes prescribed medication.

A mental health care professional can help family members to know about warning signs after treatment has started (for instance, if the person stops taking medication, seems to stop eating or sleeping, or otherwise doesn't seem to get better) and how best to understand and interact with their family member with schizophrenia.

Before Treatment Begins

Before treatment can begin, a doctor must conduct a thorough medical exam to rule out substance use or other medical illnesses that can cause psychotic symptoms. Many persons with schizophrenia may also have problems with drug use, so it may take time for the diagnosis to become clear. For a schizophrenia diagnosis, the symptoms must be present even when the person is not under the influence of a substance and has not used the substance for a long time, such as a month or more. Also, symptoms that first appear to be due to schizophrenia may later turn out to be those of a manic episode (a time of extreme energy, risky behavior, or little sleep) or depression (feeling hopeless or sad, or having little energy). The source of the problem may be *bipolar disorder* or *major depressive disorder* (see full discussions in Chapter 3, "Bipolar Disorders" and Chapter 4, "Depressive Disorders").

If a person shows signs of an alcohol or drug addiction, treatment for substance abuse should be pursued along with treatment for schizophrenia. The use of alcohol or drugs can make schizophrenia symptoms worse and cause problems with medications prescribed to treat schizophrenia. Treatment for an alcohol or drug problem is helpful and can occur along with treatment for schizophrenia.

Medications

Antipsychotic medications are used to treat schizophrenia. These medications are most often taken every day to keep symptoms under control—in the same way that many people need to take medicines every day to keep their blood pressure or cholesterol under control. Taking the medicine as prescribed helps control delusions and hallucinations and prevents them from coming back.

There are two groups of antipsychotic medications. The first group is called *first-generation* or *typical antipsychotics* (some of these have been available since the mid-1950s). Some of the more common typical antipsychotics include haloperidol, fluphenazine, and perphenazine. The other group is called *second-generation* or *atypical antipsychotics* (these became available in the 1990s). Common atypical antipsychotics include risperidone, olanzapine, and quetiapine.

Sometimes, people with symptoms of schizophrenia may not be able to understand that they have an illness. This is a symptom called "poor insight." To them, their delusions and hallucinations are real, and so they don't understand the need for medication. This can be hard for loved ones and mental health care professionals who want needed medication to be taken. It may be helpful to have a family member remind the person about the need for medicines and to make sure they are taken. In other cases, antipsychotic medicines can be given in a shot (injection) form once or twice a month to ensure the person receives treatment. Learning about the different types of medications and their effects is also helpful (see box).

Key Support Options

Once the symptoms of schizophrenia have come under control, support services can help people improve skills that may have declined during the illness or were never attained. Services can provide training to help in coping with day-to-day stresses, building social skills, learning early warning signs of relapse, and learning how to manage symptoms before they worsen.

Because schizophrenia often occurs in early adult years, those with the disorder may need support and guidance to help build life skills, complete school or training, and hold a job. For instance, supported-employment programs help people with schizophrenia prepare for, find, and keep jobs in real-world settings.

Medication Tips

The medications used for schizophrenia are each very different in their side effects. If problems arise with one of the medicines, ask the doctor about other choices. Here are some more tips:

- Take the medication as the doctor directs.
- Know what to expect with side effects (weight gain or fatigue may be common side effects with some medications). Ask about how best to cope with side effects.
- Set a helpful routine to make sure the medications are taken every day.
- Do not stop a medication right away or decrease the dose without checking with a doctor first. If some medications are stopped right away or the dose is reduced, they may cause unhealthy and unpleasant symptoms—or can make symptoms worse.
- Pay close attention to how the medicines are working or not working, even as time passes. After a while, the body can adjust to medications, symptoms can improve or worsen, and the doctor may need to adjust the dose or switch medications.
- Even when symptoms improve—or side effects are unpleasant—know that medications must continue to be taken to help symptoms improve.
- Be sure to keep in touch with your doctor. Medicines can cause health changes over time (for instance, in cholesterol, blood pressure, and blood sugar). Any of these problems can be handled safely as long as you see the doctor regularly.

Rehabilitation and community support programs can include psychological counseling, job counseling and training, teaching skills to manage money, help in using public transport, and chances to practice communication skills. Rehabilitation programs work well when they include both job training and therapy designed to improve thinking skills. Programs like this help people with schizophrenia hold jobs, remember important details, and improve their function.

Many people living with schizophrenia receive emotional and material support from their family. Therefore, families must receive education and assistance on how best to manage their loved one's illness. This type of help has been shown to help prevent relapses and improve the overall mental health of the family, as well as the person with the illness.

Cognitive-behavior therapy (CBT) is a type of psychotherapy that focuses on thinking and behavior. CBT helps people with schizophrenia to test the reality of their thoughts and perceptions, how to "not listen" to their voices, and how to manage their symptoms overall. Along with medication, CBT can help reduce the severity of symptoms and reduce the risk of relapse.

People with schizophrenia often can receive care for their illness in the community where they live. If symptoms become severe, hospital care may be needed. When living alone or with family is not an option for someone with schizophrenia, supportive housing (such as halfway houses, group homes, or care facilities) is another option.

It is important that caregivers for someone with schizophrenia get support for themselves and understand how best to help their friend or family member. Talking with a mental health care professional can benefit and comfort those caring for their loved one. Appendix C, "Helpful Resources," contains a list of organizations that focus on mental health care information and resources for the public. Some of these organizations offer support groups for friends and family members of those with mental disorders.

Schizoaffective Disorder

People with *schizoaffective disorder* suffer from a mixture of psychotic and mood symptoms. Schizoaffective disorder may begin with symptoms of delusions and hallucinations much like schizophrenia. There are also frequent episodes of depression or mania (an extreme high or euphoric mood). Most often, people with this disorder have a decline in day-to-day living skills and achieve less than they could without the disorder. How well they are able to function at work or school, relate with people, and have close ties with others varies from person to person.

Schizoaffective disorder is less common than schizophrenia. About 0.3% of people will have the disorder in their lifetime, and it is more common in women than men. Symptoms may first appear during the teen years, early adulthood, or later in life.

People with schizoaffective disorder have a 5% risk for suicide. The risk is higher for people who have depressive symptoms. This risk can be managed by getting care for the illness and appropriate treatment.

Many with the disorder are also diagnosed with other mental disorders, especially a *substance use disorder* or an *anxiety disorder.*

Schizoaffective Disorder

Schizoaffective disorder is diagnosed when someone has:

- A major depressive mood or manic mood while also having periods of time with at least one of the following symptoms of *schizophrenia:* delusions, hallucinations, disorganized speech, grossly disorganized or catatonic behavior, or negative symptoms.

- Delusions or hallucinations for at least 2 weeks without a major depressive or manic mood.

Mood symptoms must exist for more than half of the total length of the illness. The symptoms of schizoaffective disorder cannot be related to a drug, medication, or any other medical condition.

Risk Factors

The causes of schizoaffective disorder are unknown, but genes likely play a role. People with a first-degree blood relative (parent or sibling) with *schizophrenia, bipolar disorder,* or *schizoaffective disorder* may be at higher risk for schizoaffective disorder.

Treatment

Treating schizoaffective disorder is much like treating schizophrenia. Treatment may include antipsychotic medication, as well as antidepressant medication to improve depressive moods that may occur with the disorder. Often people with schizoaffective disorder also have problems with manic symptoms, so medications that stabilize mood and prevent extreme "highs" are needed. These medications may include lithium carbonate or valproate. In addition to medication, the same types of therapy and rehabilitation support used to help those with schizophrenia also enable those with schizoaffective disorder and their families to better manage the condition.

Delusional Disorder

Delusional disorder involves a false belief (delusion) in something that is not true, just as someone with schizophrenia may have. The disorder differs from schizophrenia because it does not include the other schizophrenia symptoms of hallucinations; disorganized thought, speech, or movement; or negative symptoms. Like people with schizophrenia, people with delusional disorder may have nonbizarre or bizarre delusions.

Nonbizarre delusions are false beliefs about events that could occur in real life but are unlikely. These include beliefs about being followed, poisoned, deceived, or conspired against, or that a stranger or famous person is in love with them. *Bizarre delusions* are false beliefs that are not possible to occur (for instance, a stranger has removed their organs and replaced them with someone else's without leaving any wounds or scars).

Aside from the delusion, the person with a delusional disorder may seem normal to most other people. They may not appear to be ill or strange in any way, unless they begin to talk about or act on their delusions.

Delusional disorder is less common than the other psychotic disorders—about 0.2% of adults will have it in their lifetime. Because people with the disorder often do not have other severe schizophrenia symptoms aside from their false beliefs, they are more likely to hold a job and may not seek care for their problem. Delusional disorder can occur in young people but seems to occur more often in middle to late adult life. It affects men and women equally. The mental health care professional should ask about faith and culture to assess whether the belief is a part of these systems or is a delusion.

 Delusional Disorder

Delusional disorder is diagnosed when someone:

- Has one or more delusions that have lasted at least 1 month.
- Does not have hallucinations, disorganized speech, disorganized behavior, or negative symptoms.

Although the person has delusions and may have problems relating with others due to the false beliefs, in general the person can do fine in day-to-day life and does not show bizarre or odd behavior. Other symptoms such as depression or manic symptoms tend not to occur along with delusional disorder. If they do occur, these symptoms would be only a brief part of the illness, because the delusions are the main problem. The disorder also cannot be caused by a drug, medication, another medical condition, or another mental disorder, such as *obsessive-compulsive disorder*.

Risk Factors

The cause of delusional disorder is unknown, although risk may be increased if there are family members who have either *schizophrenia* or *schizotypal personality disorder*.

Treatment

Getting someone with a delusional disorder to accept treatment can be very hard. Those with the disorder often don't believe they have a problem and can mistrust other people and their motives. If they agree to treatment, one-on-one psychotherapy may help them notice and change their false beliefs and manage stressful feelings. Antipsychotic medications are prescribed if the person is willing to take them, but they often do not reduce the delusions. For most persons, the delusions persist and never fully go away.

Other Psychotic Disorders

This brief review of other psychotic disorders that can occur (but are less common than schizophrenia) includes *brief psychotic disorder, schizophreniform disorder,* and *catatonia.* These disorders differ in their symptom profiles. Catatonia is a medical emergency and can occur with other medical and mental disorders.

Brief Psychotic Disorder

People with *brief psychotic disorder* have sudden, short periods of psychotic behavior that last at least 1 day but less than 1 month. They often recover quickly afterward, and the symptoms fully go away. Symptoms may appear to be like *schizophrenia.* People with brief psychotic disorder may be greatly confused and upset, and have extreme moods that change quickly. They have severe problems with self-care and with home, school, work, and life function. Because of delusions or hallucinations, they may be at risk for suicide and have poor judgment.

Antipsychotic medications may be used, but only for a short time until the episode is over. Once the brief episode is over, often within a few days, the person returns to their daily life, and there is no longer any sign of a problem. At least one of the first three symptoms below must be present for at least 1 day but less than 1 month:

- Delusions
- Hallucinations
- Disorganized speech
- Grossly disorganized behavior or catatonic behavior

The disorder is not due to any drug or medication, another medical condition, or *major depressive, bipolar,* or *other psychotic disorders.*

Schizophreniform Disorder

Schizophreniform disorder has the same key symptoms as *schizophrenia*, but the symptoms last for a shorter time—at least 1 month, but less than 6 months. Once the symptoms last at least 6 months, the diagnosis is changed from schizophreniform disorder to schizophrenia. With schizophreniform disorder, the person often loses daily living skills, may be confused, and often begins having problems with school or work. They may stop joining in usual activities, stop caring for themselves, and have problems interacting with others. Most often, schizophreniform disorder is diagnosed when someone may have schizophrenia, but 6 months have not yet passed to meet the schizophrenia diagnosis. Key symptoms are at least two of the items below. At least one of the symptoms must be delusions, hallucinations, or disorganized speech:

- Delusions
- Hallucinations
- Disorganized speech
- Grossly disorganized behavior or catatonic behavior
- Negative symptoms

The disorder is not due to any drug or medication, another medical condition, or *major depressive, bipolar,* or *other psychotic disorders.*

Catatonia

Catatonia can occur as a symptom of other medical conditions (such as head trauma and brain diseases) and several mental disorders, such as *neurodevelopmental, psychotic, bipolar,* and *depressive disorders.* It can occur at any age. Most of the time, it happens fairly quickly, over a few days or weeks. The problem is often very serious and requires treatment in a hospital. The main features include decreased response to others and decreased, extreme, or strange movement. Symptoms may switch between decreased and extreme movement. In severe stages, safety measures and watching are needed to prevent harm to self or others. A person with catatonia has at least three of the following symptoms:

- Stupor (that is, unable to move, not responding to the settings around them)
- Rigid muscles or fixed posture
- Waxy flexibility (a person's limbs stay in any position they are put in by another person)

- No or little verbal response to others
- Extreme resistance (not responding to instructions)
- Sudden holding of a position for a long time against gravity
- Strange movements or mannerisms
- Frequent, repeating movements that do not have a purpose
- Agitation (restless movement, moving in an excited manner)
- Grimacing (face shows pain, disgust, or displeasure)
- Repeating someone else's words
- Copying someone else's movements

People with catatonia cannot respond to their surroundings and may stop eating and drinking. Treatment for catatonia varies based on other illnesses that may be present. Sometimes getting fluids and nutrition in the hospital is needed to maintain health until the best treatment is decided. Treatments such as electroconvulsive therapy (ECT) can sometimes improve symptoms quickly. The person begins to "wake up," respond to others, and be aware of what is going on around them after a short time of treatment. (See Chapter 20, "Treatment Essentials," for more about ECT.)

Key Points

- People with a *psychotic disorder* lose touch with reality, and they have problems knowing what is real and thinking clearly. With treatment, they usually improve, and many can work and live on their own.
- People with symptoms of *schizophrenia and other psychotic disorders* may not be able to understand that they have an illness. They experience their delusions and hallucinations as real, and for that reason they do not see a need for treatment.
- Family members and loved ones play a key role in helping someone with schizophrenia or another psychotic disorder get and stay better. Along with the person who has the disorder, they should learn as much as possible about the disease. With the help of a mental health care professional, family members and loved ones can learn coping strategies and problem-solving skills. When needed, they can help make sure needed treatment is received.
- A doctor should be contacted at any time with concerns or questions about medications or side effects. If some medications are stopped right away or the dose is reduced, they may cause unhealthy and unpleasant symptoms—or can make symptoms worse. Alcohol or drug use also makes symptoms worse and can disrupt the way medications work.

- Mental health care professionals can help people with these disorders better handle their feelings. They can teach how to test the reality of thoughts and perceptions, how to "not listen" to voices, and how to manage their symptoms in all parts of life. Psychotherapy can help reduce the risk of relapse.

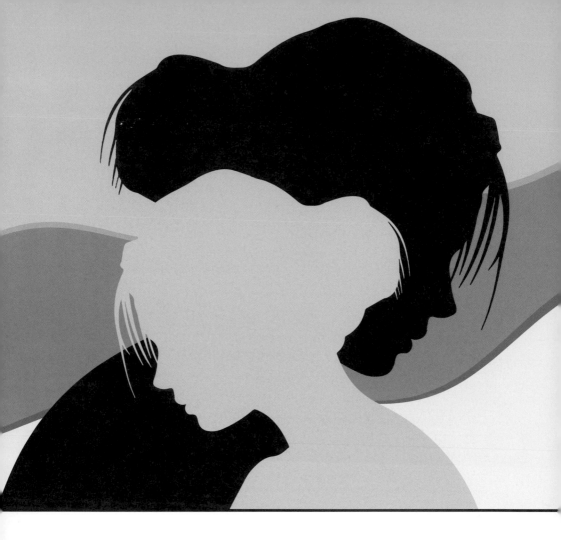

Bipolar I Disorder
Bipolar II Disorder
Cyclothymic Disorder

For a complete list of DSM-5-TR disorders, see Appendix A.

CHAPTER 3

Bipolar Disorders

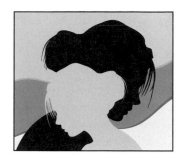

*B*ipolar disorders cause marked shifts in a person's mood, energy, and ability to function. People with these disorders have extreme and intense emotional states that occur in distinct periods called *mood episodes*. These differ from the normal ups and downs in mood that occur in daily life.

The symptoms of bipolar disorder can damage relationships, cause problems with work or school, and even lead to suicide. People with the disorder may feel out of control or ruled by their extreme moods and behaviors. Although there may be periods of normal mood as well, people with a bipolar disorder will often continue to have these mood episodes if the condition is left untreated.

More than 9 million Americans suffer from a bipolar disorder each year. The bipolar disorder class includes three different conditions: *bipolar I, bipolar II,* and *cyclothymic disorder.* They share many of the same symptoms but differ in severity and intensity, and thus need somewhat different treatments.

Although these disorders tend to be lifelong once they begin, treatment can relieve symptoms and bring hope. People with these disorders benefit most from a combination of medications, psychotherapy ("talk therapy"), and healthy lifestyle habits. With the right treatment, people with bipolar disorders can lead full and productive lives.

Bipolar I Disorder

Bipolar I disorder can cause dramatic and wild mood swings—from high spirits that lead the person to feel on top of the world, to being quickly annoyed or angry, to feeling sad and hopeless, often with periods of normal moods in between. The high spells are called episodes of *mania*, and the low spells are episodes of *depression*. *Hypomanic* episodes can also occur. These are like manic episodes but only last a few days and are not as intense as a manic episode.

An older name for bipolar disorder is "manic-depressive disorder." It is normal for most people to have a very good mood some of the time and a lower mood at other times. For those with bipolar disorder, severe mood swings create major problems in their day-to-day life. These mood symptoms affect their relationships and their ability to function at work or school.

More than 90% of people who have one manic episode will have more episodes. Sometimes manic episodes happen right after a major depressive episode, but the reverse can also be true. Four or more major depressive, manic, or hypomanic episodes in the same year are a form of bipolar I disorder known as *rapid cycling.*

Bipolar I disorder affects about 1.5% of the U.S. population each year. The average age for a person to have a first manic or depressive episode is 22 years, although the illness can start in early childhood or older adulthood, such as in the 60s and 70s. Men and women are just as likely to have bipolar I disorder. Women may be more likely than men to have rapid cycling and depressive symptoms. There is an increased risk for manic or depressive episodes in women with bipolar I disorder who have just had a baby.

It is common to have other mental disorders along with bipolar I disorder, such as an anxiety disorder (*panic disorder, social anxiety disorder*), *attention-deficit/hyperactivity disorder* (ADHD), or a *substance use disorder*. In fact, more than half of the people with a bipolar I disorder also have an alcohol or drug use disorder. (As noted in Chapter 20, "Treatment Essentials," using alcohol or drugs to try to lessen symptoms does the opposite and makes any mental disorder worse.) Severe and untreated medical conditions are also common, such as heart, sleep, and migraine problems that affect quality of life and shorten life span.

The risk of suicide is estimated to be about 20–30 times higher in people with bipolar I disorder than in the general population. Having an alcohol use disorder and bipolar disorder increases the risk for a suicide attempt even more. Getting proper treatment for bipolar disorder can help the person feel more in control of their emotions and their life, as well as build on their strengths. Proper treatment can also help the sense of shame a person may have about the disorder, which has been found to worsen function.

 ## Bipolar I Disorder

Bipolar I disorder is diagnosed when a person has had a manic episode. The manic episode can come before or after a hypomanic episode or a major depressive episode. The symptoms are not due to psychotic disorders such as *schizoaffective disorder, schizophrenia, schizophreniform disorder,* or *delusional disorder.*

Manic Episode

A *manic episode* is a distinct period lasting at least 1 week (or less if the symptoms require hospital care) in which a person is oddly very happy or excited, in high spirits, or irritable in an extreme way nearly every day for most of the day; is much more active or hyper or has more energy than usual; and has at least three of the following symptoms that reflect a clear change in behavior:

- Inflated self-esteem or grandiosity (such as believing they are better than others and deserve special treatment, believing they have a special talent that does not exist).

- Less need for sleep (for instance, feels rested or full of energy after only 3 hours of sleep).

- Talking more than usual (for instance, talking loudly and quickly, without stopping or concern for others' wishes).

- Racing thoughts or quickly changing ideas or topics that don't have any link to each other.

- Being easily distracted (for instance, not able to block out minor details such as someone's clothes or background noise, so that they cannot talk with others or follow instructions).

- Doing many activities at once (for instance, planning more events in the day than can be done or taking on new projects that overlap each other, often with little knowledge of the topic and at strange hours of the day).

- Increased risky behavior (reckless driving, spending sprees, out-of-character or careless sex).

Symptoms are severe enough to cause problems with social or work function. People with these symptoms may require hospital care to prevent harm to self or others. The changes are obvious to friends and family members. (For instance, those who know the person well have told them that this is not their normal way of acting.) Symptoms are not due to the effects of a drug of abuse, a medication, or another medical condition.

Hypomanic Episode

A *hypomanic episode* is similar to a manic episode, but the symptoms last at least 4 days in a row (rather than at least 1 week with mania). The key difference between mania and hypomania is that while the mood changes are noticed by others, the hypomanic symptoms are not severe enough to cause the person such problems as getting arrested for speeding, getting into fights, or losing a valued relationship because of something reckless they said or did—and the symptoms are not severe enough to require hospital care. Symptoms are not due to the effects of a drug of abuse or a medication.

Major Depressive Episode

A person with a *major depressive episode* has at least five of the following symptoms for 2 weeks, has a decline in normal social or work function, and must have one of the first two symptoms on the list:

- Depressed mood or sadness lasting most of the day, nearly every day (feels sad, empty, or hopeless).
- Great loss of interest or pleasure in all or almost all activities that were once enjoyed.
- Sudden change in appetite, with weight gain or loss.
- Insomnia or hypersomnia (sleeping too little or too much).
- Feeling restless or agitated (as seen in pacing or hand-wringing) or having slowed speech and movements (behavior must be noticed by others).
- Fatigue or loss of energy.
- Feeling worthless or guilty.
- Trouble keeping focused or making decisions.
- Frequent thoughts of death or suicide, a suicide plan, or suicide attempt.

These depressive symptoms cause extreme distress or impair social or work function. They are not due to the effects of a drug of abuse, a medication, or another medical condition.

Risk Factors

A family history of bipolar I disorder is a strong risk factor. The risk is 10 times higher than in the general population in adults who have first-degree blood relatives (parents, siblings) with bipolar I or bipolar II disorder.

Early childhood trauma (such as abuse or violence) has been found to be a risk factor for the disorder. Cannabis and other drugs of abuse have been linked with the onset of manic symptoms, as well as making manic symptoms worse.

Anthony's Story

Anthony, a man in his 30s, was brought to a city emergency room (ER) by the police. He spoke rapidly and referred to himself as the "New Jesus." He declined to offer another name.

He refused to remain in his exam room and kept walking into the special desk area for nurses and doctors. He became upset when he was led back to his exam room, raised his voice, and kept talking rapidly to the ER staff.

When asked when he last slept, he said he no longer needed sleep, saying that he had been "touched by heaven." The doctors took blood samples and gave him a drug test. They also noticed blisters on his feet. A review of his electronic medical record showed he had behaved this way 2 years earlier. At that time, a drug test was negative.

Anthony's sister soon arrived and said he had seemed strange a week ago. He had argued all night about religion with relatives at a holiday party, which he had never done before. She knew their father had bipolar disorder, but she had not seen their father since she was a child. She said that Anthony did not use drugs. She told the ER team that Anthony was a middle school math teacher who had just finished a semester of teaching.

Over the next 24 hours, Anthony became calmer, but he still spoke rapidly and loudly. His thoughts jumped from idea to idea. When the blood and drug tests came back, they showed that he had not been using drugs or alcohol.

Anthony was diagnosed with *bipolar I disorder* and with having a *current, severe manic episode.* He arrived at the ER with classic symptoms of mania: irritable mood, grandiosity, less need for sleep, racing thoughts, and restless movement. The blisters on his feet showed that he had likely been walking nonstop when he was brought to the ER. His symptoms fully met DSM-5-TR criteria for a manic episode.

Treatment

Bipolar I disorder is very treatable. In almost all cases, treatment must be maintained throughout life to avoid relapse. Symptoms improve and can change over time, so keeping in touch with a mental health care provider will ensure the treatment that best suits the person and their life and needs.

Medications

Medications called *mood stabilizers* are often prescribed to help control bipolar disorder. Lithium, the oldest and best-known mood stabilizer, is still widely used. *Anticonvulsant medications* (often prescribed for epilepsy seizures) are also used as mood stabilizers and include valproate, lamotrigine, and carbamazepine. For most people with bipolar disorder, treatment with medication is a daily need in the same way that people take medicine every day to lower high blood pressure.

If people with bipolar disorder stop taking their prescribed medications, the risk for another episode of mania or depression is high. These medications can work so well that some people with bipolar disorder sometimes believe the medication is no longer needed. They stop taking the medication even when they know they had severe episodes in the past. They may do well for a while at work or school, but at some point they are likely to have another disabling episode.

People with bipolar disorder should always check with their doctor or other mental health care provider before changing or stopping medication. For information about medication and treatment, see Chapter 20, "Treatment Essentials."

Psychotherapy

Like all major illnesses, bipolar disorder can disrupt life and relationships with others, especially with spouses and family members. People receiving medication for bipolar disorder often benefit from psychotherapy. They can learn more about the illness, work on the problems the illness has created, and renew close bonds damaged by the illness.

Several forms of psychotherapy focus on people with bipolar disorder. These include family-focused therapy, interpersonal and social rhythm therapy, a life goals program, and cognitive-behavior therapy. These forms of therapy share a number of common elements. They involve education about the illness, setting sleep and other daily routines, and a focus on the present and future. These therapies have been shown to help bipolar depression and prevent the return of symptoms.

Electroconvulsive Therapy

In severe cases of bipolar I disorder, when medication and psychotherapy have not helped, a treatment known as *electroconvulsive therapy* (ECT) can be used. With modern techniques, ECT is safely used to help relieve severe episodes of illness. For more information on ECT, see Chapter 20, "Treatment Essentials."

Family Therapy and Support Groups

Bipolar disorder can create a stressful home life and cause serious trouble not just for people with the illness, but for those they love. The whole family may benefit from mental health care services, either through formal family therapy or through a mental health advocacy or support group. Families can learn how best to cope with the illness and its impact. They can become an active part in their loved one's treatment. For people with bipolar I disorder who are married, marriage counseling can help repair the damage caused by the illness.

A Healthy Mind and Body

Along with treatment, a healthy lifestyle can also help ease some of the symptoms of bipolar I disorder:

- **Keep a regular routine.** Getting out of bed, eating meals, and going to sleep at just about the same time every day, 7 days a week, have been shown to help maintain wellness in those with bipolar disorder.
- **Make healthy choices.** Eating well-balanced meals, exercising, and getting plenty of sleep can improve mood.
- **Connect with peers.** Getting support from people who are coping with similar challenges is a key part of feeling better. A treatment center or mental health care provider can provide a referral to a local group, or one can be found online at the Depression and Bipolar Support Alliance Web site (www.dbsalliance.org).
- **Learn personal warning signs.** Figure out what symptoms signal the start of a manic or depressive episode and notify your mental health care provider when they appear.

Bipolar II Disorder

People with *bipolar II disorder* have had at least one major depressive episode and at least one hypomanic episode (see definitions in "Bipolar I Disorder"). The main difference between bipolar I and bipolar II disorder is that there is no period of mania in bipolar II disorder.

Hypomanic episodes do not cause as many problems as manic episodes. For instance, they do not require hospital care (if so, the diagnosis changes from a hypomanic episode to a manic episode). Many people with bipolar II disorder return to full function between episodes.

Hypomanic symptoms can cause random mood changes, disrupt social or work function, or change the person's normal behavior in ways that others notice. But they do not greatly impair the person, as can occur with mania. Close friends or family can provide useful information to help the mental health care provider conclude whether a hypomanic episode is present or has occurred.

Although bipolar II disorder most often begins in the mid-20s, it can begin in the late teens or adulthood, even later in life. The average age at onset is a bit later than bipolar I disorder.

Bipolar II disorder affects 0.8% of people in the United States each year. The disorder tends to begin with a major depressive episode. It is often not clear until later that the person has bipolar II disorder—when the hypomanic symptoms first appear. In 12% of people with *major depressive disorder,* hypomanic symptoms appear later, and the diagnosis becomes bipolar II disorder.

People with bipolar II disorder often first seek treatment from a mental health care provider because of depressive symptoms (feeling low, worthless, or guilty), which can be quite severe. The depressive symptoms tend to cause more problems than symptoms of hypomania, which may not bother them. People with bipolar II disorder tend to have longer episodes of depression than those with bipolar I disorder. The depressive symptoms can cause problems with relationships and work function.

Other disorders often occur with bipolar II disorder. These include *anxiety disorders* (such as *social anxiety disorder, specific phobia, generalized anxiety disorder*); *substance use disorders* (from alcohol or cannabis use), *eating disorders* (such as *binge-eating disorder*), and other medical conditions (such as heart disease or migraines). Premenstrual syndrome and *premenstrual dysphoric disorder* are common in women with bipolar II disorder, and mood symptoms may be more severe during those times. About 60% of people with bipolar II disorder have three or more other mental disorders.

Another concern for those with bipolar II disorder is the risk of suicide. They may be more prone to acting on impulse, which can increase risk. About one-third of people with the illness will attempt suicide at least once. Getting help for any symptom of bipolar II disorder is vital to improve quality of life and reduce the risk of suicide.

 Bipolar II Disorder

In bipolar II disorder, at least one hypomanic and one major depressive episode have occurred (as described for *bipolar I disorder*). Hypomanic symptoms do not lead to the major problems (such as arrests, broken relationships, lost jobs) that mania often causes. A manic episode has never occurred for this diagnosis. Someone with bipolar II disorder has had:

- A hypomanic episode lasting at least 4 days in a row.
- An episode of major depression lasting at least 2 weeks.

The symptoms are not due to the effects of a drug of abuse, a medication, another medical condition, or other psychotic disorders such as *schizoaffective disorder, schizophrenia, schizophreniform disorder*, or *delusional disorder*.

Risk Factors

People with blood relatives who have a bipolar disorder are at highest risk of also developing the condition. In 10%–20% of women, childbirth may be a trigger for a hypomanic episode. It may occur early in the postpartum period (shortly after giving birth) and may precede a depressive episode. Being alert to this risk and getting treatment for depression can relieve symptoms.

 ### Chelsea's Story

Chelsea was a 43-year-old married librarian who came to an outpatient mental health clinic with a long history of depression. She described being depressed for a month since she began a new job. She had concerns that her new boss and colleagues thought her work was poor and slow and that she was not friendly. She had no energy or enthusiasm at home. Instead of playing with her children or talking to her husband, she watched TV for hours, overate, and slept long hours. She gained 6 pounds in just 3 weeks, which made her feel even worse about herself. She cried many times through the week, which she reported as a sign that "the depression was back." She also thought often of death but had never attempted suicide.

Chelsea said her memory about her history of depression was a little fuzzy, so she brought in her husband, who had known her since college. They agreed that she had first become depressed in her teens and that she had had at least five different periods of depression as an adult. These episodes involved depressed mood, lack of energy, deep feelings of guilt, loss of interest in sex, and some thoughts that life wasn't worth living. Chelsea also sometimes had periods of "too much" energy, irritability, and racing thoughts. These episodes of excess energy could last hours, days, or a couple of weeks.

Chelsea's husband also described times when Chelsea seemed excited, happy, and self-confident—"like a different person." She would talk fast, seem full of energy and good cheer, do all the daily chores, and start (and often finish) new projects. She would need little sleep and still be up the next day.

Because of her periods of low mood and thoughts of death, she had seen mental health care providers since her mid-teen years. Psychotherapy had helped somewhat. Chelsea said that it "worked okay"—until she had another depressive episode. Then she could not attend sessions and would just quit. She had tried three antidepressants. Each gave short-term relief from the depression, followed by a relapse. An aunt and grandfather had been in the hospital for mania, although Chelsea was quick to point out that she was "not at all like them."

Chelsea was diagnosed with *bipolar II disorder* and as having a *current depressive episode.* Her husband's information about her moments of hypomania helped in making the diagnosis.

Treatment

Bipolar II disorder often responds to many of the same treatments as *bipolar I disorder* (see the "Treatment" section for that disorder). The medications for bipolar I disorder are often used to steady moods, and these medications can help prevent episodes of hypomania. These include either mood stabilizers or antidepressant medications. The symptoms that are the most serious in the current hypomanic or depressive episode will affect which medication is chosen.

Checking with the doctor about how long to keep taking the medication is important. It may be safest to take the medications daily for a long time to prevent more episodes. Each person is unique, and the doctor and patient should talk about the person's needs and symptoms to find the best course. Stopping or changing the dose of medication without checking with a doctor first can cause problems and make symptoms worse.

People with bipolar II disorder can have severe depressive episodes. Treatment for these severe depressions can require care in a hospital. If medications cannot relieve depression, then ECT may be chosen as needed.

Some of the same types of psychotherapy and the healthy lifestyle tips that ease bipolar I disorder symptoms can help those with bipolar II disorder. The goal is to live a full and meaningful life, prevent relapse, and improve coping when symptoms are present.

Cyclothymic Disorder

Cyclothymic disorder is a less common, milder form of bipolar illness in which many mood swings with hypomania and depressive symptoms occur often and on a fairly constant basis. There are not enough symptoms to be full hypomanic and major depressive episodes (as defined in

"Bipolar I Disorder"). People with this disorder may appear to others as moody. Even though the symptoms are not severe enough to require care in a hospital, the disorder can cause great distress and impair social, work, and other key aspects of function. It often begins in the teen or early adult years. Those with the disorder may seek treatment to help reduce their constant mood swings.

 ## Cyclothymic Disorder

Cyclothymic disorder occurs when:

- For at least 2 years (or 1 year in children and teens), many periods of hypomanic symptoms and depressive symptoms have occurred. These have never reached the guidelines that define hypomanic and major depressive episodes (as defined in *bipolar I disorder*).

- During the same 2 years (or 1 year in children and teens), the hypomanic and depressive mood swings have lasted for at least half the time (1 year for adults, 6 months for children and teens). Symptoms have never stopped for more than 2 months.

- Manic episodes have never occurred (as defined in *bipolar I disorder*).

The symptoms cause great distress and problems with social, work, and other key aspects of function. They are not due to the effects of a drug of abuse, a medication, another medical condition (such as thyroid problems), or psychotic disorders such as *schizoaffective disorder, schizophrenia, schizophreniform disorder,* or *delusional disorder*.

Treatment

Treatments that are helpful for bipolar I disorder are also helpful for cyclothymic disorder: psychotherapy, family and support groups, medicine, and lifestyle changes. These lifestyle habits include keeping regular daily routines; getting regular sleep, daily exercise, and careful sunlight exposure; having a healthy diet; and avoiding use of drugs and alcohol.

Key Points

- People with *bipolar disorders* have extreme and intense moods (for instance, switching between being very happy and active—or feeling very low and out of energy). These are unlike the normal ups and downs in mood that occur in daily life.

- People with these disorders may feel out of control or ruled by their extreme moods and behaviors. The disorder can damage relationships, cause problems with work or school, and even lead to suicide.
- The bipolar disorder class includes three different conditions: *bipolar I, bipolar II,* and *cyclothymic disorder.* They share many of the same symptoms but differ in severity and intensity, and thus need somewhat different treatment.
- Although these disorders are lifelong once they begin, they are very treatable. People with these disorders benefit most from a combination of medications, psychotherapy ("talk therapy"), and healthy lifestyle habits. With the right treatment, people with bipolar disorders can lead full and productive lives.
- Symptoms improve and can change over time, so keeping in touch with a mental health care provider will ensure that treatment best suits the person and their life and needs.

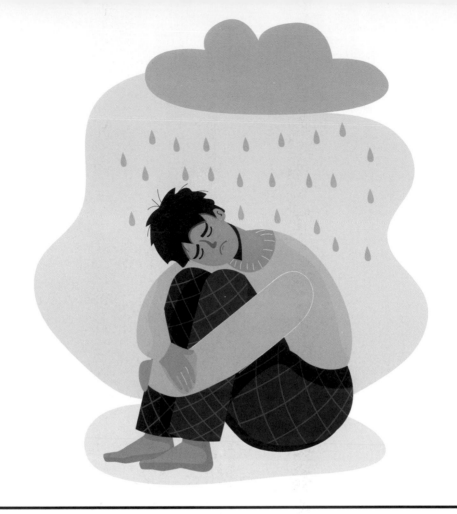

Major Depressive Disorder

Persistent Depressive Disorder

Premenstrual Dysphoric Disorder

Disruptive Mood Dysregulation Disorder

For a complete list of DSM-5-TR disorders, see Appendix A.

CHAPTER 4

Depressive Disorders

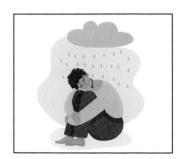

I n everyday life, the words "depression" and "depressed" are often used to express when someone is unhappy or sad for a moment. For example, people might say "I'm depressed" when they feel let down that their sports team lost a game. In contrast, real depression is a major medical problem that can have a deep and profound impact on a person's safety and well-being. *Depressive disorders* share the common feature of causing a person to feel sad, empty, or irritable (easily annoyed or in a bad mood). Someone with depression may have trouble sleeping, thinking, or doing once-normal daily functions. The disorders in this group differ in how long symptoms last, when they arise, and their causes.

Depressive disorders include *major depressive disorder, persistent depressive disorder, premenstrual dysphoric disorder,* and *disruptive mood dysregulation disorder.* Depressive disorders can sometimes be caused by certain medications, alcohol and other drugs, and some medical conditions, such as thyroid disease.

Depression is not the same as normal sadness and grief. The death of a loved one, the loss of a job, or the ending of a relationship may be painful to endure, but they do not trigger major depression in most people. Depression can cause someone to feel hopeless, worthless, or guilty for weeks, months, and even years. The good news is that depression is often relieved with treatment. About 80%–90% of those with depression gain some relief from symptoms with treatment. Treatment can include medication, psychotherapy ("talk therapy"), or both. For many people, both treatments combined have shown to work better than either one alone. Some people may need to try several different medications before finding what works best for them.

Major Depressive Disorder

Major depressive disorder is a serious illness that causes a person to feel deeply sad (or wholly absent of feeling) most of the day, nearly every day, for at least 2 weeks. This disorder is different from "the blues," which last for just a few days. Many people feel blue (a little sad or low) from time to time, but people with major depressive disorder often lose interest in what they once enjoyed. They may have problems with sleep, find it hard to think or focus, and feel worthless or hopeless. People with a major depressive disorder may describe it as "feeling down in the dumps" almost all the time, and they are not able to simply shake it off.

About 7% of people in the United States have a major depressive disorder in any given year. Young adults ages 18–29 are three times more likely to have the disorder than people over age 60.

More women than men have major depressive disorder. Starting in the early teen years, the chance that women will have the disorder is two times higher than for men, but the symptoms and how they are treated are the same for both men and women.

Anyone with symptoms of a major depressive disorder should seek help. The mental pain and loss of hope may lead to thoughts of suicide or even suicide attempts. There is a great risk for suicide for those with this disorder. In the United States, anyone can call or text 988 if they are having thoughts of suicide or care about someone who is. The line is open 24 hours a day, 7 days a week for any mental health crisis.

Major depressive disorder often occurs along with other disorders. These include *substance use disorders* (sometimes called "addictive disorders"), *panic disorder, obsessive-compulsive disorder, anorexia nervosa,* and *bulimia nervosa.*

Major Depressive Disorder

Major depressive disorder occurs when a person has five or more of the symptoms below almost every day for at least 2 weeks:

- Depressed mood or sadness.
- Loss of interest or pleasure in activities that were once enjoyed.
- Sudden or recent weight gain, weight loss, or change in appetite.
- Insomnia (trouble sleeping) or hypersomnia (sleeping too much).
- Feeling restless or stirred up (such as pacing or hand-wringing), or having slowed speech and movements.
- Fatigue or loss of energy.
- Feeling worthless or guilty.
- Trouble staying focused or making decisions.
- Regular thoughts of death or suicide, planned suicide, or attempted suicide.

One of the first two symptoms above must be present, and the changes in behavior cause great distress or impair social, work, or other key aspects of function. Children and teens may be irritable instead of sad. The symptoms cannot be caused by a drug, medication, *psychotic disorder,* or any other medical condition. A manic or hypomanic episode (see Chapter 3, "Bipolar Disorders," for more detail) has never occurred. The disorder may be mild, moderate, or severe, based on the number of symptoms and level of impaired function. Although a major loss may cause feelings like those of depression, normal grieving differs from depression (see box).

Risk Factors

Although major depressive disorder can affect anyone, several factors can play a role:

- **Temperament.** People who tend to have frequent fear, sadness, guilt, shame, distress, low self-esteem, or trouble coping with stress in daily life may be at more risk for the disorder.
- **Environment.** A stressful childhood or life events such as violence, neglect, abuse, or low income can lead to major depressive disorder.
- **Genetics.** A person with a close blood relative with major depressive disorder (such as a parent, sibling, or child) has a two to four times higher risk of also having the disorder.

Grieving the death of a loved one can cause feelings of emptiness and loss that often come in waves. These feelings become less frequent and severe as weeks and months pass. These waves of feelings, sometimes called "pangs of grief," are focused on the lost loved one. Often, there are also moments of good thoughts, humor, and happy memories.

In contrast to grief, someone with *major depressive disorder* has feelings of sadness and despair that touch all aspects of life. They have few, if any, pleasant or enjoyable thoughts.

- Grief usually does not cause the sense of low self-worth or guilt that often occurs with major depressive disorder.
- If these feelings are present with grief, they may focus on how the person might have failed the deceased, such as not visiting often enough or not telling the deceased how much they were loved. In this case, the guilty feelings are about certain actions not taken, not a total sense of low self-worth and despair that occurs in depression.
- A person's frequent thoughts of their own death and wishing to die because of feeling worthless or hopeless do not often happen during grief as they do with major depressive disorder.

For some people, grief might cause an episode of depression or worsen it if they already have the disorder. When a grieving person has had at least four or five symptoms of major depressive disorder for at least 2 weeks, the person should think about seeing a doctor.

Other problems might occur with grief that do not occur with major depressive disorder. See Chapter 7, "Trauma and Stress Disorders," for information about *prolonged grief disorder*.

Trish's Story

Trish, a 42-year-old homemaker, came to a clinic seeking "someone to talk to" about hopeless feelings that had increased over the past 8–10 months. She was upset about frequent marital conflict and "pacing and yelling" at her husband "all the time."

Trish said she had begun to wake before dawn, feeling down and tearful. She had a hard time getting out of bed, completing her usual household tasks, and keeping up with her usual parenting activities for their two preteen children. At times, she felt guilty for not being her "usual self." She became easily irritated with her husband for minor issues that would not have bothered her in the past.

Trish worries that she has become a burden to her husband. He has helped to pick up the slack when she couldn't do her usual household and parenting duties because of her lack of energy. In the past few months, she had lost 13 pounds without dieting. While usually friendly, she now rarely talks to her own mother and sisters, much less her friends. She denied current suicidal thoughts, saying she "would never do something like that," but acknowledged having thought that she "should just give up" and that she "would be better off dead." She decided to make an appointment after she attended her good friend's wedding and found she did not enjoy any of it.

For 8–10 months, Trish has had a depressed mood, loss of interest or pleasure, diminished appetite with weight loss, poor sleep, loss of energy, and thoughts of death. She was diagnosed with *major depressive disorder.*

Treatment

Major depressive disorder is among the most treatable of mental disorders. Most people respond well to treatment and almost all gain some relief from their symptoms.

Before doctors suggest a certain treatment, they will fully assess the problem and the symptoms the person is having. This includes asking questions about the problem and symptoms. A physical exam or discussion with the person's primary care doctor may also occur. Psychotherapy and medication are useful in treating moderate and severe major depressive disorder. Mild cases of major depressive disorder often can be treated with psychotherapy alone.

See Chapter 20, "Treatment Essentials," to learn more about the types of treatments discussed below. The chapter has information on recovery-focused care, which can be a part of any type of treatment. This approach focuses on the person's strengths and goals.

Psychotherapy, or "talk therapy," may be one-on-one with the mental health care provider or may include others. Certain types of psychotherapy have been shown useful in the treatment of major depressive disorder and include the following:

- *Interpersonal therapy* aims to enhance relationships and interpersonal skills.
- *Supportive psychotherapy* aims to maintain or restore the highest level of function possible with problem solving, advice, and other methods.
- *Cognitive-behavior therapy* finds and changes patterns in unhelpful thinking and behavior.
- *Family or couples therapy* may help address issues that can arise within families or couples.
- *Group therapy* involves people who have similar illnesses.

Medications also help reduce the symptoms of major depressive disorder. Antidepressants may be used to adjust the chemicals in the brain that affect mood and depression. The types of antidepressants most often used are as follows:

- Selective serotonin reuptake inhibitors (SSRIs)
- Serotonin-norepinephrine reuptake inhibitors (SNRIs)
- Dopamine-norepinephrine reuptake inhibitors

Two older classes of antidepressants are rarely used now, but remain effective options instead of newer medications. They have many more side effects and can be dangerous or even fatal in overdose.

- Tricyclics
- Monoamine oxidase inhibitors (MAOIs)

These antidepressant classes work in slightly different ways. When choosing one that will likely work best, the doctor will look at factors such as a person's symptoms, other health issues, special concerns (such as weight gain), side effects, and cost.

Antidepressants can cause some side effects, such as nausea, weight gain, tiredness, and loss of sexual desire. Side effects may go away or lessen as the body adjusts to the medication. The doctor can change the dose or type of medication if these side effects become a problem. The doctor may prescribe a few different medications before finding one that works best, and can advise on the benefits and risks. Stopping an antidepressant or reducing its dose should be discussed with a doctor or other mental health care provider. With some antidepressants, the amount of medicine must be slowly reduced because sudden stopping can worsen depression or cause withdrawal side effects.

Most people start feeling better 2–4 weeks after starting treatment. Full benefits of the medication may not be felt for 2–3 months, or even longer. If there is little or no progress after several weeks, the doctor may change the dose of the medication or will add or replace it with another antidepressant. It is important to keep taking the medication as prescribed and allow it time to work, even after symptoms start to improve, to prevent depression from returning. Doctors often recommend that patients keep taking the medication for 6 months or more once symptoms have improved.

Having one episode of depression greatly increases the risk of having another one, but treatment can reduce this risk. Psychotherapy may lessen the chance of depression coming back or being as intense if it recurs. For those who have had at least two episodes of depression, taking the medication after the second episode lowers the risk that depression will return. After two or three episodes of major depression, long-term maintenance treatment may be suggested.

Unlike the first stage of treatment, which aims to help the person get well, the goal of *maintenance treatment* is to keep the person well. This can be done using medication, psychotherapy, or both. With any of these approaches, during maintenance treatment, the person sees their mental health care provider less often, while the person and their family members and friends remain alert for signs of possible relapse between visits.

A Healthy Mind and Body

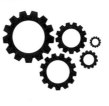

- **Support** of family and friends can help someone to prevent or overcome depression. They can encourage a depressed loved one to stay with treatment and practice the coping techniques and problem-solving skills learned in therapy.
- A **healthy lifestyle** also can help ease some of the suffering from major depressive disorder.
  - **Exercise.** Although it can be very hard for people with major depression to feel motivated to exercise, regular exercise can help in coping with depression. Most types of exercise, such as walking, jogging, dancing, and yoga, improve the body's ability to fight pain and can reduce stress, boost self-esteem, and improve sleep in people of all ages.
  - **Eat healthy.** Eating well-balanced meals is key to staying healthy during treatment. Meals with vegetables, fruits, and low-fat protein supply good nutrition and can help offset some of the side effects of treatment. Drinking alcohol can worsen depression. While alcohol may first take the edge off the anxiety that often goes along with depression, it later makes the anxiety worse. It also disrupts the deep middle-of-the-night sleep needed to relieve depression.
  - **Be social.** Although being alone may feel more comfortable, isolation and loneliness make depression even worse. Close ties with family and friends can provide comfort, and being involved in social activities offers a way to have some pleasure or fun.
- **Join a support group.** Being with others dealing with depression can go a long way in reducing the feeling of being "all alone." Support group members can encourage each other, get advice on how to cope, and

Depressive Disorders

share similar experiences. A treatment center or doctor can provide a referral to a local group, or one can be found online at the Depression and Bipolar Support Alliance's Web site (www.dbsalliance.org).

- **Get virtual help.** Attending in-person support group meetings may not suit everyone. Some organizations offer support for patients and family members who prefer to meet with others in online forums. The National Alliance on Mental Illness (www.nami.org) and the Depression and Bipolar Support Alliance offer virtual community groups and classes that teach coping skills for depression.

Persistent Depressive Disorder

Persistent depressive disorder refers to a chronic or long-lasting type of depression in which a person's moods are often low for a long time. Symptoms last for at least 2 years—and can last much longer. Persistent depressive disorder can begin early in childhood or in the teen or early adult years. If these symptoms become a part of a person's day-to-day life, they may not tell loved ones or mental health care providers about the feelings, assuming that's just how life is.

In any given year, about 1.5% of adults in the United States have persistent depressive disorder. Those with the disorder may also have an *anxiety, substance use,* or *personality disorder*. These disorders can be treated along with persistent depressive disorder.

 Persistent Depressive Disorder

Persistent depressive disorder occurs when symptoms for *major depressive disorder* are often present for 2 years. The disorder also is likely when a person:
- Has a depressed mood on most days for at least 2 years.
- While depressed, has two or more of the symptoms below:
  - Poor eating habits: eating too much or too little.
  - Trouble sleeping or sleeping too much.
  - Low energy.
  - Low self-esteem.
  - Difficulty staying focused or making decisions.
  - Feeling hopeless.
- Has symptoms without any relief for more than 2 months at a time.

The symptoms cause great distress or impair social, work, or other key aspects of function. Children and teens may be irritable instead of depressed, and their symptoms last for at least 1 year. The symptoms are not caused by a drug, medication, *psychotic disorder,* or any other medical condition. A manic or hypomanic episode or *cyclothymic disorder* (see Chapter 3, "Bipolar Disorders," for more detail) has never occurred. The disorder may be mild, moderate, or severe, based on the number of symptoms and level of impaired function.

Risk Factors

Factors that play a role in persistent depressive disorder are:

- **Temperament.** People who tend to have frequent fear, sadness, guilt, shame, distress, low self-esteem, trouble coping with stress in daily life, or problems with social or work life (such as no or few friends, not able to work or keep a job, trouble getting along with others) have a higher risk for long-term depression.
- **Environment.** Stressful childhood events, such as abuse, neglect, or death of a parent, are risk factors for the disorder.
- **Genetics.** A person with a close blood relative with *persistent depressive disorder* (such as a parent, sibling, or child) is more likely to also have the disorder.

Heather's Story

Heather, 35, was referred to psychiatric treatment by her employer after she became tearful while being mildly criticized during an otherwise positive annual performance review. She told the psychiatrist that she had been "feeling low for years." Hearing what she felt were negative comments about her work had been "just too much." Heather left graduate school before getting her doctoral degree in chemistry and began work as a laboratory technician. She felt frustrated with her job, which she saw as a "dead end," yet feared that she lacked the talent to find more satisfying work. As a result, she struggled with guilty feelings that she "hadn't done much" with her life. Heather at times had trouble falling asleep. Although her romantic relationships tended to "not last long," she felt that her sex drive was normal. She noted that her symptoms would increase and decrease over the years, but they had been unchanged for the past 3 years. Growing up, Heather had a close relationship with her father. She became depressed for the first time in high school when he was often in the hospital for leukemia treatment. At that time, she was treated with psychotherapy and responded well.

Heather was diagnosed with *persistent depressive disorder.* Her symptoms had lasted for more than 2 years and were harming both her social and work life. After several months of treatment, she revealed that she had been sexually abused by a family friend during her childhood. It also emerged that she had few women friends and a pattern of unhealthy relationships with men, who often abused her.

Treatment

As with *major depressive disorder,* the two main treatments for persistent depressive disorder are medications and psychotherapy.

Most people start feeling better 2–4 weeks after starting medication. Full effects of the medication, however, may not be felt for 2–3 months, or longer in older adults. If there is little or no progress after several weeks, the doctor may change the dose of the medication or may add or replace it with another antidepressant. The person should keep taking the medication even when symptoms start to improve.

Psychotherapy can also be a key tool in getting better. A special form of cognitive-behavior therapy has been shown to be of great help to those with persistent depressive disorder. Other kinds of psychotherapy may also be useful (see Chapter 20, "Treatment Essentials").

The nature of persistent depressive disorder is that it can last for years. While many people fully recover, others may still have some symptoms—even with treatment. The best way to cope with the disorder is to stay with the treatment plan developed by the mental health care provider. Meanwhile, people who have persistent depressive disorder can practice some of the same lifestyle tips that help improve mental and physical health in those who have major depressive disorder.

Premenstrual Dysphoric Disorder

A woman with *premenstrual dysphoric disorder* (PMDD) has severe symptoms of depression, irritability, and tension 1 week before menstruation (bleeding) begins. These symptoms lessen a few days after menstruation begins, and they end 1 week after menstruation stops. The main symptoms include problems with mood, anxiety, and sleep. Women with the disorder can also have physical symptoms, such as breast tenderness or bloating.

PMDD can arise at any point during a teen or adult woman's menstruating years. At least 1.3% of adult women have the disorder, and some say their symptoms get worse as they near menopause. Symptoms stop once a woman's menstrual cycles end at menopause.

Some women may have premenstrual syndrome (PMS). This condition describes a range of broad emotional and physical symptoms that occur before menstruation, but these symptoms are not severe enough to disrupt daily life. In contrast, a diagnosis of PMDD requires that a number of certain symptoms be severe enough to lead to problems with relationships and work, school, or social function.

 ## Premenstrual Dysphoric Disorder

Women with PMDD have five of the symptoms below (at least one of the first four must be present):
- Sudden mood swings.
- Irritability, anger, or increased conflict with others.
- Depressed mood or feelings of hopelessness.
- Anxiety or tension.
- Decreased interest in usual activities.
- Difficulty staying focused in attention or thinking.
- Fatigue.
- Change in appetite, or food cravings.
- Trouble sleeping or sleeping more than usual.
- Feeling overwhelmed or out of control.
- Physical symptoms, such as breast tenderness, joint or muscle pain, weight gain, and bloating.

The diagnosis requires that symptoms have occurred for most menstrual cycles in the preceding year. Symptoms occur during the week before the start of menstruation (the day bleeding begins) and start to get better a few days after menstruation begins. They should go away the week after menstruation stops. The symptoms must cause great distress or greatly disrupt work, school, usual activities, or relationships, and must not be due to the worsening of another disorder, such as *major depressive disorder*. The diagnosis can be confirmed by daily self-ratings of symptoms noted for at least two menstrual cycles, such as depressed mood, anxiety or tension, feeling moody or irritable, lack of energy, and sleep changes.

Risk Factors

The risk of PMDD is increased by:

- **Environment.** Stress, history of trauma, seasonal changes, and cultural beliefs about distinct roles for women.
- **Genetics.** Between 30% and 80% of those with premenstrual symptoms have a close relative who has also had them.

Treatment

Antidepressants may be used to relieve the mood symptoms. In many cases, women find relief from psychotherapy to learn how to best cope with the stress and anxiety caused by the disorder. Oral contraceptives and other hormone treatments may be helpful for some women.

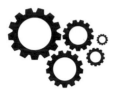 ## A Healthy Mind and Body

During treatment, changes in lifestyle may help relieve symptoms:

- **Eat healthy.** Making diet changes to reduce the intake of caffeine, salt, and sugar may help relieve symptoms.
- **Try over-the-counter relief.** Pain relievers such as aspirin and ibuprofen may help ease breast tenderness, backache, and cramping. Diuretics, or water pills, can help with bloating.
- **Exercise.** Although it's unclear whether exercise can relieve more severe symptoms of PMDD (and it may be hard to exercise when symptoms are at their worst), regular aerobic exercise—such as walking or bicycling—can help ease fatigue, boost moods, and improve sleep.
- **Keep a diary.** Writing down the type of symptoms, how severe they are, and how long they last can help the health care provider diagnose the disorder and choose the best treatment.

Disruptive Mood Dysregulation Disorder

Disruptive mood dysregulation disorder is diagnosed in children who are severely irritable or angry and have frequent temper outbursts. The disorder often occurs along with other disorders such as *major depressive disorder, attention-deficit/hyperactivity disorder, conduct disorder,* or a *substance use disorder*.

Children with disruptive mood dysregulation disorder have temper outbursts that are unique and differ from a normal temper tantrum. These outbursts are of greater force and length than the type of situation that triggers them. With disruptive mood dysregulation disorder, these outbursts happen as often as three times a week for over a year. People who are in close contact with the child witness the behavior. The symptoms often cause problems with how the child relates with family and friends, as well as the child's conduct at school. When not having an outburst, children with the disorder are still irritable or angry nearly every day.

Symptoms of the disorder must start before the child reaches age 10. It is only diagnosed for the first time in children who are at least 6 years old but not yet age 18. The disorder is more common in boys and younger children than in girls and teens.

 Disruptive Mood Dysregulation Disorder

Disruptive mood dysregulation disorder is diagnosed when a child has the symptoms below for at least 12 months:

- Severe and frequent temper outbursts, such as verbal rages and physical aggression toward people or property.
- Outbursts that are inappropriate for the child's developmental stage.
- Outbursts that occur about three times or more each week.
- Irritable or angry mood almost every day.
- Temper outbursts and angry mood occur in two different settings, such as at home, at school, and with friends.

During the year of temper outbursts and angry mood, the child must not have gone 3 or more months in a row without these symptoms. The symptoms are not due to a drug, medication, or other medical condition. Parents should be aware that some of the symptoms of disruptive mood dysregulation disorder may look like those of other disorders, such as *major depressive disorder, bipolar disorder,* and *oppositional defiant disorder.* Some children with disruptive mood dysregulation disorder also have another disorder, such as problems with attention or anxiety.

Treatment

If a child is having symptoms of disruptive mood dysregulation disorder, parents should seek help for the child from a mental health care provider as soon as possible. Getting a diagnosis and starting treatment are key to the child's future normal development. A positive family relationship also helps support treatment.

Treatment of disruptive mood dysregulation disorder usually consists of both psychotherapy and medication. Psychotherapy as the first step may be with the child alone or with the family. Medication can sometimes help to address certain symptoms, such as symptoms of *major depressive disorder* or *attention deficit/hyperactivity disorder.* Parents should seek the advice of a mental health care provider regarding use of medication. The support of parents and other family members is key to the relief of symptoms and learning how to cope with behavior problems.

Ways to Cope

- Having a child with disruptive mood dysregulation disorder can be challenging. The best way to help the child cope with the condition is to follow the treatment plan set by the mental health care provider. It can also help to:
    - **Learn as much as possible.** Ask the provider for any information that may be available about the condition, including good sources of information to learn more. Do not delay asking questions if you have concerns about the risks and benefits of specific treatment options before deciding which is best.
    - **Talk to other parents.** Joining a support group with other parents can help you feel less alone. Sharing experiences and getting advice from each other can go a long way in easing the stress and frustration in your home. If a support group is not offered in your area, try finding a virtual group that connects online. The National Alliance on Mental Illness (www.nami.org) offers support for parents and family members of children with mental illness.

Key Points

- Depression is more than "the blues" that all people feel from time to time. Depression can cause someone to feel hopeless, worthless, or guilty for weeks, months, and even years. It is a major medical problem—but it is also among the most treatable of mental disorders.
- Finding help quickly can prevent the disorder from getting worse or lasting longer. Treatments often found to be helpful include psychotherapy ("talk therapy"), medications, or both.
- Common symptoms of *depressive disorders* include loss of pleasure in what the person once enjoyed, sleep problems (too much or too little), eating too much or too little, low energy or feeling tired, problems staying focused, and often feeling worthless, sad, or guilty.
- Someone with depression may not seem sad or hopeless. Children, teens, or older adults may seem worried, angry, or irritated much of the time.

- Being social, building close bonds with friends and family, eating healthy foods, and getting exercise can all help improve depression. Although it can be very hard for someone with a depressive disorder to engage in these healthy lifestyle habits, even small steps can benefit health. Drinking alcohol can worsen depression.

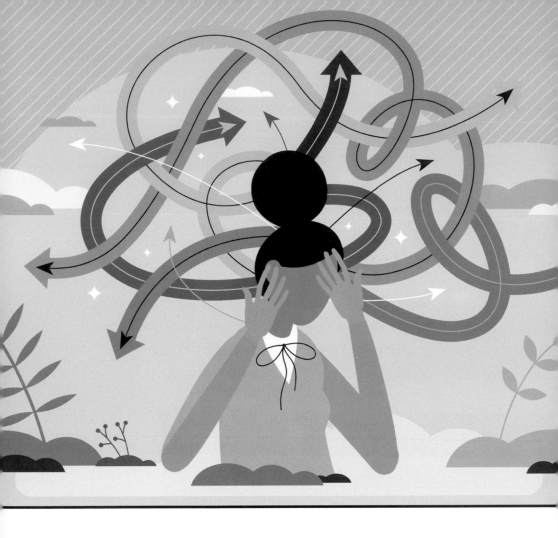

Panic Disorder

Agoraphobia

Generalized Anxiety Disorder

Specific Phobia

Social Anxiety Disorder

Separation Anxiety Disorder

For a complete list of DSM-5-TR disorders, see Appendix A.

CHAPTER 5

Anxiety Disorders

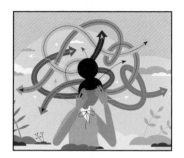

Everyone has worried during brief times of stress—or can be nervous or anxious at first when going to a party or facing new situations. Children may have normal fears when they are away from parents that often subside after a short time. *Anxiety disorders* differ from these normal feelings of at times being worried, ill at ease, or afraid. People with these disorders have extreme fear or worry that impairs their life function and goes beyond what is normal for their age or the setting.

The most common anxiety disorders are discussed in this chapter: *panic disorder, agoraphobia, generalized anxiety disorder, specific phobia, social anxiety disorder,* and *separation anxiety disorder.* The anxiety disorders differ from one another in the types of objects or settings that cause intense fear or anxiety. Unlike brief times of stress and worry, symptoms for anxiety disorders often last for 6 months or more. People may limit their job choices, prospects for promotion, daily routines, social life, and where they live because of their fears.

All anxiety disorders share symptoms of extreme fear and anxiety. The symptoms may be felt strongly even if the real threat or danger is slight. At times, there may be no true danger at all. States of fear and anxiety overlap, but they also differ:

- *Anxiety* is felt when someone expects future danger. Symptoms often include muscle tension, a feeling of dread, or a sense of being alert or getting ready for the future danger. Sometimes people with anxiety will tend to avoid settings that trigger or worsen their symptoms, such as being in public places alone.

- *Fear* is felt when there is danger. Fear is often focused on escape and is linked with a surge of physical symptoms that involve the *fight-or-flight response*. This response occurs with a real or perceived threat to life or safety. It causes a faster heartbeat, faster breathing, and sweating. The surge of physical fear symptoms differs from anxiety symptoms, which are more sustained.
- *Panic attacks* are a type of fear response. They involve a rapid flood of intense fear that peaks within minutes. They can occur with anxiety and other mental disorders or on their own.

Panic Disorder

The core symptoms of *panic disorder* are panic attacks that recur without warning. *Panic attacks* are sudden spells of intense fear and discomfort that can include chest pains and shortness of breath. They can occur whether someone is calm or anxious and may at first seem like a heart attack. When the first panic attack strikes, it causes great alarm and often a rushed visit to the emergency room (ER). At the hospital, tests show normal results. Panic attacks sometimes wake someone from sleep. They often peak within a few minutes of their onset.

People often first seek care for panic attacks for the physical symptoms, which mimic those that can threaten life, such as a heart attack. When the panic attacks recur, they cause many types of distress. This includes social concerns from being embarrassed by the symptoms, concerns about mental function (fears of "going crazy"), concerns about being able to function at work, and changing routines to avoid being in public if an attack should occur.

How often panic attacks occur varies widely. They can occur once per week for months at a time, or happen every day for a few weeks and then months may pass without any attacks.

Panic disorder affects about 2%–3% of American adults and teens and is twice as common in women as in men. Panic attacks often begin between ages 20 and 24 years. They are rare before age 14 and after age 55. Although panic attacks are the main symptom for the disorder, not everyone who has a panic attack will go on to have panic disorder. Many people have just one attack and never have another. Panic disorder is diagnosed when there is more than one panic attack that occurs without warning.

People with panic disorder are more likely to have other mental disorders, such as other *anxiety disorders, major depressive disorder,* and *bipolar I disorder* or *bipolar II disorder*.

Panic Disorder

The disorder is diagnosed when the following occur:

- More than one panic attack that recurs without warning. A panic attack is a sudden surge of intense fear or discomfort. During an attack, at least four of the following symptoms occur:
  - Pounding heart
  - Sweating
  - Trembling or shaking
  - Shortness of breath
  - Feelings of choking
  - Chest pain
  - Nausea or abdominal pain
  - Dizziness or feeling light-headed
  - Chills or hot flashes
  - Numbness
  - Feeling unreal or disconnected
  - Fear of losing control or "going crazy"
  - Fear of dying
- After a sudden panic attack, a person has at least 1 month of one or both of the following:
  - Constant worry about having another attack and what will happen when it does (such as concern about losing control, "going crazy").
  - A major change in normal behavior in an effort to avoid having another attack (such as no longer exercising or going to unknown places).

The panic attacks are not due to another medical condition; the use of a drug, alcohol, or medication; or another mental disorder, such as *obsessive-compulsive disorder, posttraumatic stress disorder,* and other *anxiety disorders*.

Risk Factors

The causes of panic disorder are unknown. The following factors may increase risk:

- **Temperament.** People who often have fear or anxiety about unknown people or settings and who then tend to avoid or withdraw from such situations; who often worry or expect the worst to happen; who perceive harm in anxiety symptoms; or who often feel sadness, guilt, shame, distress, or low self-esteem have a greater risk for panic attacks.
- **Environment.** People with panic disorder often had physical or sexual abuse in their childhood. Smoking increases the risk for panic attacks and panic disorder, as does having few financial resources. Stressful life events linked to physical health and well-being (such as the illness or death of a loved one) may also increase risk for a panic attack.
- **Genetics.** There is an increased risk for children whose parents have an *anxiety, depressive,* or *bipolar disorder*.

Laura's Story

Laura was a 23-year-old single woman who was referred for psychiatric evaluation by her cardiologist. In the past 2 months, she went to the ER four times with complaints of heart pounding, shortness of breath, sweating, and the fear that she was about to die. Each of these events had a sudden start. The symptoms peaked within minutes, leaving Laura scared, exhausted, and convinced she had just had a heart attack. In the ER, all the exams and lab results came back as normal.

Laura said she had had five of these attacks in the last 3 months, while at work, at home, and driving a car. During the attacks, she was certain that her health was in danger because she could feel the symptoms of a heart attack. When the symptoms ended and she saw the normal test results, she knew that she was not in danger and felt embarrassed that she had hurried to the ER. Because the attacks were so scary, she became afraid of having other attacks, which led her to take many days off work and to avoid exercise, driving, and drinking coffee. When she had been wakened from sleep by a panic attack in the middle of the night, she agreed to see a psychiatrist.

Laura said she had no history of psychiatric disorders except for a history of anxiety during childhood that had been diagnosed as a "school phobia." Also when Laura was a child, her mother had been in the hospital with major depressive disorder. Her mother continues to take medication for depression and sees a mental health care professional for treatment on a regular basis. Laura denied having symptoms of depression but worried about how these attacks might affect her career and job function.

Laura was diagnosed with *panic disorder.* She has panic attacks, and she has 5 out of 13 panic symptoms: pounding heart, sweating, trembling, chest pain, and a fear of dying. The diagnosis of panic disorder also requires that the panic attacks affect the person between episodes. Not only does Laura have frequent worries about another panic attack, she avoids settings and tasks that might trigger another one. She also has a childhood history of anxiety and "school phobia." Her mother's long-term depression also would have had an effect on Laura.

Agoraphobia

People with *agoraphobia* have intense fear or anxiety about real or expected problems that might occur in a wide range of places outside their homes. This includes places where they fear escape may be hard, they may not receive help, or they may have embarrassing health or panic symptoms (see "Panic Disorder" for symptoms). They begin to avoid settings that trigger their fear, such as public transportation, open spaces (such as parking lots or bridges), or crowds. They often change their daily lives to avoid being in these settings.

Without treatment, people who have agoraphobia can have symptoms so severe that they may refuse to leave their home. They then depend on others for basic tasks, such as grocery shopping. They often can venture into the feared setting with a trusted friend or a mental health care professional.

If they have another medical condition, such as inflammatory bowel disease or Parkinson's disease, the fear or avoidance is very extreme. In the case of bowel diseases, they may avoid leaving their homes due to an extreme fear that they may be unable to reach a restroom when needed and may lose control of their bowels in public. If they have Parkinson's disease, they may fear being away from medication in the event of a "freezing" episode from the disease. Or they may fear being unable to move quickly enough to depart a bus or train at the right exit.

Every year about 1%–1.7% of teens and adults in the United States are diagnosed with agoraphobia. Women are twice as likely to have the disorder than men. Most cases of agoraphobia start before age 35, with the highest risk for first symptoms in the late teen and early adult years. Agoraphobia rarely starts in childhood.

Most people with agoraphobia also have other mental disorders, such as other *anxiety disorders, depressive disorders, posttraumatic stress disorder,* and *alcohol use disorder.*

Agoraphobia

The disorder is diagnosed when the following symptoms occur:

- Intense fear or anxiety about at least two of the following:
    - Using public transportation (cars, trains, ships, planes)
    - Being in open spaces (parking lots, bridges)
    - Being in enclosed spaces (shops, theaters)
    - Standing in line or being in a crowd
    - Being outside of the home alone
- The person fears or avoids these settings because of concern that escape might be hard or help not ready in the event of embarrassing health (vomiting, losing bladder control) or panic (sweating, shaking) symptoms.
- The settings require the presence of a trusted companion or are endured with intense fear or anxiety.
- The fear or anxiety exceeds the true risk of danger in the setting.

The fear, anxiety, or avoidance must persist, often for at least 6 months, before a diagnosis is made. The symptoms of fear, anxiety, or avoidance cause major distress and impair social, work, or other key aspects of function. If the person has a medical condition, the fear, anxiety, or avoidance clearly exceeds the normal range of concerns. The symptoms cannot result from another mental disorder, such as other *anxiety disorders* or *obsessive-compulsive disorder*.

Risk Factors

The following factors may increase risk of agoraphobia:

- **Temperament.** People who often withdraw from or avoid unknown settings; who worry often; who perceive harm in anxiety symptoms; or who often have fear, sadness, guilt, shame, distress, low self-esteem, or trouble coping with stress may have an increased risk for the disorder.
- **Environment.** Childhood adverse events (such as death of a parent), other adverse life events (such as being attacked or mugged), or a childhood home life with little warmth and high levels of parental control may increase risk.
- **Genetics.** Agoraphobia has a strong genetic link; 61% of people with agoraphobia also have parents with the disorder.

Generalized Anxiety Disorder

Unlike minor worries that may arise from time to time about something specific and that quickly end or fade into the background, *generalized anxiety disorder* involves severe and continued anxiety or worry about many topics, events, or tasks. These frequent and intense worries exceed the real impact of the expected events. The constant worries disrupt daily function, making it hard to focus on tasks. People with the disorder feel unable to control these worries. The worries mix and shift from one concern to another and may include worries about their job, family, health, and money matters. The disorder often occurs with trouble sleeping, muscle aches and tension, and headaches.

About 0.9% of adolescents and 2.9% of adults in the United States have symptoms of generalized anxiety disorder each year. Women and teen girls are twice as likely as men and teen boys to be affected. Although symptoms may be experienced earlier, the disorder often is not diagnosed until people are in their mid-30s. It occurs rarely before the teenage years. When it does, the worries tend to focus on doing well in schoolwork and sports.

The symptoms of generalized anxiety disorder can begin slowly. Symptoms can come and go throughout life. The key symptoms of feeling worried differ in how they are expressed across cultures. For instance, some people may express more symptoms linked to worried thoughts and fears. Others may express more physical symptoms linked to lack of sleep or muscle tension when the disorder is first diagnosed. People with generalized anxiety disorder are more likely to have another *anxiety disorder* or *major depressive disorder*. The disorder also may overlap with physical symptoms that are common in middle age and older adults, such as poor sleep.

 Generalized Anxiety Disorder

The disorder is diagnosed when the following symptoms occur:

- Severe anxiety or worry about a number of topics, events, or tasks (such as health, family, and work) that occurs most days for at least 6 months.

- The person finds it hard to control the worry.

- The anxiety or worry occurs with at least three of the following symptoms for most days in the past 6 months (only one symptom is needed for children):

- Restlessness
- Fatigue
- Trouble keeping thoughts focused
- Irritability
- Muscle tension
- Sleep problems

The anxiety, worry, or physical symptoms cause major distress or impair social, work, or other key aspects of function. The symptoms are not due to another medical condition; the use of a drug, alcohol, or medication; or another mental disorder, such as other *anxiety disorders, obsessive-compulsive disorder, posttraumatic stress disorder, anorexia nervosa,* or *delusional disorder.*

Risk Factors

The following factors may increase the risk for generalized anxiety disorder:

- **Temperament.** People who often withdraw from or avoid unknown settings and who often have fear, sadness, guilt, shame, distress, low self-esteem, or trouble coping with stress in daily life may be at higher risk.
- **Environment.** Adverse childhood events and overprotective parenting may have occurred in those with generalized anxiety disorder.
- **Genetics.** People with a first-degree blood relative (parents, siblings) with *anxiety* or *depressive disorders* have an increased risk for generalized anxiety disorder.

Specific Phobia

People with a *specific phobia* have an extreme fear of a certain object, place, or setting that is often not as harmful as they perceive. They may know their fear exceeds any real danger, but they have trouble calming it.

Specific phobias can focus on a fear of animals, insects, heights, thunder, needles (or getting a shot), flying, and elevators. While many people may feel uneasy during an airplane takeoff, people with a specific phobia may refuse to travel by plane. The intense fear causes people with the disorder to change their lives and daily routines to avoid the fear of being in the setting or near the object. For instance, someone with a phobia for flying may decline job offers if the work requires air travel. Others may move away or commute longer routes to avoid the feared object.

While specific phobias can occur after a traumatic event (such as nearly choking or drowning), many people with the disorder cannot recall why the phobias started. For most, specific phobias began before age 10. Fleeting fears are common in children as a part of normal growth, but the extreme fears in a phobia are long-lasting.

About 8%–12% of adults in the United States have a specific phobia. Women are two times more likely than men to be affected. About 5% of children and 16% of teens (ages 13–17) have a specific phobia. Specific phobias also occur in 3%–5% of older adults in the United States. In this group, phobias are more likely to center on fear of natural disasters (such as storms, floods, or fire), falling, and medical concerns, such as breathing problems and choking. These extreme fears combined with medical illness can greatly reduce their quality of life. These phobias may cause the elderly person to avoid eating, as well as to stop or greatly reduce social outings and physical activity or tasks.

About 75% of people with a specific phobia have more than one feared object or setting (such as fear of thunderstorms and fear of flying). People with four or more specific phobias are at risk for a reduced quality of life. The fear from combined phobias can reduce how well they function at work and in social relationships.

Those with specific phobia are also at increased risk for other disorders, such as *depressive disorders, substance-related disorders,* and other *anxiety disorders.* These other disorders may explain the greater risk of thoughts about suicide and suicide attempts in those with specific phobias. These facts are good reasons to seek mental health care.

 ## Specific Phobia

The disorder is diagnosed when the following symptoms occur:

- Extreme fear or anxiety about a certain object (such as needles or animals) or setting (such as flying or heights). Children may cry, have tantrums, freeze, or cling to an adult.
- Instant fear or anxiety almost always occurs with the feared object or setting.
- The feared object or setting is strongly avoided, or endured with intense fear or anxiety.
- The fear or anxiety exceeds the true risk of danger.

The fear, anxiety, or avoidance must persist, often for at least 6 months, before a diagnosis is made. The symptoms of fear, anxiety, or avoidance

Anxiety Disorders   **83**

cause major distress and impair school, work, or other key aspects of function. The symptoms are not due to another mental disorder, such as *agoraphobia, separation anxiety disorder, social anxiety disorder, obsessive-compulsive disorder,* or *posttraumatic stress disorder.*

Risk Factors

The following factors may increase risk for the disorder:

- **Temperament.** People who often withdraw from or avoid unknown settings, who worry often, or who tend to have fear, sadness, guilt, shame, distress, low self-esteem, or trouble coping with stress in daily life may be at risk for a specific phobia.
- **Environment.** Being raised by overprotective parents, losing a parent to death or separation, or experiencing physical or sexual abuse can increase risk for the disorder. Traumatic events that involve the feared object or setting may also lead to a specific phobia.
- **Genetics.** People with a first-degree blood relative (parent or sibling) with a specific phobia are more likely to have that same phobia.

Social Anxiety Disorder

People with *social anxiety disorder* have an intense fear of social settings in which others may watch, study, or judge them. This can involve public speaking, meeting new people, eating with others, or using public restrooms. Those with the disorder fear they may offend others, be embarrassed, or be looked down upon. They have an intense concern that others will reject them or not like them. These fears include thinking that others will find them to be nervous, weak, crazy, stupid, boring, or dirty. The degree of fear exceeds the real risk or result of any such negative judgments.

Because of these intense fears, people with the disorder often avoid social settings where they fear such judgments. This behavior can limit the fullness of their life because of fewer choices in activities they will do (such as not going to parties or other social events) and a reduced range of friendships. They may avoid jobs that require meeting people or giving talks—or endure these tasks with great dread and anxiety. They may have few close friendships and romantic relationships.

About 7% of American adults have social anxiety disorder. The average age for the first symptom to appear is age 13, and 75% of people have their first symptoms between ages 8–15. Women are up to two times more likely to have the disorder than men. In adults older than age 65, rates of the disorder are 2%–5% and may be linked to reduced eyesight or hearing, shame about medical issues such as a tremor, or fear of forgetting people's names.

Social anxiety disorder sometimes occurs in people who are shy or have endured a stressful or embarrassing event, such as being bullied or vomiting during a public speech. The disorder also can occur more slowly, with symptoms building over time. In adults, it occurs more rarely. It is linked to major role changes, such as a higher-level job or marrying someone from a higher social class. Those with the disorder are more likely to also have other *anxiety disorders* and *substance use disorders*. (For instance, drinking before a party to calm nerves may lead to drinking in excess to dampen frequent social fears.) With social anxiety disorder, being often alone and without support can lead to *major depressive disorder*.

 ## Social Anxiety Disorder

The disorder is diagnosed when the following symptoms occur:

- Extreme fear or anxiety about one or more social settings in which others may watch, study, or judge the person. This may include talking with others, meeting new people, eating with others, or giving a speech. Children will show symptoms with their peers and not just with adults. They may cry, have tantrums, freeze, or cling to an adult.

- Fear of acting in a way or showing anxiety symptoms (such as sweating or shaking) that will lead to being ashamed, embarrassed, or rejected by others.

- The social settings almost always cause fear or anxiety.

- The social settings are avoided or endured with intense fear or anxiety.

- The fear or anxiety exceeds the real threat posed by the social setting.

The fear, anxiety, or avoidance must persist, often for at least 6 months, before a diagnosis is made. The symptoms of fear, anxiety, or avoidance cause major distress and impair social, work, or other key aspects of function. The symptoms are not due to another medical condition; the use of a drug, alcohol, or medication; or another mental disorder, such as *panic disorder, body dysmorphic disorder,* or *autism spectrum disorder.*

Risk Factors

The following factors may increase risk for social anxiety disorder:

- **Temperament.** People who often withdraw from or avoid unknown settings are at higher risk, as well as those who often have a high degree of fear, sadness, guilt, shame, distress, low self-esteem, or trouble coping with stress in daily life.
- **Environment.** Childhood abuse, neglect, being bullied, experiencing racism or discrimination, or other adverse life events are linked to risk for the disorder.
- **Genetics.** People with a first-degree blood relative (parent, sibling) with a social anxiety disorder are two to six times more likely to also have the disorder.

Separation Anxiety Disorder

Separation anxiety is the feeling of discomfort children have when separated—or when they expect separation—from a loved one, such as a parent or other caregiver. This anxiety is a normal part of growth in very young children who are ages 10–15 months. When the fear is extreme and occurs in an older child, teen, or adult, and it impairs normal life or family function, it may be a more severe *separation anxiety disorder.*

Children with separation anxiety disorder may cling to the parent and be unable to go or stay in a room by themselves. They may have trouble sleeping alone at bedtime and want a parent to stay with them until they fall asleep. They also may refuse to go to school for fear of being away from their parent.

Teens and adults with the disorder may have fears of harm that might endanger their family or themselves while away from each other, such as being robbed, being kidnapped, or being in car or plane crashes. They may feel great discomfort if they travel alone. Some with separation anxiety also become homesick and filled with grief when away from home. Some young adults may choose not to attend college because of their anxiety. Adults with the disorder may have constant concern for their children's welfare and check in on them throughout the day. This disrupts their workday and the daily life of their children.

Separation anxiety affects about 4% of boys and girls younger than age 12 in the United States. It is less common in teens and occurs in only about 1.6%. Between 1% and 2% of adults also have the disorder.

Children with separation anxiety disorder are more likely to also have *generalized anxiety disorder* and *specific phobia.* Adults with the disorder can also have other disorders, such as other *anxiety disorders, obsessive-compulsive disorder, posttraumatic stress disorder,* and *depressive, bipolar,* and *personality disorders.*

 ## Separation Anxiety Disorder

The disorder is diagnosed when at least three of the following symptoms occur, beyond what is normal for the person's age:

- Frequent and extreme distress when separated, or expecting separation, from home or a loved one (parent or other caregiver).
- Frequent and extreme worry about losing a loved one or possible harm to the loved one, such as illness or death.
- Frequent and extreme worry about a harmful or traumatic event that will cause separation from a loved one, such as getting lost or being kidnapped.
- Firm refusal or being unwilling to go away from home because of fear of separation, such as going to school or work.
- Frequent and extreme fear of being alone without the loved one at home or other settings.
- Firm refusal or being unwilling to sleep away from home or go to sleep without being near the loved one.
- Frequent nightmares about being separated.
- Frequent complaints of physical symptoms because of fear of separation, such as headaches and stomachaches.

The fear, anxiety, or avoidance must persist, lasting at least 4 weeks in children and teens and at least 6 months in adults, before a diagnosis is made. The symptoms cause major distress and impair social, school, work, or other key aspects of function. Symptoms are not due to another mental disorder, such as *autism spectrum disorder, psychotic disorders, generalized anxiety disorder, illness anxiety disorder,* or *agoraphobia.*

Risk Factors

The following factors may increase risk for the disorder:

- **Environment.** Separation anxiety disorder often occurs after stressful life events that involve separation from a loved one. This includes the death of a relative or pet, a change in schools, parents' divorce, being bullied during childhood, a natural disaster, or a move to a new neighborhood or country. In young adults, the life stress may involve leaving the parents' home or becoming a parent. Overprotective or intrusive parenting styles may also increase risk for the disorder.

- **Genetics.** The disorder runs in families. Those with relatives with anxiety disorders may be at higher risk.

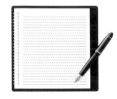

Joey's Story

Joey was a 12-year-old boy who was referred to mental health care for long-standing anxiety about losing his parents. He had begun to have anxieties as a young child and had great trouble starting kindergarten. He had been scared of being away from home for school. He was also briefly bullied in third grade, which made his anxieties worse.

Joey's parents noted that he "always seemed to have a new worry." His most constant fear revolved around his parents' safety. He often was fine when both were at work or home, but when they were in transit or elsewhere, he was afraid that they would die in an accident. When the parents were late from work or when they tried to go out together, Joey became frantic, constantly calling and texting them. Joey was mostly concerned about his mother's safety, and she had gradually reduced her solo activities to a minimum. She said that it felt like "he would like to follow me into the toilet." Joey was less demanding toward his father, who said, "When we comfort him all the time or stay at home, he'll never become independent." He believed his wife had been too soft and overprotective.

Joey's grades were good. His teachers agreed that he was quiet but had a number of friends and worked well with other children. They noted that he seemed sensitive to any hint that he was being picked on.

Joey was diagnosed with *separation anxiety disorder.* He has at least four of the eight symptoms: long-standing, extreme fears of anticipated separations, harm to his parents, events that could lead to separations, and being left alone. Joey's mother has a history of *panic disorder, agoraphobia,* and *social anxiety disorder,* and both parents agree that her own worries have affected her parenting style. His grandmother was described as being as anxious as Joey's mother. Joey's fears appear to be rewarded: the parents stay home, rarely leave Joey alone, and respond quickly to all his calls and text messages.

Treatment

Most anxiety disorders respond well to treatment. Treatment for anxiety disorders usually involves a mix of psychotherapy ("talk therapy") and medications. Treatment can improve symptoms and teach the person healthy coping skills, but it may not always provide complete relief. People with anxiety disorders also benefit from healthy lifestyle habits. See the section "A Healthy Mind and Body" on the next page for tips.

Cognitive-Behavior Therapy

This form of psychotherapy (also called CBT) involves helping the person to change unhealthy thinking and behavior patterns. The mental health care professional may work with the person to develop a plan of action to help reduce fears and improve habits of thinking. CBT may include relaxation methods, breathing exercises, and ways to distract or refocus worries and fears. Many anxiety symptoms can improve greatly with CBT. People may learn how to stop avoiding feared situations by going into settings that frighten them, under the guidance of the mental health care professional. When a person has a certain fear, such as seeing spiders or being in high places (described in "Specific Phobia"), CBT may include techniques to practice being near the feared object. This method can help someone manage a fear response when there is no urgent danger.

Medications

Treatment with medication often requires several weeks or more before people begin to get relief from their symptoms. The doctor needs to follow the person's progress with care and adjust the medication as needed.

Antidepressants that are used to treat *major depressive disorder* are also used to treat anxiety disorders. Several different types of antidepressants can be prescribed. These include selective serotonin reuptake inhibitors (SSRIs), such as fluoxetine and paroxetine, and serotonin-norepinephrine reuptake inhibitors (SNRIs), such as venlafaxine.

Other types of medications may be used for anxiety symptoms because they have a stronger "calming" effect that can reduce the symptoms of fear, panic, anxiety, tension, and stress. These are the *benzodiazepines,* such as alprazolam, diazepam, and lorazepam. Because these can become habit-forming, the doctor may prescribe them only for short-term use. (As noted in Chapter 20, "Treatment Essentials," care should be taken with these medications, which should not be stopped suddenly. Harmful and unpleasant side effects can occur and symptoms can worsen if a medication is stopped suddenly. Seek a doctor's care and follow instructions before changing how these medications are taken.)

A Healthy Mind and Body

Making these healthy lifestyle choices can help ease some of the suffering caused by anxiety disorders:

- **Learn basic relaxation techniques.** Relaxation may help in the treatment of phobias and panic disorder. Several types of techniques help people cope with stress, such as meditation, visualization, and massage. These techniques may be included in a CBT program.
- **Exercise.** Regular aerobic exercise (walking, biking, dancing) is one of the best ways to reduce symptoms of anxiety and stress. People who are physically active have lower rates of anxiety and depression than people who are less active. Yoga is a popular mind-body exercise that can also help with relaxation and stress management.
- **Limit or avoid caffeine.** The caffeine found in coffee, tea, cola drinks, and even some over-the-counter cold medications can make anxiety symptoms worse.
- **Join a support group.** Being with others who have anxiety disorders can be very helpful. Support group members can encourage each other, get advice on how to cope, and share similar experiences.

Key Points

- *Anxiety disorders* differ from normal feelings of being worried, ill at ease, or afraid at certain brief times. People with anxiety disorders have extreme fear or worry that impairs their life function and goes beyond what is normal for their age or the setting. Unlike brief times of stress and worry, the symptoms of anxiety disorders often last for 6 months or more.
- Most anxiety disorders respond well to treatment. Often treatment for anxiety disorders involves a mix of psychotherapy ("talk therapy") and medications. Treatment can provide great relief from symptoms and teach healthy coping skills, but it may not always provide a complete cure.
- Cognitive-behavior therapy (CBT) involves helping to change unhealthy thinking and behavior patterns. The mental health care professional may work with the person to develop a plan of action to help reduce fears and improve habits of thinking.
- Medicines that treat depression also can help anxiety disorders. These medications include antidepressants, such as selective serotonin re-

uptake inhibitors (SSRIs) and serotonin-norepinephrine reuptake inhibitors (SNRIs). Benzodiazepines calm fear, panic, and anxiety. Benzodiazepines can only be used for a short time.

- People with anxiety disorders also benefit from healthy lifestyle habits. Learning relaxation techniques, exercise, limiting caffeine, and joining a support group can boost efforts to cope and reduce symptoms.

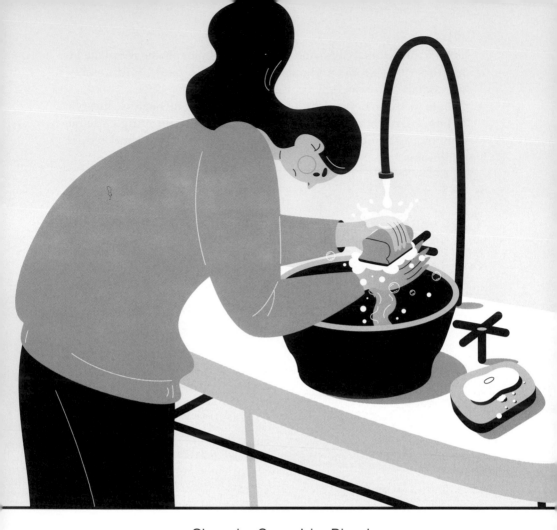

Obsessive-Compulsive Disorder

Body Dysmorphic Disorder

Hoarding Disorder

Other Obsessive-Compulsive Disorders

    Hair-Pulling Disorder

    Skin-Picking Disorder

For a complete list of DSM-5-TR disorders, see Appendix A.

CHAPTER 6

Obsessive-Compulsive Disorders

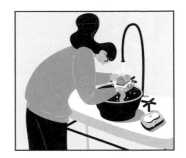

Obsessive-compulsive disorders involve frequent fears, worries, urges, or thoughts *(obsessions)* that distract and distress the people who have them. These obsessions often lead to ritualistic behaviors *(compulsions)* that are repeated in an intense attempt to deal with the unwanted obsessions. Other related disorders in this group involve repeated body-focused behaviors (such as hair pulling or skin picking) despite the person's attempts to decrease or stop them.

These disorders include *obsessive-compulsive disorder* (OCD), *body dysmorphic disorder, hoarding disorder, hair-pulling disorder,* and *skin-picking disorder*. Although anxiety is a frequent symptom of these disorders, the obsessions and compulsions are unique features that cause these disorders to be grouped in their own chapter.

At times, people may double-check a locked door, dislike a new facial wrinkle, save a few special items, pull out a stray gray hair, or pick at a blemish. This normal behavior is part of life from time to time, and the checking or saving does not have an impact on their daily life. In contrast, people with obsessive-compulsive and related disorders often are held captive by their obsessions and compulsions. Their repeated behaviors and extreme concerns can take over their daily lives, cause health problems, and impair their ability to work, attend school, or to interact with others.

Treatment can help relieve and control obsessions and compulsions and prevent disorders from getting worse. Treatment often involves both medication and psychotherapy ("talk therapy"). Most people with these disorders can go on to live full and satisfying lives with treatment.

 **A Healthy Mind and Body**
Keeping a healthy lifestyle is important in coping with obsessive-compulsive and related disorders. In addition to following the treatment set by the mental health care professional, these tips can help:

- **Learn basic relaxation techniques.** Relaxation helps ease the stress and anxiety caused by these disorders. Several types of relaxation techniques help relieve stress and worry. These include meditation, visualization, yoga, and massage.
- **Be aware of warning signs.** Learn what triggers obsessive-compulsive symptoms and what to do if they return.
- **Avoid drugs and alcohol.** Using these substances can make obsessive symptoms worse and can delay the success of treatment.

Obsessive-Compulsive Disorder

Most people with OCD have both obsessions and compulsions throughout their day. These disrupt their daily routine, making it hard to go to school, work, or have a normal social life. Many people with OCD know or suspect that their obsessions are likely not true. This awareness is called *insight*. Others with OCD may think that their beliefs could be true (poor insight), or they may be strongly convinced that their beliefs are in fact true (no insight). Despite their level of insight, people with OCD have a hard time keeping their focus off their strong obsessions and stopping their compulsions.

The worry or stress caused by the obsession (a thought, urge, or image that causes distress) leads to an attempt to ignore or suppress it by another thought or action (that is, by doing a compulsion). Common obsessions include concerns about harm to self or others, fear of getting sick from dirt or germs, and having forbidden or taboo thoughts about topics such as sex or religion. Compulsions can include constant checking (such as locks on doors), frequent hand washing until skin is raw, and counting, praying, or saying words silently over and over.

The compulsions also can be done with the goal of preventing a feared event. (Children with OCD may not be able to explain the purpose for their compulsions.) The acts cannot prevent the feared event in real life (such as placing objects on a shelf in a certain order to prevent parents from being in a car accident). Sometimes the acts are clearly extreme (for instance, checking that the door is locked 30 times before leaving for work). These acts are performed in the belief that they will counter or render harmless the thought, urge, or fear. Although compulsions may bring some brief relief to the worry and stress of an obsession, the obsession returns, and the cycle of obsessions and compulsions repeats again and again. People with OCD feel driven to perform their compulsions.

While most people will at times have concerned thoughts or repeated behaviors ("Did I check that lock?"), these tend not to disrupt living and only cause concern for a brief time. For many people, minor routines add needed structure to their day and make certain tasks easy. These routines are helpful and are easy to change with new events, such as a guest's visit. For people with OCD, their routines are rigid, and they have great distress if they try not to do them. Their compulsions can become a way of life.

OCD affects 1.2% of the U.S. population. In childhood, it affects more boys, but more women are affected than men in adult years. The average age when symptoms first appear is 19 years. Onset in childhood or teen years can lead to a lifetime of OCD symptoms that can be managed with treatment. In 40% of those with onset in childhood or teen years, there may be no symptoms by early adult years. It is rare for the disorder to first appear after age 35.

People with OCD also may have a *tic disorder, anxiety disorder,* or *major depressive disorder.* Any other mental disorder that occurs with OCD will need to be considered when planning treatment.

 ## Obsessive-Compulsive Disorder

OCD is diagnosed when the following symptoms occur:

- Obsessions, compulsions, or both.
- Obsessions or compulsions that are time-consuming (take more than 1 hour per day), cause major distress, or impair social, work, or other key aspects of function.

The symptoms are not due to another medical condition, the use of a drug or medication, or another mental disorder, such as an *anxiety disorder,* another *obsessive-compulsive disorder,* an *eating disorder,* or *major depressive disorder.*

Risk Factors

Certain factors may increase a person's risk for OCD:

- **Temperament.** People who tended to withdraw from unknown settings as a child or who often have fear, worry, sadness, guilt, shame, distress, low self-esteem, or trouble coping with stress in daily life may be at more risk for the disorder.
- **Environment.** Low birth weight, early birth, being born to a mother who smoked while pregnant, and being exposed to physical or sexual abuse or other stressful events in childhood increase the risk of OCD. Some children have a sudden onset of OCD after they have been exposed to a strep infection, such as strep throat or scarlet fever.
- **Genetics.** People with a first-degree blood relative (parent, sibling) with OCD are at 2 times greater risk for the disorder than are people who have no close relative with OCD. The risk is 10 times higher in relatives of those who have OCD in childhood or teen years.

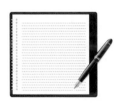

Allen's Story

Allen, a 22-year-old gay man, came to a mental health clinic for treatment of anxiety. He worked full-time as a janitor and engaged in very few activities outside of work. When asked about anxiety, Allen said he was worried about contracting diseases such as HIV.

Aware of a strong disinfectant smell, the mental health care professional asked Allen if he had any special cleaning behaviors linked to his concern about getting HIV. Allen said that he avoided touching almost anything outside of his home. He said that if he even came close to things that he thought might have been in contact with the virus, he had to wash his hands many times with bleach. He often washed his hands up to 30 times a day, spending hours on this routine. Physical contact was quite difficult. Shopping for groceries and taking the subway were big problems, and he had almost given up trying to go to social events or engage in romantic relationships.

When asked if he had other worries, Allen said that he was bothered by sudden images of hitting someone, fears that he would say things that might be offensive or wrong, and concerns about upsetting his neighbors. To ease the anxiety caused by these thoughts, he often replayed prior conversations in his mind, kept diaries to record what he said, and often apologized for fear he might have sounded offensive. When he showered, he made sure the water in the tub only reached a certain level. He was afraid that if he was not careful, he would flood his neighbors.

Allen used gloves at work and performed well. He spent most of his free time at home. Although he enjoyed the company of others, the fear of having to touch something if he was invited to a meal or to another person's home was too much for him to handle. He knew that his fears and urges were "kinda crazy," but he felt they were out of his control.

Allen was diagnosed with *obsessive-compulsive disorder* (OCD). He had many obsessions, including ones related to contamination (fear of contracting HIV), aggression (intrusive images of hitting someone), and symmetry (exactness in the level of water). These caused Allen to spend hours on his OCD routines and to avoid leaving his apartment, engaging in social relationships, and performing basic errands.

He also had many compulsions: excessive hand washing, checking (keeping diaries), repeating (often clarifying what he said), and mental compulsions (replaying prior conversations in his mind).

These symptoms also got in the way of Allen's normal daily tasks. Even though he was able to work, his job choice may have been swayed by his symptoms (few other jobs would allow him to always wear gloves and use bleach). Not only did his symptoms consume much of his time, but he appeared to be a lonely, isolated man whose quality of life has been greatly affected by his OCD.

Treatment

Treatments for OCD often combine both medication and psychotherapy. The medications most often prescribed to treat OCD are the *selective serotonin reuptake inhibitors* (SSRIs) and clomipramine. These antidepressant medications are widely used to treat depression, anxiety, and other conditions, and work well in the treatment of OCD. Although all these medications work well, some people have a better response to one than to another. If one medication is not working, talking with the doctor is key to finding another medication that can improve symptoms. Clomipramine is rarely used because of its many side effects. Response to the medication often takes at least 6 to 12 weeks, longer than the response when used to treat *major depressive disorder*. People with OCD who are treated with medication will note that the obsessions are not as bothersome, they spend less time on compulsions, and they are better able to exert control over the disorder, though some symptoms will often remain.

Medications are often combined with *cognitive-behavior therapy* (CBT). With CBT, the mental health care professional will teach the patient to fight the obsessions more effectively and to challenge the ritualistic behaviors. During treatment sessions, people may be exposed to the obsessions that create anxiety and provoke the compulsions. They may write a "script" in which the obsessions are described, and then read the script over and over. This technique works well for people whose compulsions cause great problems. For instance, with extreme hand washing, the mental health care professional might have the person touch a "dirty" object such as a doorknob, and then not allow the person to wash their hands. This *exposure and response prevention therapy* has been proved useful. It briefly exposes the person to what is feared, in greater amounts of time, and the person's urge to do a compulsion in response to the fear is delayed or blocked. With very anxious people, the mental health care professional might begin with having them think of touching a doorknob, and then not washing their hands. The exposure and response prevention methods teach people with OCD to decrease and then stop the rituals that affect their lives.

People with OCD who receive proper treatment function better and improve their quality of life. Effective treatment may improve people's ability to attend school, function at work, build and enjoy relationships, and pursue leisure activities.

Body Dysmorphic Disorder

People with *body dysmorphic disorder* are obsessed with what they think are flaws or defects in how they look. They think these flaws make them ugly, unattractive, or deformed. However, other people do not see these defects or see them as only being minor.

People with the disorder find it hard to stop or control their negative thoughts. They don't believe people who tell them they look fine. Their extreme concerns can focus on one or many body parts, often the skin, hair, or nose. Any body part can be the focus: the eyes, eyebrows, teeth, weight, stomach, face size or shape, and so on. If they can afford plastic surgery, they may have repeated surgery to correct the perceived flaw— but are rarely pleased with the results. Some people with the disorder, often men or teen boys, believe their bodies are too small or not lean or muscular enough, even when they appear normal or even quite fit and muscular. These ideas cause them to diet, exercise, or lift weights to excess, causing injury or harm to their bodies.

For people with body dysmorphic disorder, obsessions about their appearance can cause severe distress lasting for hours, or even all day. They feel driven to repeat certain behaviors to try to hide or improve the flaws. These frequent behaviors only add to their stress and anxiety. Examples of repetitive behaviors are as follows:

- Constant checking in a mirror
- Constant grooming
- Hiding or covering certain body parts or perceived flaws (frequent use of makeup or choosing certain types of clothing, hairstyles, hats, etc.)
- Comparing their body part to that of others

Body dysmorphic disorder affects about 2.4% of U.S. adults and affects women and men at about the same rate. For most people with the disorder, the first symptoms appear before age 18. The most common age for the disorder to begin is 12–13 years.

The disorder can cause low self-esteem. People with the disorder may avoid social settings. Some may drop out of school because of their extreme concerns. Thoughts of suicide and suicide attempts are high in those with the disorder, based on distress about their appearance.

Although the disorder can last for many years, treatment can relieve symptoms (see the "Treatment" section). People with body dysmorphic disorder also may have *major depressive disorder, social anxiety disorder, OCD,* or *substance use disorder.*

 ## Body Dysmorphic Disorder

Body dysmorphic disorder is diagnosed when the following symptoms occur:

- Frequent and intense focus on one or more perceived or slight defects in appearance that are not seen by others or are seen as minor.
- Repeats behavior to try to hide or improve the "flaws" or performs mental acts (for instance, compares self to others) in response to intense concerns.

The symptoms cause major distress or impair social, work, or other key aspects of function. They are not due to concerns about body weight or body fat that come with an *eating disorder.*

Risk Factors

The following factors may increase the risk for this disorder:

- **Environment.** Childhood neglect, abuse, or trauma are often linked with the disorder.
- **Genetics.** People who have a first-degree blood relative (parent or sibling) with OCD have a higher risk of body dysmorphic disorder.

Treatment

As with OCD, treatment for body dysmorphic disorder relies on CBT, SSRI antidepressants, or a mix of the two. With treatment, the symptoms can be reduced and have less effect on the person's life over time.

Those with the disorder also can benefit from the "Healthy Mind and Body" lifestyle tips noted near the start of this chapter.

Hoarding Disorder

Hoarding disorder is marked by long-standing problems throwing away or giving up possessions, regardless of whether the objects have any value ("hoarding"). People who hoard often save items because they believe they will need these items in the future or the items will have value in the future. They also may be strongly attached to the items. People who hoard have great distress (such as regret, sadness, fear, guilt, worry) when an item is thrown out, recycled, sold, or given away.

The most common items that people save are newspapers, magazines, clothing, bags, books, junk mail, and paperwork. Any item can be hoarded. Items of value may be mixed with items having little or no value.

Hoarding is not the same as collecting. Collectors look for specific items of clear, known value, such as stamps or coins. These items are neatly ordered and sometimes displayed. In contrast, people who hoard often save random items and store them without any sense of order.

In the homes of people with hoarding disorder, the countertops, desks, tabletops, hallways, stairways, and most of the floor space cannot be used because of the clutter. *Clutter* refers to large piles of mixed objects filling spaces designed for other use. Clutter can be so great that the living spaces of the home cannot be used. For instance, the person may not be able to cook in the kitchen, sleep in bed, or sit in a chair. As the clutter grows, so does the stress and impaired function. People with the disorder may not report their distress, but it is clear to those who know them or see their living spaces.

When severe, the disorder can threaten the safety of those who live in the home. Fires, falls, uncleaned spaces, and rotting food are some of the health risks that can occur. It can disrupt family relationships and cause discord with neighbors and local authorities.

Hoarding disorder occurs in about 2%–6% of the U.S. population and affects both men and women. Hoarding habits may begin early in life—and become noticed when the person is between ages 15 and 19 years. It then starts to disrupt daily function by the mid-20s and causes impaired function by the mid-30s. It often becomes more severe as a person grows older. The disorder is almost three times more common in adults over age 65.

About 75% of people with hoarding disorder also have depressive or anxiety disorders. The most common are *major depressive disorder, so-*

cial anxiety disorder, and *generalized anxiety disorder.* About 20% of those who hoard also have *OCD*.

 Hoarding Disorder

Hoarding disorder is diagnosed when the following symptoms occur:

- Lasting problems with throwing out or giving away possessions, regardless of their actual value.
- The problems are due to a perceived need to save the items and to distress linked to parting with them.
- Objects fill, block, and clutter active living spaces so they cannot be used, or use is hampered by the large amount of items (if living spaces are clear, it is only because of the efforts of others, such as family members or cleaners).

The symptoms cause major distress or impair social, work, or other key aspects of function. They are not due to another medical condition (such as brain injury) or another mental disorder (such as *OCD, major depressive disorder, schizophrenia,* or *autism spectrum disorder*).

Risk Factors

The following factors may increase the risk for this disorder:

- **Temperament.** People who have trouble making decisions are prone to hoarding.
- **Environment.** A stressful or traumatic life event can trigger hoarding, such as the death of a loved one, divorce, or eviction.
- **Genetics.** More than half of the people who hoard have a family member who also hoards.

Animal Hoarding

Some people who hoard objects also hoard animals. Animal hoarding involves collecting and owning a large number of animals but failing to provide proper care for them. The living spaces and yards of people hoarding animals become very messy with animal waste. The animals are often crowded, neglected, starving, ill, or diseased, or have died. People who hoard animals rarely seek treatment on their own and need family and friends to get involved and notify authorities.

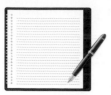

Lainie's Story

Lainie was a 47-year-old single woman referred to a community mental health team for treatment of *depression* and *anxiety.* She had never taken any psychiatric medication but had undergone CBT for depression 5 years earlier.

Lainie had a college degree and worked as a part-time sales assistant in a charity thrift shop. She said she had dated in college but had "somehow been too busy" in recent years. She was clearly in a down mood. She complained about poor concentration and problems getting organized. She said she hadn't abused any substance.

The mental health care professional noticed that Lainie's purse was filled with bills and other papers. When asked, she first shrugged it off, saying that she "carried around my office." But when asked again, Lainie admitted she had a hard time throwing away business papers, newspapers, and magazines for as long as she could remember. She felt that it all started when her mother got rid of her old toys when she was 12 years old. Now, many years later, Lainie's apartment had become filled with books, stationery, crafts, plastic packages, cardboard boxes, and all sorts of other things. She said she knew it was a little crazy, but these items could be handy one day. She also stated that many of her possessions were beautiful, unique, and irreplaceable, or had strong sentimental value. The thought of throwing out any of these items caused her great distress.

Over a series of interviews, the mental health care professional learned that rooms in Lainie's apartment had begun to fill when she was in her early 30s, and by the time of the interview, she had little room to live. Her kitchen was almost entirely full, so she used a mini-fridge and a toaster oven that she had wedged between piles of paper in the hallway. She ate her meals in the only open chair. At night, she moved a pile of papers from the bed onto that chair so she could sleep. Lainie kept buying items from the charity thrift store where she worked and also picked up daily free newspapers that she planned to read in the future.

Ashamed by the state of her apartment, she had told no one about her behavior and had invited no one into her apartment for at least 15 years. She also avoided social functions and dating, because—despite being friendly and very lonely—she knew she could not invite anyone into her apartment. She did not want the mental health care professional to visit her at home but showed some photographs from her phone's camera. The pictures showed furniture, papers, boxes, and clothes piled from floor to ceiling.

Lainie was diagnosed with *hoarding disorder.* She has had problems throwing away possessions for as long as she can recall, which have resulted in a home that she can barely live in.

Treatment

Treatment can help people with hoarding disorder decrease their saving and collecting of items and live safer, more enjoyable lives. Severe hoarding is very hard for people to fully stop and may endure despite treatment. Symptoms can be reduced with regular help. Those with the disorder also can benefit from the "Healthy Mind and Body" lifestyle tips noted near the start of this chapter. Psychotherapy is often combined with an SSRI antidepressant to help curb the hoarding behavior.

Some people can benefit from hiring a professional organizer to help "declutter" their homes. Because people who hoard tend to have great problems parting with saved items, they must trust the organizer. Because hoarding can last even after the cleanup, the organizer should return from time to time to help keep the person's home tidy.

Other Obsessive-Compulsive Disorders

People with *hair-pulling disorder* or *skin-picking disorder* often feel shame and a loss of control about their extreme acts of hair pulling or skin picking. They may avoid social and other public settings where the results of these acts may be noticed. They cover the body regions where hair has been lost due to pulling or skin is damaged from picking. Hair pulling and skin picking often are not done in front of other people, except family members. These acts cause great distress or impaired social, work, or other key aspects of function. These disorders are not diagnosed if the symptoms are due to another medical condition or another mental disorder. These disorders can come and go for weeks, months, or years if untreated. They are more common in women: hair pulling is 10 times more common in women than men, and 75% of those with skin-picking disorder are women. Both disorders may occur together, and those with either disorder may also have *major depressive disorder*.

Hair-Pulling Disorder

People with *hair-pulling disorder* often pull out the hair from their scalp, eyelashes, eyebrows, or other parts of the body—that is, any region where hair grows. The places where hair is pulled from can change over time. Most people with hair-pulling disorder pull enough scalp hair that they have bald spots, which they may try to cover with hairstyles, scarves, wigs, or makeup.

Often the behavior is a reflex, done without purpose or thought. At other times, it is on purpose or planned. The disorder is diagnosed when the following symptoms occur:

- Frequently pulling out of one's hair, causing hair loss
- Repeated attempts to decrease or stop hair pulling

The hair pulling can lead to lasting damage to hair growth and hair quality. If often swallowed, hair may collect in the stomach, which can lead to anemia (low iron), stomach pain, nausea, vomiting, bowel blockage, and even bowel tears in the most severe cases.

Treatment often consists of a mix of medication and CBT. SSRI antidepressants are often used and can help curb the urge to pull hair. With psychotherapy, people learn to become more aware of their hair pulling. They also may learn helpful techniques of *habit reversal*. This includes learning to replace hair pulling with less harmful acts, such as squeezing a ball. Some also improve by learning to prevent hair pulling by wearing gloves or a hat.

Skin-Picking Disorder

People with *skin-picking disorder* often pick, rub, and scratch their skin. They might pick at healthy skin, pimples, calluses, or scabs. Many people with the disorder spend at least 1 hour per day picking their skin, thinking about it, or trying to resist the urge.

The face, arms, and hands are the most common sites of picking, but skin picking may occur at any body site or more than one place on the body. Fingernails, knives, tweezers, or pins may be used in the process. Picking may result in scars, major tissue damage, and medical problems, such as skin or blood infections.

Skin picking most often begins during teen years, and acne may be a trigger for the symptoms. The picking may occur when a person feels anxious or bored. The picking can lead to a sense of relief or pleasure. It can last for several hours each day. The disorder is diagnosed when the following occurs:

- Frequent skin picking that results in skin lesions or sores
- Repeated attempts to stop or lessen skin picking

Because of the amount of time spent picking, people report missing or being late for work, school, or social functions. The problem also can distract people from their work or school tasks.

Treatment for skin-picking disorder is similar to that for hair-pulling disorder. SSRI antidepressants may help reduce urges and increase control over the picking. Through therapy, people can learn to become more aware of their picking behavior and learn how to stop.

Key Points

- People with *obsessive-compulsive disorders* have disturbing fears, worries, urges, or thoughts (obsessions) that fill their mind. These are often combined with behaviors (compulsions) that are repeated in an intense attempt to deal with the unwanted obsessions.
- Obsessions and compulsions often rule people with these disorders. Their repeated behaviors and extreme concerns take over their lives and impair their ability to work, attend school, or interact with others.
- Similar treatments can help people with these disorders. This involves both antidepressant medication and psychotherapy ("talk therapy"). Most people with these disorders can go on to live full and satisfying lives with treatment.
- Cognitive-behavior therapy (CBT) helps people with these disorders learn how to reduce their symptoms. The medications most often prescribed to treat these disorders are antidepressants known as selective serotonin reuptake inhibitors (SSRIs).
- Keeping a healthy lifestyle is important in coping with these disorders. The following tips can help: learn basic relaxation techniques to ease stress and anxiety, be aware of warning signs, and avoid drugs and alcohol, which can worsen symptoms.

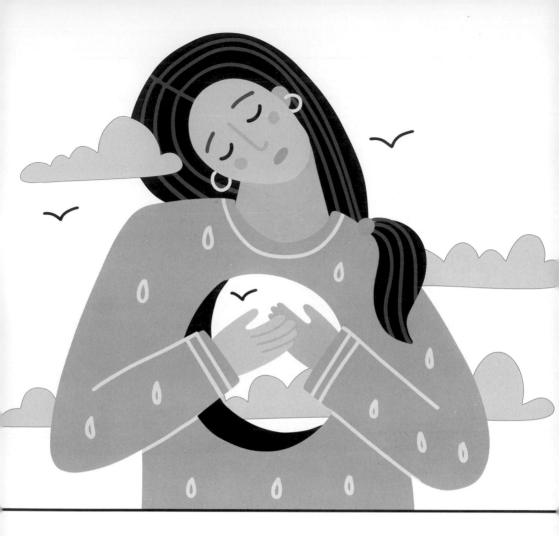

Posttraumatic Stress Disorder

Acute Stress Disorder

Adjustment Disorders

Prolonged Grief Disorder

Other Trauma and Stress Disorders

    Reactive Attachment Disorder

    Disinhibited Social Engagement Disorder

For a complete list of DSM-5-TR disorders, see Appendix A.

CHAPTER 7

Trauma and Stress Disorders

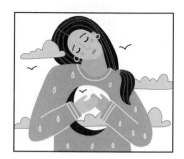

A *traumatic event* is something greatly distressing that people have lived through or seen in person. It upsets, scares, and disturbs those who survive and close friends or family who learn about what their loved one experienced. *Stress* is a common experience and involves feeling tense or pressured. For some, major stress can lead to feeling overwhelmed and unable to cope.

About 60% of men and 50% of women live through one or more traumatic events in their lives, such as accidents, physical assault, sexual abuse, natural disasters, and war combat. People of all ages react to trauma in different ways. They can have strong emotions, such as feeling very sad, frightened, guilty, ashamed, or angry. Others have a loss of emotions and energy. Such feelings can subside with time, but some people have more lasting problems for weeks, months, or years. About 30% of disaster survivors have mental or emotional symptoms, as do 30% of women who have reported rape and sexual abuse.

Trauma and stress disorders are caused by events or circumstances that overwhelm the person. *Posttraumatic stress disorder* and *acute stress disorder* are triggered by traumatic events that lead to distressing symptoms such as nightmares, flashbacks, and vivid upsetting memories. An *adjustment disorder* is a response to a stressful life event that is not life threatening, such as divorce, bankruptcy, or a spouse having an affair.

Prolonged grief disorder is a new diagnosis added to DSM-5-TR. Intense and painful prolonged grief (over 1 year) after the death of a loved one or significant other person may cause sustained problems in function for the person grieving.

Two disorders in this chapter are diagnosed in children only. *Reactive attachment disorder* and *disinhibited social engagement disorder* can occur in children who have been subject to severe abuse or neglect, and both disorders can have lifelong effects.

Posttraumatic Stress Disorder

People with *posttraumatic stress disorder* (PTSD) have a range of symptoms because of a traumatic event. PTSD symptoms may vary from person to person. A person may not appear sad or afraid, but may be angry, reckless, moody, withdrawn, jumpy, forgetful, or hard to talk to and get along with. PTSD is diagnosed when the person has had symptoms for longer than 1 month.

For the diagnosis of PTSD, the *traumatic event* must involve the person's real or threatened death, severe injury, or sexual assault (such as rape). Learning that such a trauma happened to a family member or close friend can count toward the diagnosis. Learning about a family member's death that was due to natural causes (such as a heart attack) does not meet the standards for a PTSD diagnosis, but learning of a family member's death that was due to violence or accident counts toward the diagnosis. Watching a terrorist attack on the evening news does not meet the standards for the PTSD diagnosis. PTSD can affect soldiers who have returned from combat, as well as men, women, and children who have lived through other traumatic events.

People with PTSD often relive the experience through sudden disturbing memories that repeat and involve what they saw, felt, heard, or smelled, as if the event were happening again. They may have distressing dreams, intense fear, helplessness, horror, nightmares, and problems sleeping, and feel detached or distant. Sights, sounds, and other settings may trigger symptoms, and these triggers are often avoided. Up to 30%–50% of people who have experienced trauma will develop PTSD.

Others with the disorder may have changes in thinking and mood. They may make negative statements about themselves, others, or the future, such as "Bad things will always happen to me"; "My life is ruined"; or "I can't trust anyone ever again." They may blame themselves or others for the trauma. PTSD is linked with reduced quality of life, health problems, poor social and family relationships, problems with work function, and lower levels of success in school and work.

PTSD can occur at any age. Symptoms of PTSD often begin within the first 3 months after the trauma, but they may appear even later. Those with PTSD often have a first response to trauma that meets the guidelines for *acute stress disorder*, which lasts no longer than 1 month. About one-half of adults who have PTSD will fully recover within 3 months, while some have symptoms longer than a year and sometimes for more than 50 years.

Children can also develop PTSD and at first may be restless or confused after the traumatic event. They also may show intense fear and sadness. Their play often reflects the trauma they lived through or witnessed. DSM-5-TR has set forth guidelines to detect the unique symptoms of children age 6 and younger who have this disorder.

In the United States, PTSD is found about two times more often in women than men. The increased lifetime risk of women's exposure to violence and sexual assault, including during childhood, may account in part for this difference. Traumatic events in childhood increase risk for suicide, and PTSD is linked with suicidal thoughts, attempts, and deaths. Most people with PTSD have at least one other mental disorder. The most common are *depressive, bipolar, anxiety,* and *substance use disorders.*

 Posttraumatic Stress Disorder

PTSD is diagnosed when the following symptoms occur in adults, teens, and children older than age 6 years (see the symptom list for children age 6 years and younger on later pages):

- Being exposed to threatened or real death, severe injury, or sexual assault in at least one of the following ways:
  - Living through the traumatic event.
  - Seeing the event in person as it happens to others.
  - Learning the traumatic event happened to a family member or close friend. In the threatened or real death of a family member or friend, the event must be violent or due to accident.
  - Being exposed to horrible details of trauma again and again (such as medics collecting body parts or police officers exposed to details of child abuse cases). Watching events via computers, TV, movies, or pictures does not apply unless it is work related.
- Having at least one of the following symptoms of *intrusion* for 1 month or more after the traumatic event:

- Memories of the trauma recur without warning and cause distress ("intrude" into current life). In children older than age 6, play may repeat with themes or aspects of the trauma expressed.
- Nightmares that reflect details or feelings during the trauma. (In children, scary dreams may not have content that is clearly tied to the trauma.)
- Flashbacks that cause the person to feel or act as though the trauma is happening again. (In children, this may be expressed in play.)
- Intense or lasting distress when exposed to thoughts, memories, or other reminders that reflect aspects of the trauma, such as objects, sounds, and sights.
- Physical responses (such as rapid heartbeat, feeling dizzy, sweating) to thoughts, memories, or other reminders that reflect aspects of the trauma, such as objects, sounds, and sights.
- Frequent *avoidance* of any reminder of the event for 1 month or more, shown by one or both of the following:
  - Avoids or tries to avoid memories, thoughts, or feelings about the event.
  - Avoids or tries to avoid settings or tasks that are reminders of the event (such as people, places, objects, or conversations).
- Showing at least two of the following negative changes in beliefs and feelings for 1 month or more, which began or became worse after the trauma:
  - Cannot recall key parts of the event (not due to head injury, alcohol, or drugs).
  - Frequent and extreme negative beliefs about self, others, or the world ("I am bad"; "No one can be trusted").
  - Lasting distorted thoughts about the cause or results of the trauma that lead to blaming self or others.
  - Frequent and lasting fear, horror, anger, guilt, or shame.
  - Greatly decreased interest or not taking part in activities once enjoyed.
  - Feeling detached or distant from others.
  - Often does not feel positive, happy, pleased, content, or loving.
- Showing at least two major changes in *arousal* (being keyed up) and response for 1 month or more, which began or became worse after the trauma:

- Irritable or angry outbursts (even when not provoked) often shown as verbal or physical anger toward people or objects.
- Reckless or self-destructive behavior.
- Hypervigilance (being on high alert for threats or danger, constant scanning of surroundings).
- Greatly startled by loud noise or surprise.
- Problems staying focused in thoughts or attention.
- Trouble sleeping (such as problems falling asleep or staying asleep; having restless sleep).

These symptoms cause major distress and impair social, work, or other key aspects of function. They are not due to a drug, alcohol, medication, or another medical condition. Some people with PTSD may have *dissociative symptoms*: They feel like an outside observer to their own thoughts or body, as if in a dream. They also may feel as if the world around them is unreal, dreamlike, or distant. Dissociative symptoms also include flashbacks and not being able to recall key parts of the traumatic event (as described in the guidelines above).

 ## Posttraumatic Stress Disorder for Children 6 Years and Younger

A PTSD diagnosis for young children age 6 years and under includes the following features:

- Being exposed to threatened or real death, severe injury, or sexual assault in at least one of the following ways:
  - Living through the traumatic event.
  - Seeing the event in person as it happens to others, such as parents or key caregivers (doesn't include events seen via computers, TV, movies, or pictures).
  - Learning the traumatic event happened to a parent or caregiver.
- Having at least one of the following symptoms of *intrusion* for 1 month or more after the traumatic event:
  - Memories of the trauma recur without warning and cause distress ("intrude" into current life). (Sudden memories may not cause distress in some children and may be expressed in play.)
  - Nightmares that reflect details or feelings during the trauma. (In children, scary dreams may not have content that is clearly tied to the trauma.)

- Flashbacks that cause the child to feel or act as though the trauma is happening again. This may be expressed in play.

- Intense or lasting distress when exposed to thoughts, memories, or other reminders that reflect aspects of the trauma, such as objects, sounds, and sights.

- Physical symptoms (such as rapid heartbeat, feeling dizzy, sweating) in response to reminders of the trauma.

- At least one of the following symptoms is present and reflects frequent efforts to avoid reminders of the trauma or negative changes in thinking and mood. These symptoms began or became worse after the trauma and have lasted for 1 month or more:

  - Avoids or tries to avoid activities, places, or objects that bring back memories of the event.

  - Avoids or tries to avoid people, conversations, or settings that are reminders of the event.

  - More frequent feelings of fear, guilt, sadness, shame, or confusion.

  - Greatly reduced interest or not taking part in activities once enjoyed, such as less play.

  - Withdraws from others.

  - Seldom shows happy, positive, or loving feelings.

- Showing at least two major changes in *arousal* (being keyed up) and response for 1 month or more, which began or became worse after the trauma:

  - Irritable or angry outbursts (even when not provoked) often shown as verbal or physical anger toward people or objects (such as in extreme temper tantrums).

  - Hypervigilance (being on high alert for threats or danger, constant scanning of surroundings).

  - Greatly startled by loud noise or surprise.

  - Problems staying focused in thoughts or attention.

  - Trouble sleeping (such as problems falling asleep or staying asleep; having restless sleep).

These symptoms cause major distress; impair ties with parents, siblings, friends, or other caregivers; or impact school behavior. They are not due to a drug, alcohol, medication, or another medical condition. Some children with PTSD may have *dissociative symptoms*: They feel like an outside observer to their own thoughts or body, as if in a dream.

They also may feel as if the world around them is unreal, dreamlike, or distant. Dissociative symptoms in children also include flashbacks (as described in the guidelines above).

Risk Factors

The risk factors for PTSD are divided into three categories: pretraumatic (before the trauma), peritraumatic (at the time of the trauma), and post-traumatic (after the trauma). Social support and a stable family for children help to protect from or lessen risk of the disorder.

Pretraumatic Factors

- *Temperament.* Increased risks for the disorder include childhood emotional problems before age 6, frequent anxiety or depressed mood, and a prior mental disorder before the trauma, such as *panic disorder, major depressive disorder, substance use disorder,* or *obsessive-compulsive disorder.*
- *Environment.* A background of lower income level and educational achievement; past history of trauma, divorce, or death in the family; and a family history of mental health problems or substance use may increase risk.
- *Genetics.* A person with a close blood relative (such as a parent or sibling) who has had PTSD has an increased risk for the disorder after a traumatic event.

Peritraumatic Factors

- *Temperament.* Dissociative symptoms, fear, or panic during the trauma and lasting after the trauma increase risk.
- *Environment.* The chances of developing PTSD are higher based on how severe the event was in terms of perceived life threat, harm to self, and degree of violence between persons. For instance, a child being harmed by a parent or a soldier killing an enemy or seeing the death of a fellow soldier is at increased risk.

Posttraumatic Factors

- *Temperament.* Those without healthy coping skills or who develop acute stress disorder may have an increased risk.
- *Environment.* Being around constant reminders of the event, high levels of daily stress, further life crises, and financial or other losses from the trauma increases risk for PTSD. Exposure to racial and ethnic discrimination is linked with a lasting duration of symptoms in adults.

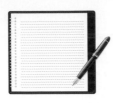

Jared's Story

Jared was a 36-year-old married veteran who had returned from Afghanistan, where he had served as an officer. He went to the Veterans Affairs outpatient mental health clinic complaining of having "a short fuse" and being "easily triggered."

Jared's symptoms involved out-of-control rage when startled, constant thoughts and memories of death-related events, weekly vivid nightmares of combat that caused trouble sleeping, anxiety, and a loss of interest in hobbies he once enjoyed with friends.

Although these symptoms were very distressing, Jared was most worried about his extreme anger. His "hair-trigger temper" caused fights with drivers who cut him off, cursing at strangers who stood too close in checkout lines, and shifts into "attack mode" when coworkers startled him by accident. In a recent visit to the doctor, he was drifting off to sleep on the exam table. A nurse brushed by his foot, and he leapt up, cursing and threatening her—scaring both the nurse and himself.

He kept a handgun in his car for self-protection, but Jared had no intent to harm others. He had deep remorse after an incident in which he threatened someone and worried that he might accidentally hurt another person.

These moments reminded him of a time in the military when he was on guard at the front gate. While he was dozing, an enemy mortar round stunned him into action.

Jared was raised in a loving family that struggled to make ends meet as Midwestern farmers. At age 20, he joined the U.S. Army and deployed to Afghanistan. He described himself as having been upbeat and happy before his army service. He said he enjoyed basic training and his first few weeks in Afghanistan, until one of his comrades got killed. At that point, all he cared about was getting his best friend and himself home alive, even if it meant killing others. His personality changed, he said, from that of a happy-go-lucky farm boy to a frightened, overprotective soldier.

When he returned to civilian life, he got a college degree and a graduate business degree. He chose to work as a self-employed plumber because of his need to stay alone in his work. He had been married for 7 years and was the father of two young daughters. In his retirement, he looked forward to woodworking, reading, and getting some "peace and quiet."

Jared was diagnosed with *posttraumatic stress disorder.* His main concerns were due to his symptoms of fear, and his aggression when startled by someone. Jared was jittery and always on the lookout for danger. He also had intrusive memories, nightmares, and flashbacks.

Jared's attempts to reduce the risk of conflict has reduced his social and career opportunities. For instance, his decision to work as a plumber rather than to use his M.B.A. seemed based largely on his effort to control his personal space.

Treatment

People with PTSD may require different types of help at different stages. Some recover with the help of family, friends, or clergy. But many will benefit from mental health treatment. Psychiatrists and other mental health care providers have good success in treating the painful effects of PTSD. A range of treatment methods are used to help people with this disorder work through their trauma and pain (see Chapter 20, "Treatment Essentials," for more detail). Medication combined with psychotherapy tends to be more helpful than either treatment alone.

- **Medication.** The selective serotonin reuptake inhibitor (SSRI) antidepressants, such as paroxetine and sertraline, can help in treating the symptoms of PTSD, such as nightmares and flashbacks.
- **Cognitive-behavior therapy (CBT).** This form of psychotherapy focuses on changing painful patterns of behavior and intrusive thoughts by teaching relaxation techniques. CBT also pinpoints, reviews, and challenges the thoughts that are causing problems.
- **Cognitive processing therapy (CPT).** This form of therapy teaches how to think about and change upsetting thoughts from trauma, such as feeling guilty or to blame for what happened. CPT teaches a new way to handle these upsetting thoughts. In CPT, people with PTSD learn skills that can help them decide whether there are more helpful ways to think about their trauma.
- **Prolonged exposure therapy.** This type of CBT uses careful, repeated, detailed reliving of the trauma (exposure) to "trigger" symptoms in a safe, controlled context. This helps the survivor face and gain control of the extreme fear and distress from the trauma. In some cases, trauma memories can be faced all at once (known as "flooding"). In others, it is better to work up to the most severe trauma slowly or by taking the trauma one piece at a time (known as "desensitization").
- **Eye movement desensitization and reprocessing (EMDR).** EMDR is a type of psychotherapy that can help to process upsetting memories, thoughts, and feelings related to the trauma. It involves focusing on a back-and-forth movement or sound while calling to mind the upsetting memory. This approach causes shifts in processing these experiences that can help people with PTSD to get relief from their symptoms.

For Service Members and Their Families: Coping With PTSD

Talk about it.
- Seek support from family members.
- Speak to other service members who have been through similar situations.
- Speak to a mental health care provider (either one-on-one or as a family). See Appendix C, "Helpful Resources," for support services, such as **Give an Hour**.
- Get advice from people you trust or respect.

Strive for balance.
- Avoid extremes in personal behavior, such as drinking too much alcohol.
- Seek out people who are supportive and positive.

Take care of yourself.
- Engage in healthy behaviors, such as getting exercise, adequate rest, and a balanced diet.
- Avoid alcohol and drugs. They won't improve your symptoms, but only mask them for a short time.

Take care of your loved ones.
- Spend more time with your romantic partner, children, or other family members.
- Focus some of your energy on helping your family cope with their problems.

Give yourself a break.
- Limit your exposure to distressing news reports and violent movies or games.
- Focus more time on what you enjoy.

Help others.
- Provide aid to other service members or families who are coping with trauma.
- Helping others will also help you to cope. Find and get engaged in volunteer activities you enjoy.

For more help:
See the **National Center for PTSD** website (www.ptsd.va.gov) for these tools and more:
- A good overview of PTSD and effective treatment options
- Self-help tools, including PTSD apps and videos
  - Offer support for coping with sadness, anxiety, and other symptoms.
  - Can help you relax when you feel stressed, improve your mood, learn how to tackle difficult problems, and help change thinking patterns.

When children experience a trauma or stressful event, they are often afraid it will happen again. Parents can help children and teens feel supported and safe in the following ways:

- Let them know that feeling upset after a bad or scary event is normal.
- Allow them to express how they feel. Don't ignore or make light of their feelings.
- Protect them from further exposure to the trauma, as much as possible.
- Return to normal routines as much as possible, such as meal times and going to school.

Getting early treatment and help is essential. Psychotherapy sessions alone or with other family members can also help children to speak, play, draw, or write about the event and work through their fears.

Just knowing a parent is there to listen and give attention, love, and time is helpful to the child. The **American Academy of Child and Adolescent Psychiatry** (www.aacap.org) offers resources for families about coping with life crises, as well as how to find a local child and adolescent psychiatrist. The website contains helpful tips such as avoiding violent or upsetting TV images and setting routines to help the child feel safe.

A Healthy Mind and Body

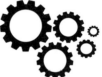

Taking care of your body and emotions can go a long way in helping to ease the stress and anxiety caused by a traumatic event. A few lifestyle changes can help:

- **Stay connected with family and friends.** Try to keep close contact through talking and being with loved ones who can offer emotional support as you work through PTSD.
- **Join a support group of trauma survivors.** Group therapy or discussion groups encourage survivors of similar events to share their experiences and reactions to them. Group members help one another realize that many people would have done the same thing and felt the same emotions. (See Appendix C, "Helpful Resources," for groups that can help.)
- **Exercise.** Almost any type of physical activity, such as walking, jogging, biking, and weight lifting, can boost mood, reduce tension, and improve self-esteem.
- **Avoid drugs and alcohol.** Many who suffer from PTSD symptoms turn to alcohol and drugs for relief. These only make the symptoms worse and delay the success of treatment.

Acute Stress Disorder

Acute stress disorder occurs in some people after traumatic events. Traumatic events that can cause acute stress disorder are the same as those that can cause PTSD. These include threatened or real death, serious accidents, violent personal attack, sexual assault or abuse, disasters, and war combat. The symptoms for acute stress disorder last for a shorter time than for PTSD.

Traumatic events cause strong feelings of anxiety, fear, helplessness, or horror. People with acute stress disorder often may relive the trauma. They may feel extreme guilt for their response, feel ashamed for not getting over the trauma more quickly, or be very focused on future harm. Some may have *dissociative symptoms*: They feel numb, dazed, or detached from themselves. They may see things happen in slow motion.

The disorder lasts from 3 days to 1 month after the traumatic event. When symptoms last longer than 1 month, the disorder may progress to PTSD. Studies show that about 50% of people with acute stress disorder may go on to have PTSD. For others, the stress response may end shortly after 1 month.

The number of people who have acute stress disorder varies for different types of trauma. Survivors of trauma that did not involve personal assault (such as car accidents or severe burns), have rates lower than 20%. Those who survive assault, rape, or mass shootings have higher rates, between 19% and 50%.

Women are diagnosed with acute stress disorder more often than men. The higher numbers in women may be due to the higher rates of personal violence they experience.

 Acute Stress Disorder

The following must occur for a diagnosis of acute stress disorder:

- Being exposed to threatened or real death, severe injury, or sexual assault in at least one of the following ways:
    - Living through the traumatic event.
    - Seeing the event in person as it happens to others.
    - Learning the traumatic event happened to a family member or close friend. In the threatened or real death of a family member or friend, the event must be violent or due to accident.
    - Being exposed to horrible details of trauma again and again (such as medics collecting body parts or police officers exposed

to details of child abuse cases). Watching events via computers, TV, movies, or pictures does not apply unless it is work related.

- Having at least nine of the following symptoms from any of the five categories below. Symptoms begin or become worse after the traumatic event. They last for at least 3 days and up to 1 month after the trauma:

Intrusion Symptoms

- Memories of the trauma recur without warning and cause distress. In children, play may repeat with themes or aspects of the trauma expressed.
- Nightmares that reflect details or feelings during the trauma. (In children, scary dreams may not have content that is clearly tied to the trauma.)
- Flashbacks that cause the person to feel or act as though the trauma is happening again. (In children, this may be expressed in play.)
- Intense or lasting distress when exposed to thoughts, memories, or other reminders that reflect aspects of the trauma, such as objects, sounds, and sights.

Negative Mood

- Often does not feel positive, happy, pleased, content, or loving.

Dissociative Symptoms

- An altered sense of what is real in one's surroundings or self (such as seeing oneself as if watching from the other side of the room, being in a daze).
- Cannot recall key aspects of the trauma (not because of head injury, alcohol, or drugs).

Avoidance Symptoms

- Tries to avoid memories, thoughts, or feelings about the event.
- Tries to avoid reminders (such as people, places, objects, tasks, or conversations) that raise memories, thoughts, or feelings about the event.

Arousal Symptoms

- Trouble sleeping (such as problems falling asleep or staying asleep; having restless sleep).
- Irritable or angry outbursts (even when not provoked) often shown as verbal or physical anger toward people or objects.

- Hypervigilance (being on high alert for threats or danger, constant scanning of surroundings).
- Problems staying focused in thoughts or attention.
- Greatly startled by loud noise or surprise.

These symptoms cause major distress or impair social, work, or other key aspects of function. They are not due to a drug, alcohol, medication, another medical condition, or *brief psychotic disorder.*

Risk Factors

Several factors can increase a person's risk of developing acute stress disorder:

- **Temperament.** Those who have had another mental disorder, who have a coping style based on avoiding thoughts and feelings, or who often feel fear, sadness, guilt, anxiety, shame, or distress have an increased risk for this disorder. People who fear the worst after the trauma are also at greater risk for the disorder.
- **Environment.** Being exposed to prior trauma.

Mary's and Robert's Stories

Traumatic Event
Mary went to a theater to see a movie premiere. As she settled into her seat, a young man in a ski mask suddenly appeared in front of the screen. Holding an assault rifle, he fired into the crowd. She saw many people get shot, including the woman sitting next to her. People all around began screaming, and there was a confused stampede for the exit door. Terrified, she somehow fought her way to the exit. She escaped, uninjured, to the parking lot, just as police cars arrived.

Robert was in the same movie theater at the same time. He too feared for his life. Hiding behind a row of seats, he was able to crawl to the aisle and quickly sprint to the exit. Although covered in blood, he escaped without physical injury.

Two days later, both Mary and Robert considered themselves "nervous wrecks." Grateful that they were alive and uninjured, they still found themselves very anxious and on edge. They jumped at the slightest noise. They kept watching TV for the latest news about the shooting. Every time there was real video of the event, they had panic attacks, broke out into a sweat, were unable to calm down, and could not stop thinking about the trauma. They could not sleep at night because of nightmares, and during the day they had constant intrusive and unwelcome memories of gunshots, screams, and their own personal terror during the event.

Mary—Two Weeks Later

Mary was feeling and behaving like her normal self within 2 weeks. Although reminders of the shooting sometimes led to a brief panic or physical reaction, they did not dominate her waking hours. She no longer had nightmares. She knew that she would never forget what happened in that movie theater, but for the most part, her life was returning to normal.

Robert—Two Weeks Later

Robert had not recovered 2 weeks later. He felt unable to express his feelings and to have pleasant or positive feelings. He jumped at the slightest sound and was unable to focus on his work, and he had nightmares. He tried to avoid any reminders of the shootings but still remembered the sound of gunfire, the screams, and the sticky feel of the blood pouring out of his neighbor's chest and onto him as he hid behind the seats. He felt disconnected from his surroundings and from himself. He viewed his life as having been changed by this trauma.

Diagnosis

Two weeks after the shooting, Mary did not have symptoms that met criteria for a trauma diagnosis. Right after a traumatic event, almost everyone is upset, but most will often start feeling better within 2–3 days and have a normal recovery. Mary's response right after the shooting was normal for the trauma: shock, fear, grief, confusion, trouble staying focused, fatigue, trouble sleeping, easily startled, racing pulse, nausea, and loss of appetite. These symptoms had gone away after about 2 weeks.

Robert was diagnosed with acute stress disorder. This involved more intense symptoms during the month after the shooting. He had at least 9 of 14 possible symptoms, including nightmares, flashbacks, trouble sleeping, and hypervigilance.

Treatment

The same types of treatments used for PTSD can help those with acute stress disorder. CBT has shown the most success for treating people with acute stress disorder. It can help people learn to control their symptoms and may keep symptoms from getting worse. The other therapies described for PTSD can also be used.

Medication may ease symptoms of anxiety and stress on a short-term basis. These include the SSRI antidepressants and the benzodiazepine tranquilizers. Some patients may benefit from medication to help them sleep at night.

Adjustment Disorders

Changes in life often cause stress—whether it's a single event, such as starting a new job or going away to school, or a series of events, such as marital and work problems. Stressful change also can be an ongoing problem, such as with a newly diagnosed serious illness or a child living in different homes of parents who have just divorced.

Some people adjust to such changes, but others will develop symptoms of an *adjustment disorder*. Those with an adjustment disorder may have a range of symptoms that include depressed mood, thoughts of suicide, anxiety, and impaired work or school function. These "walking wounded" may have symptoms that are severe enough to require treatment or care. Adjustment disorders are linked with an increased risk of suicide attempts and suicide.

After the stressful event or circumstance occurs, signs of adjustment disorder begin within 3 months of the event and go away 6 months after the event has resolved. Between 5% and 20% of people in the United States seeking mental health treatment have symptoms of the disorder.

Sometimes the person's symptoms lead to a more specific disorder, such as *major depressive disorder*. If so, that diagnosis will be given even if a stressor appears to have caused the symptoms.

 Adjustment Disorders

The disorder is diagnosed when one or both of the following symptoms occur within 3 months after the stressful event began:

- Extreme and lasting distress that exceeds the type of stressor. This includes depressed mood, anxiety, or a mix of anxiety with depressed mood.
- Major problems in social, work, or other key aspects of function.

These symptoms are not due to another mental disorder. They do not reflect normal grieving over a loved one's death. Once the stressful event has passed, symptoms do not last for more than another 6 months.

Risk Factors

People who may have a higher risk for adjustment disorders are those from disadvantaged surroundings (such as being poor, having been in foster care, or having less education). They are faced with many stressful life events that may increase risk.

Treatment

Most people with adjustment disorders do well and may need treatment for only a short time. There are two main types of treatment for adjustment disorders—psychotherapy (counseling or "talk therapy") and medications.

Brief psychotherapy, either alone or in a group, helps people learn why the stressful event had such a great impact on them. Putting painful feelings and fears into words lessens the pressure caused by the stressor and helps people with the disorder to cope better. As they see this connection, they also learn coping skills to help deal with any future stressful events.

Group therapy involves people with similar problems. In the group, people can learn more about their problem, gain a fresh view of it, face emotional issues, release pent-up feelings, and feel less alone.

Medications also may reduce symptoms and can be used for a short time. Antidepressant and anti-anxiety medications are usually prescribed. Medication to help a person sleep may also be prescribed.

Prolonged Grief Disorder

The death of a loved one or significant other often leaves those who are mourning with intense and painful feelings of grief in the first few weeks and months after the loss. This is normal and part of the natural process of grieving and healing. While grief is expressed and felt in different ways, the symptoms of *prolonged grief disorder* can occur in anyone and in all social and cultural groups.

In prolonged grief disorder, after at least 1 year (or 6 months in children and teens), severe grief continues beyond what is expected by the grieving person's culture and religion. For nearly every day, those with prolonged grief disorder may have an intense longing for the person who has died, and may be unable to stop thinking about the person, sometimes along with feelings of intense sorrow and frequent crying. They may have thoughts throughout the day about how the death happened. People with prolonged grief disorder feel disbelief that the person has died; avoid reminders that the person is truly dead; often feel emotionally numb or removed from others; and may often feel angry, bitter, or filled with sorrow about the death of this loved one or significant other. It is hard for them to take part in social activities with family members and friends, and activities enjoyed before the death no longer provide enjoyment or comfort. They feel that life no longer has meaning and are extremely lonely.

For older children and teens with prolonged grief disorder, feeling that life has no meaning without the person who died may include giving up on their life goals ("It's not worth trying if they can't be here"), not caring about risky behavior ("So what if I get hurt or die?"), or feeling that their future is "ruined."

People who were very close to and relied on the deceased person a great deal are at risk of developing prolonged grief disorder. Those with symptoms of prolonged grief disorder are also at high risk for suicidal thoughts, especially when they feel shame or distress. Risk for both the disorder and suicidal thoughts is increased if the cause of death was suicide, if the mourner feels cut off from others, and if the mourner lacks or avoids friends, family, and community support.

Prolonged grief disorder often occurs along with other mental disorders, such as *major depressive disorder, posttraumatic stress disorder,* and *substance use disorders.*

 Prolonged Grief Disorder

For a diagnosis of prolonged grief disorder, the loss of a loved one or significant other person must have occurred at least 1 year ago for adults and at least 6 months ago for children and adolescents.

Since the death, one or both symptoms below have been present most days to a great degree, nearly every day for at least the last month:

- Intense yearning or longing for the deceased person.
- Constant thoughts or memories of the deceased person (in children and adolescents, constant thoughts may focus on the details of the death).

Since the death, at least three of the symptoms below occur nearly every day for at least the last month:

- Identity disruption (for example, feeling as though part of oneself has died).
- Strong disbelief about the death.
- Avoidance of reminders that the person is dead.
- Intense emotional pain (such as anger, bitterness, or sorrow) related to the death.
- Problems engaging with friends, pursuing interests, and planning for the future.
- Feeling emotionally numb.
- Feeling that life has no meaning.
- Intense loneliness (that is, feeling alone or removed from others).

These symptoms cause major distress or impair social, work, or other key aspects of function. In addition, the person's grief lasts longer than what is thought to be a natural grief response for their culture and religion. The symptoms are not better explained by another mental disorder, such as *major depressive disorder* or *posttraumatic stress disorder*, and are not due a substance (such as medication or alcohol) or another medical condition.

Risk Factors

Risks for prolonged grief disorder include the death of a spouse, partner, or child; the violent or unexpected death of the loved one or significant person; and the deceased person was the main source of financial, practical, or emotional support. Changing caregivers or lack of supportive caregivers increases the risk for bereaved children. Those who experience the death of a child, especially if the child is younger than 25 years old, are more likely to have prolonged grief disorder symptoms linked to suicidal thoughts.

Shawna's Story

Shawna, a 46-year-old married woman, lost her 22-year-old daughter, Keisha, in a car accident over 14 months ago. She and Keisha's father, James, had been married for 23 years. Keisha was their only child. Shawna's mother died when she was 8 years old, after which Shawna developed separation anxiety symptoms. She still had difficulty leaving home as a teen and young adult until she met James. She and James grew close, married quickly, and had Keisha soon after they were married.

Keisha became the center of Shawna's world, and given the early loss of her own mother, Shawna prided herself on being an involved and devoted caregiver to Keisha. James worked as an electrician while Shawna was a stay-at-home mother. Although Shawna and James struggled to make ends meet, they tried hard to make a comfortable life for Keisha, including buying her a car when she was 19 years old. Keisha was just about to graduate from college when she died in a car accident while driving alone at 1 A.M. back to her parents' home, where she still lived. There were rumors that Keisha fell asleep at the wheel because she was worn out from studying for finals.

For over 14 months since Keisha's death, Shawna has tried to keep busy with household tasks to distract herself from her painful longing for Keisha and sorrow over her death. At times she thinks she was a failure as a mother. She feels guilty for buying Keisha a car and for being alive when her daughter is not. She has become withdrawn from everyone, including her husband. Their marriage has been strained because Shawna has become distant and consumed by grief and despair. She does not care if she lives or dies. She finds that being with other parents is very hard for her. She has trouble listening to others speak about their children and avoids most of her former friends because when they talk of their children, it upsets her. Aside from the separation anxiety Shawna felt as a child, she has no history of other mood, anxiety, alcohol, or substance use disorders; is not currently drinking or using other drugs; has no medical conditions that might be contributing to the symptoms she describes; and has never seen a mental health professional.

Treatment

Prolonged grief disorder treatment uses elements of CBT to help the mourner accept the loss and achieve a sense of inner peace. It helps the mourner come to terms with the loss and realize that life can continue without the loved one or significant other. CBT can be effective with children and teens as well. *Meaning-centered therapy* has also been shown to benefit those with prolonged grief disorder.

Grief support groups can also provide a useful source of social connection and care. They can help people feel less alone, thus reducing the isolation that could increase the risk for prolonged grief disorder. While medications are not commonly prescribed for people with prolonged grief disorder, antidepressants may be helpful for those with depressive or anxiety symptoms. More information on treatment is available from The Center for Prolonged Grief (https://prolongedgrief.columbia.edu/for-the-public).

Other Trauma and Stress Disorders

Two disorders describe how some children respond to the distress of severe neglect (that is, not receiving enough needed love and care when they were infants or very young children). Even though these disorders share the same cause, they reflect whether the child's response is inward (*reactive attachment disorder*) or outward (*disinhibited social engagement disorder*). These disorders are diagnosed when symptoms have occurred in a child older than 9 months for more than 1 year.

These disorders also can occur along with malnutrition and delays in language and thinking skills. They have one key feature in common—the child has had an extreme lack of needed care as shown by at least one of the following:

- Social neglect (lack of comfort, relating, and affection from parents or caregivers).
- Frequent changes of main caregivers, such as in foster care. This limits being able to form stable attachments (connections) with known caregivers.

- Being raised in a setting that greatly limits chances to closely attach to certain caregivers (such as institutions with many children and few caregivers).

Family therapy and parenting skills can help parents and caregivers give more frequent, stable, and loving care, such as holding the child often. A healthy, caring bond with the child and a mental health care provider can also help.

Reactive Attachment Disorder

Reactive attachment disorder affects infants and very young children. The key feature is absent or very little attachment between the child and key adults who provide care. When distressed, children with the disorder rarely turn to these adults for comfort, support, nurture, or protection. When given comfort, the child does not seem to respond or responds very little. The child shows withdrawn behavior, depressive symptoms, and few happy feelings. Without normal comfort, holding, and relating with the child, signs of the disorder may last for years. The disorder occurs in less than 10% of children in foster care or institutions. It must be diagnosed with caution in children older than 5 years. The behavior is not due to *autism spectrum disorder*, and the following symptoms appear before age 5:

- A frequent pattern of withdrawn and restrained behavior toward parents or other adult caregivers, as shown by the following:
  - Rare or little effort to seek comfort when distressed.
  - Rare or little response to comfort when distressed.
- Frequent social and emotional problems shown by at least two of the following:
  - Little social and emotional response to others.
  - Little positive emotion (such as smiling).
  - Sudden moments of irritable, sad, or fearful behavior when no threat or harm exists with adult caregivers.

Disinhibited Social Engagement Disorder

Children with *disinhibited social engagement disorder* relate to strangers in the same way they relate with their parents or other adult caregivers. They aren't shy or hesitant—and are too friendly—around strange adults. The disorder is rare and may occur with *autism spectrum disorder* or *attention-deficit/hyperactivity disorder*. When the disorder lasts into teen years, social ties may be on a surface level, with more risk for peer conflicts. Symptoms include the following:

- A frequent pattern in which the child approaches and interacts with strangers, showing at least two of the following:
  - Little or no shyness in approaching and interacting with unknown adults.
  - Very talkative or physical (cuddly) with strangers.
  - Little or no checking back with the parent or caregiver after venturing off, even in unknown settings.
  - Willing to go off with an unknown adult with little or no caution.

Key Points

- A *traumatic event* is something greatly distressing that people have lived through or seen in person. It upsets, scares, and disturbs those who survive and close friends or family who learn about what their loved one experienced. *Stress* is a common experience and involves feeling tense or pressured. For some, major stress can lead to feeling overwhelmed and unable to cope. Intense and painful *prolonged grief* (over 1 year) after the death of a loved one or significant other person may cause sustained problems in function for the person grieving.
- People of all ages react to trauma in different ways. They can have strong emotions, such as feeling very sad, frightened, guilty, ashamed, or angry. Others have a loss of emotions and energy. Such feelings can subside with time, but some people have more lasting problems for weeks, months, or years. *Trauma and stress disorders* are caused by events or circumstances that overwhelm the person.
- Those with trauma disorders should be encouraged to stay connected with family and friends, join support groups of trauma survivors, get exercise, and avoid drugs and alcohol. Treatment can help relieve symptoms and improve the person's ability to function.
- A number of treatment options can help those with trauma disorders. These include medication (such as antidepressants, anti-anxiety medications, and medications to help sleep and reduce nightmares), cognitive-behavior therapy (CBT), prolonged exposure therapy, and eye movement desensitization and reprocessing (EMDR).
- When children go through a trauma or stressful event, they are often afraid it will happen again. Let them know that feeling upset after a bad or scary event is normal. Allow them to express how they feel, and don't ignore or make light of their feelings. The American Academy of Child and Adolescent Psychiatry (www.aacap.org) offers resources for families who are coping with life crises, as well as information on how to find a local child and adolescent psychiatrist.

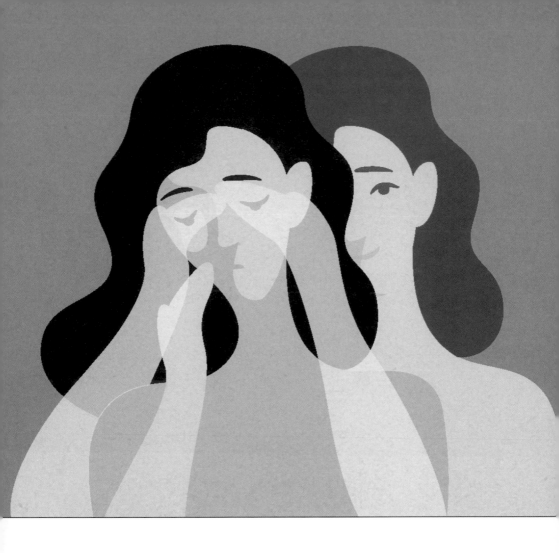

Dissociative Identity Disorder

Dissociative Amnesia

Depersonalization/Derealization Disorder

For a complete list of DSM-5-TR disorders, see Appendix A.

CHAPTER 8

Dissociative Disorders

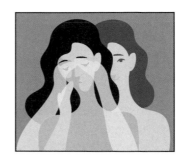

Dissociative disorders cause problems in people's normal sense of awareness and affect their sense of identity, memory, or consciousness. *Dissociation* is a change in awareness that alters a person's sense of identity or self. It affects the person's ability to connect memories and perceptions. In dissociative disorders, events that would be linked in normal memory are separated from one another. Dissociative disorders differ from normal behaviors (for example, it is normal from time to time to get lost in thought or drive somewhere and not recall the details). Instead, dissociative disorders involve major changes in a person's mental state that can sometimes cause gaps in memory for what they experience or for certain time periods or personal information. These changes can become an unhealthy way for the person to avoid reality.

There are three types of dissociative disorders discussed in this chapter: *dissociative identity disorder, dissociative amnesia*, and *depersonalization/ derealization disorder*. People may keep the symptoms of these disorders secret because they feel embarrassed or confused. Trauma (such as constant or extreme abuse or violence, whether recent or in the past) is a risk factor for all these disorders. People with dissociative identity disorder or dissociative amnesia are at increased risk for suicide.

Several different types of treatment are available for dissociative disorders. There is not a single, standard treatment, and treatment is tailored to each person. Treatment should always be guided by a mental health care provider who understands the life events and stresses that the person has endured, as well as the person's environment and personality. These treatments include psychotherapy and medications to relieve anxiety symptoms. Anxiety or mood problems may occur at the same time as the dissociative symptoms. Particularly helpful medications may include the selective serotonin reuptake inhibitors (SSRIs) that are commonly prescribed for depression.

Dissociative Identity Disorder

In the past, this disorder was known as "multiple personality disorder." People with *dissociative identity disorder* behave and feel as if they have more than one "identity." These identities may feel like different people within the person that influence the way the person thinks and interacts with others.

Some people with dissociative identity disorder may feel they have suddenly become outside observers of their own speech, thoughts, and actions, which they may feel powerless to stop. These symptoms impair their sense of self and sense of their own will.

More women than men are diagnosed with dissociative identity disorder among those seeking treatment for its symptoms. About 70% of people with the disorder have attempted suicide. Severe early and later life trauma and other mental disorders (such as *posttraumatic stress disorder, depressive disorders,* and *substance use disorders*) that can occur with this disorder may worsen symptoms.

 Dissociative Identity Disorder

Dissociative identity disorder is diagnosed when:

- There is a presence of at least two distinct identities (or "personality states") that control the person's behavior. Changes in emotions, behavior, memory, and thinking differ from the person's sense of self and sense of will.
- Ongoing gaps occur in recall of daily events, personal information, or traumatic events that are beyond normal forgetting.
- The symptoms cause distress or impair social, work, school, or other key aspects of function.

Dissociative identity disorder is not diagnosed if the behavior is part of a widely accepted practice in someone's culture or religion, and when the practice does not cause distress or disrupt daily life. (For instance, some cultures or religions accept that a spiritual presence or "possession" can guide a person's thoughts and behaviors.) The disorder is also not diagnosed when gaps in memory are due to medications, medical conditions, or use of drugs, such as alcohol. The disorder is not diagnosed in children who have imaginary friends or other pretend play.

When ongoing changes in personality and awareness cause problems with school, work, or relationships, then it is vital to seek help from a mental health care provider. Along with psychotherapy ("talk therapy"), antidepressants may relieve depressive symptoms and anxiety, if present.

Dissociative Amnesia

Dissociative amnesia involves extreme memory loss in which the person cannot remember personal information that is normal to know or recall. The *amnesia,* or memory loss, can be so severe that the person cannot recall their own name. The memory loss is often short-term and exceeds the range of normal forgetting. The person is often confused and perplexed. Dissociative amnesia can occur in children, teens, or adults. They may not know, or be only slightly aware, of the memory problems. This disorder disrupts the ability to form and keep relationships.

There are different types of dissociative amnesia:

- *Localized amnesia* is most common and prevents people from recalling events that happened during a certain time frame.
- *Selective amnesia* blocks memory of some but not all of the events during a certain time. Or the person may recall only parts of the event.
- *Generalized dissociative amnesia* causes people to have a complete loss of memory for most or all of their entire life history.
- *Systematized amnesia* is memory loss for a certain type of information (such as all events linked to a single person).
- *Continuous amnesia* involves forgetting each new event as it occurs.
- *Retrospective memory loss* includes not only lost memories of the trauma but of the person's daily life before any trauma occurred.

Dissociative Amnesia

Dissociative amnesia is diagnosed when:

- A person cannot recall personal information, often of a traumatic or stressful nature. This lack of recall is beyond normal forgetting.

- The symptoms cause distress or impair social, work, school, or other key aspects of function.

The disorder is not diagnosed if the amnesia is caused by an injury or illness that causes changes in the brain. Medications or drug use, other medical conditions, or another mental disorder, such as *acute stress disorder, posttraumatic stress disorder,* or *major or mild neurocognitive disorder,* can sometimes cause amnesia. Dissociative amnesia is not diagnosed if the amnesia results from any of these causes.

Extreme mental stress (such as military combat) may bring on the disorder. The amnesia may end on its own, and safe settings may foster recovery. A return of memories may bring great distress, an increased risk for suicidal behavior, or *posttraumatic stress disorder.* When memories return, mental health care providers can help people to manage any stressful symptoms, understand the reason for their memory loss, and learn healthy ways of coping.

Depersonalization/Derealization Disorder

People with *depersonalization/derealization disorder* feel detached or separated from themselves or their surroundings, as though they were an outside observer to their lives. This feeling is ongoing and causes much distress.

Depersonalization is a sense of being cut off from one's whole self ("I am no one"), thoughts, feelings, body, or actions. Some people feel as if they are in a dream. Others may feel like robots. They may appear stiff and without feeling to others, despite having great inner pain.

Depersonalization may occur with *derealization,* which is a sense of detachment from the outside world. Time may seem to slow down and the outside world may seem unreal.

People with depersonalization/derealization symptoms may feel that they go through their daily lives as if they are someone watching a movie. They can see people and events happening around them, but they are not part of the movie.

Episodes of depersonalization/derealization can be brief (a few hours or days) or may come and go for weeks, months, or years. The disorder tends not to occur after age 40. It can be triggered by stress, mood or anxiety symptoms that worsen, new settings, or lack of sleep.

Depersonalization/Derealization Disorder

Depersonalization/derealization disorder is diagnosed when:

- There are ongoing episodes of depersonalization, derealization, or both:

    - *Depersonalization*: experiences of unreality, detachment, or being an outside observer to one's own thoughts, feelings, body, or actions.

    - *Derealization*: experiences of unreality or detachment from one's surroundings (people or objects seem unreal, dreamlike, or lifeless).

- During such episodes, the person can tell what is occurring in their mind and what is occurring in the outside world.

- The symptoms cause distress or impair social, work, school, or other key aspects of function.

People can feel detached at times in daily life from events around them, and this is normal. Depersonalization/derealization disorder is diagnosed if the feelings of unreality or detachment greatly disrupt daily living or cause severe distress or anxiety for the person having them. Some medications or drugs can cause feelings of depersonalization and derealization, such as anesthesia used for medical procedures or surgeries. Thus, the disorder is not diagnosed if there are medications or drug use, other medical conditions (such as seizures), or another mental disorder (such as *schizophrenia, major depressive disorder, panic disorder, acute stress disorder,* or *posttraumatic stress disorder*) that appears to have caused the symptoms.

Psychotherapy may help the person to understand their symptoms and how they perceive the world around them. It can help them to pinpoint and possibly avoid settings that tend to bring on symptoms. These treatment options are as follows:

- *Cognitive-behavior therapy* can help to confront distorted thoughts and challenge feelings of unreality.

Dissociative Disorders　　　　　　　　　　　　　　　　　**135**

- *Relaxation techniques,* such as progressive muscle relaxation and biofeedback, also can help. *Biofeedback* is a technique that helps a person gain control over their body functions. A desired response is learned when instruments record information such as muscle tone, skin temperature, and breathing rate. This feedback helps the person to make certain changes (such as in breathing rate) to create a desired response (such as breathing more deeply to reduce tension).
- *SSRI medications* may be helpful but also pose a risk. Depersonalization and derealization can be side effects of these medications.

Key Points

- *Dissociation* is a change in awareness that alters a person's sense of self. It disrupts the person's ability to connect memories and perceptions.
- It is normal for people to have mild dissociative behavior from time to time. For instance, a person can get lost in thought or drive somewhere and not recall the details of the trip. This is not a sign of dissociative disorder.
- *Dissociative disorders* cause severe changes in a person's mental state. Large gaps in memory may occur for what they experience or for certain time periods or personal information. When dissociative symptoms and behaviors persist or are frequent; impair social, work, school, or other functions; or trigger distress, then the person or their loved one should seek help.
- People may keep the symptoms of these disorders secret because they feel embarrassed or confused. Trauma (such as constant or extreme abuse or violence, whether recent or in the past) is a risk factor for these disorders.
- Several different types of treatment are available for dissociative disorders. Treatment should always be decided on by a mental health care provider who understands the life events and stresses that the person has endured, as well as the person's environment and personality. These treatments include psychotherapy and medications such as selective serotonin reuptake inhibitors (SSRIs) to help relieve symptoms of depression and anxiety.

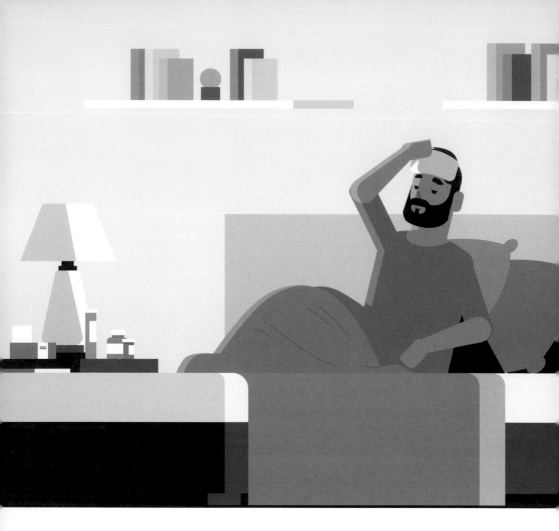

Somatic Symptom Disorder
Functional Neurological Symptom Disorder
Other Somatic Symptom Disorders
    Illness Anxiety Disorder
    Factitious Disorder

For a complete list of DSM-5-TR disorders, see Appendix A.

CHAPTER 9

Somatic (Physical) Symptom Disorders

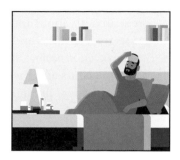

Somatic (or physical) symptom disorders involve pronounced physical problems and high levels of health concern that greatly disrupt or impair work and home life. These disorders involve abnormal thoughts, feelings, and behaviors about real, perceived, or feigned (pretend) health problems. For instance, when health problems occur, the extreme concern about them is often greater than the actual physical problem itself.

People with these disorders describe physical pain and discomfort. These symptoms are real health problems to them, not a mental health issue. These concerns can lead to medical tests, surgeries, or unneeded medications. These concerns and attempts to address them can be a source of stress and frustration for those with these disorders.

A person can have both a real medical disorder and a somatic symptom disorder at the same time. People with serious health concerns are not diagnosed with a somatic symptom disorder only because a medical cause cannot be found. For some somatic symptom disorders, the lack of a medical cause for the symptoms is still a key factor of the diagnosis. Risk factors for somatic symptom disorders include increased sensitivity to pain and early trauma or neglect.

The following somatic symptom disorders are included in DSM-5-TR: *somatic symptom disorder, functional neurological symptom disorder, illness anxiety disorder,* and *factitious disorder.* People with these disorders are more likely than others to visit a doctor, medical clinics, or hospitals instead of seeking mental health care. Each disorder is marked by a great concern for physical health:

- In *somatic symptom disorder,* the person has constant thoughts and great anxiety about their health problems. These health problems cause great distress and disrupt their lives.
- In *functional neurological symptom disorder,* a sudden, major physical problem occurs and involves a loss of ability (such as sudden paralysis or seizures) that leads to an urgent visit to an emergency room or hospital.
- In *illness anxiety disorder,* some physical discomfort may exist but the main problem is a constant worry about being sick (or about becoming sick). These mental worries impair daily life more so than any mild physical symptoms, if they exist.
- In *factious disorder,* a person seeks help for a physical complaint while aware that no physical problem exists—or hides the fact that they caused the problem on purpose.

Somatic Symptom Disorder

Somatic symptom disorder, known in the past as "somatization disorder," involves the person's great distress about physical health symptoms. These can include chronic pain, headache, and fatigue. People with the disorder have health symptoms for some time, and doctors may or may not find any health condition or disease that explains them.

People with somatic symptom disorder have high levels of worry about their health problems. They see their symptoms as harmful and think the worst about their health, even when test results show no reason for concern. For some, health concerns play a central role in their life and relationships.

Although a medical condition may not be diagnosed, they are not faking their symptoms and truly believe they are sick. The person's symptoms and pain are real to them and can linger for months or years. People with the disorder often have intense worry and anxiety that there is a cancer or infection causing their physical problems—but that their doctors are not finding it. Because of this fear, persons with somatic symptom disorder will often seek out many different doctors, hoping to find someone who can explain their symptoms and pinpoint their source.

The disorder is diagnosed more often in women. Many persons with the disorder also have medical conditions, as well as *anxiety* and *depressive disorders*. The disorder is common in people who have a diagnosed medical condition, but with symptoms that persist or go beyond what is normal for the diagnosis. For instance, a person may have a medical problem such as a stomach ulcer that needs treatment. The person with somatic symptom disorder will feel distress about their stomach and bowels that persists, consumes their life, and goes far beyond what would be normal for a stomach ulcer. More problems also may occur in daily life (such as more missed days of work) than is normal for the medical issue.

 ## Somatic Symptom Disorder

The disorder occurs when a person has the following:

- One or more physical symptoms that cause distress or much trouble with daily tasks.
- Excessive thoughts, feelings, or behaviors related to the symptoms or concerns about personal health, as shown by at least one of the following:
  - Constant thoughts about the seriousness of the symptoms.
  - Constant high level of anxiety or stress about health or symptoms.
  - Great amounts of time or energy spent thinking or worrying about these symptoms or health concerns.
- Although physical symptoms may come and go, at least one other symptom is present for more than 6 months before the diagnosis is made.

Risk Factors

The following factors are believed to raise the risk of developing somatic symptom disorder:

- **Temperament.** People who often have fear, sadness, guilt, shame, distress, or anger, or who often complain may be at increased risk.

Having anxiety or depression is also common and can make physical symptoms worse.

- **Environment.** The disorder is more common in people with few years of education and low socioeconomic status, as well as those who have recently gone through a stressful or traumatic event.

Functional Neurological Symptom Disorder

Functional neurological symptom disorder is a condition in which one or more symptoms emerge quickly and affect awareness, perception, sensation, or movement without any apparent physical cause.

People with the disorder may have multiple symptoms that affect their body movements and senses. Trouble with walking, weakness or paralysis, hearing loss, blindness, difficulty in swallowing, seizures, inability to speak, loss of consciousness, and numbness are all common symptoms of the disorder. The body shaking and loss of consciousness that happen during an epileptic seizure can also occur in functional neurological symptom disorder, except that an actual seizure is not happening in the brain. Symptoms of the disorder tend to come on quickly, and can cause an urgent visit to a clinic or emergency room. Sometimes symptoms can come and go or last for a longer time. It has been thought that because symptoms may come on quickly, they might be a response to mental stress, but in up to 50% of people with the disorder, there is no sign of a source for emotional distress.

In the United States, functional neurological symptom disorder is two to three times more common in women than in men. Symptoms often first occur in the 20s and 30s, but may start at any age. For many people, symptoms start quickly, last for only a short time, and get better without treatment, often after gentle reassurance and support from the doctor that their symptoms aren't caused by a serious problem. The symptoms can come on quickly and stop fairly quickly, and the person can return to normal daily life.

People with functional neurological symptom disorder also often have *anxiety disorders* (such as *panic disorder*) and *depressive disorders*. Other medical conditions can occur at the same time as functional neurological symptom disorder.

Functional Neurological Symptom Disorder

Functional neurological symptom disorder is diagnosed when:

- At least one symptom affects the function of the senses or body movement.
- Medical tests or a physical exam cannot find a neurological (brain-based) or other medical cause for the symptom.

The symptom is not caused by another medical condition or mental disorder. It causes great distress or problems in social, work, or other daily functions.

Risk Factors

The following factors may increase the risk of functional neurological symptom disorder:

- **Temperament.** Mood swings (rapid changes in mood) are linked with the disorder.
- **Environment.** Victims of childhood abuse and neglect may have an increased risk. A stressful life event may also increase the risk.
- **Genetics.** Having a neurological (brain) disease that causes similar symptoms. For instance, nonepileptic seizures are more common in people who also have epilepsy.

Other Somatic Symptom Disorders

Illness Anxiety Disorder

People with *illness anxiety disorder* are greatly worried about having an illness or believing they might get sick. The term "hypochondriasis" was used in the past to describe this disorder. People with illness anxiety disorder spend much time and energy worrying about their health. They feel constant anxiety and stress from these health concerns. They may also plan their life to avoid settings that might expose them to health risks or ill people, such as not traveling or visiting family members. They may be highly focused on health behaviors, such as following special diets or taking vitamins and other supplements. They may devote a lot of time and money to these behaviors. Although the results of physical exams and tests may prove negative or benign, they are rarely reassured or relieved that they are healthy. If they do have a medical condition, the symptoms are mild compared with the deep concern the person feels.

The disorder is diagnosed when the following occur:

- Extreme concern about having or getting a serious illness.
- Physical symptoms are not present or are only mild. If the person has a medical condition or a high risk of getting one, the worries about the medical condition exceed the impact of the illness itself.
- A high level of anxiety and frequent worries about their own health.
- The person obsesses over health-related behaviors, such as frequent and repeated checking of their body for signs of illness. Out of extreme fear of medical test results, the person may avoid hospitals and doctors who could confirm or dismiss the presence of health problem.
- The preoccupation with illness has lasted for at least 6 months and is not due to another mental condition, such as *panic disorder, generalized anxiety disorder,* or *body dysmorphic disorder*.

Factitious Disorder

People with *factitious disorder* produce or feign a physical or mental illness when they are not really sick. They might lie about symptoms, hurt themselves to cause symptoms, or change test results to make it look like they have an illness. For instance, people with the disorder may claim to be depressed or suicidal over a loved one's death that never happened. Sometimes people with factitious disorder have a real illness or injury, such as a wound or sore, but they might act to worsen it on purpose. For instance, they may expose their wounds to germs or do other things that prevent healing. Because of these behaviors, they may make a minor illness into a more severe problem by preventing their own recovery. They will not reveal that they acted on purpose to worsen the wound or illness.

There are two types of factitious disorders that can be diagnosed:

Factitious Disorder Imposed on Self

- Fakes physical or mental symptoms or hurts themself to cause symptoms.
- Claims to be ill or injured.

Factitious Disorder Imposed on Another

- Fakes physical or mental symptoms in another person (children, adults) or hurts another person to create symptoms.

- Tells other people that someone in their care is ill or injured.
- The person who causes these symptoms is diagnosed with the disorder, not the person (victim) who receives the acts causing their illness or injury symptoms.

In either type of factitious disorder, there is not a clear reason why the person pretends to have an illness or harms another person to create a false illness or injury. There may or may not be a benefit from the false illness or injury, such as gaining money by blaming someone else for the problem. There may be complex reasons for the person to seek medical care and attention as if they were a sick person or were caring for a sick person. Family, friends, neighbors, faith leaders, teachers, and health care workers can all be affected by the feigned illness, in terms of the time, attention, and resources given to provide support and care for the false illness. To have factitious disorder, the person must not have another mental disorder, such as *delusional disorder,* in which the person truly believes that they are sick.

Treatment

As a group, somatic symptom disorders can sometimes get better or be managed without mental health care. For some people with these disorders (except factitious disorder, discussed at the end of this section), the anxiety and stress may lessen after medical tests prove no sign of a medical illness. Others with these disorders may struggle for some time and need mental health care to return to normal function.

A major goal of treating somatic symptom disorders is to build a relationship of trust (what is known as a *therapeutic alliance*) between the doctor and patient. When this happens, the doctor makes clear that the person's discomfort is real and takes seriously their medical complaints. The doctor and patient also work toward a return to healthy daily activities. The focus of treatment should be to restore the patients' ability to function in their daily life.

Some treatment options have been found useful. *Cognitive-behavior therapy* (CBT) can address beliefs and behaviors about having an illness. The therapy may help people learn to think positively about coping with daily life even if a medical cause is not found to be the source of their physical symptoms. Therapy also teaches ways to cope with pain and learn what seems to make the pain worse. Antidepressant medications can also help reduce the pain, anxiety, irritable mood, and panic that sometimes occur with somatic symptom disorders.

People with factitious disorder rarely seek mental health treatment, and there are no research studies to guide treatment for this disorder. Psychotherapy focused on helping the person understand their need to feign a physical illness may be helpful. Medications are not needed unless the person has significant depressive or anxiety symptoms.

Key Points

- *Somatic (or physical) symptom disorders* involve abnormal thoughts, feelings, and behaviors about real or perceived health problems. One of the disorders, factitious disorder, involves feigned health problems on purpose. Each of these disorders shares some common features: People who have them are more likely to go to a medical doctor, medical clinic, or hospital instead of seeking mental health care. Each disorder is marked by a great concern for physical health.
- As a group, somatic symptom disorders can sometimes get better or be managed without mental health treatment. For some people with these disorders (except factitious disorder), the high anxiety and stress about their health may lessen after medical tests prove no sign of a medical illness.
- Other people with these disorders may struggle for some time and need mental health treatment to return to normal function. Treatment includes establishing a trusting doctor-patient relationship. The doctor acknowledges the person's distress and discomfort and takes seriously their medical complaints. The doctor and patient also work toward a return to healthy daily function.
- Cognitive-behavior therapy (CBT) can address beliefs and behaviors about having an illness. The therapy may help people learn to think positively about coping with daily life even if a medical cause is not found to be the source of their physical symptoms. Therapy also teaches ways to cope with pain and learn what seems to make the pain worse.
- Antidepressant medications can also help reduce the pain, anxiety, irritable mood, and panic that sometimes occur with somatic symptom disorders.

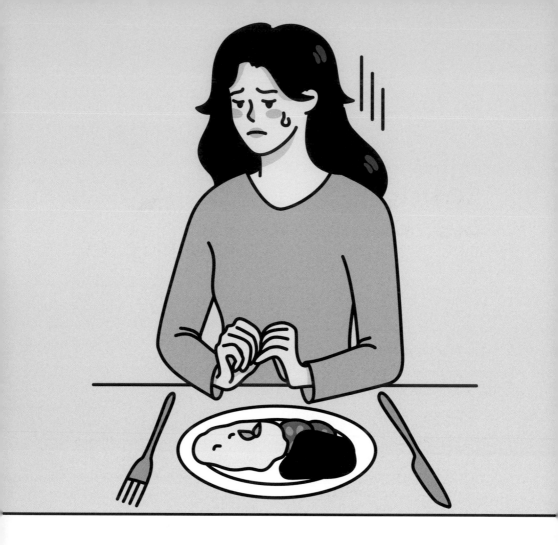

Anorexia Nervosa

Bulimia Nervosa

Binge-Eating Disorder

Other Eating Disorders

    Pica

    Rumination Disorder

    Avoidant/Restrictive Food Intake Disorder

For a complete list of DSM-5-TR disorders, see Appendix A.

CHAPTER 10

Eating Disorders

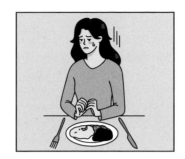

Eating disorders involve chronic problems with how someone eats food and absorbs nutrients. These disorders can greatly impair physical health and how the person thinks, feels, and relates to others. People with these disorders may be intensely concerned about their body weight and shape. Eating disorders affect millions of people each year in the United States—most often girls and women between ages 12–35.

The three main types of eating disorders are *anorexia nervosa, bulimia nervosa,* and *binge-eating disorder.* Many people believe eating disorders are somewhat new and reflect the culture's obsession with youth and beauty—yet these disorders have been noted for centuries.

In many cases, eating disorders occur with other mental disorders, such as *anxiety disorders, depressive disorders, panic disorder, obsessive-compulsive disorder,* and *substance use disorders.* Genes may play a part in why certain people develop eating disorders, but these disorders also appear in many people who have no family history.

Besides anorexia nervosa, bulimia nervosa, and binge-eating disorder, three other disorders are discussed in this chapter: *pica, rumination disorder*, and *avoidant/restrictive food intake disorder.* These are feeding disorders that often first occur in childhood.

Anorexia Nervosa

People with *anorexia nervosa* severely restrict their food intake. They have an intense fear of gaining weight or of becoming fat, even when they are starved and appear thin and gaunt to others. They see themselves as fat or overweight, and their fear is not relieved by weight loss. In fact, concern about weight gain may increase as their weight falls. They may weigh themselves often and eat very small amounts of only certain foods. People with the disorder may not accept or admit to others their fear of weight gain. Their self-esteem is based on their view of their body shape and weight.

Anorexia nervosa affects about 0.5% of girls and young women per year in the United States. The disorder is more common in girls and women than in boys and men. Body mass index (BMI) is a useful measure to assess body weight for height (see box "What Is a Healthy Weight?"). The DSM-5-TR diagnosis of anorexia nervosa uses BMI levels for thinness derived from the World Health Organization to show how severe the disorder is.

Instead of weight loss in children and teens with the disorder, there may be a failure to gain a healthy or normal weight or to maintain healthy development (such as growth). As with adults, weight history, body build, and physical health also are reviewed for a diagnosis.

There are two types of anorexia nervosa. With the *restricting type*, people maintain weight loss by dieting, fasting, or exercising in excess. They might consume only a few hundred calories a day or just water. With the *binge-eating/purging type*, people have *binge episodes* (eating large amounts of food in a short period of time) and then *purge* (vomit or use laxatives, diuretics, or enemas) to counteract the effect of the binge.

Anorexia nervosa begins in the teens or 20s for most persons, but rarely after age 40 years. It often starts after a stressful life event, such as leaving home for college. Some people who have anorexia nervosa recover with treatment after only one episode, but others may improve only to relapse into unhealthy eating behaviors. Those with the more chronic form of anorexia nervosa may struggle with the illness for years and have severe health problems. In very severe cases, people can die from the medical effects of self-starvation.

Other mental disorders can occur with anorexia nervosa. These most often include *bipolar, depressive*, and *anxiety disorders*. People with anorexia nervosa are at high risk for suicide.

 Anorexia Nervosa

Anorexia nervosa is diagnosed when a person has:
- Limited food intake that leads to marked, low body weight below the normal minimum for their age and height.
- Intense fear of gaining weight or being fat, even though underweight; or frequent behavior that obstructs weight gain.
- Body image problems or a denial that their low body weight is serious.

Thinness is linked with how severe the disorder is. The following ratings are based on BMI and derived from the World Health Organization levels of thinness for adults. The level of thinness for children and teens is based on the BMI of others their same age and sex. Problems with work, school, family, or friendships can increase the rating:
- Mild: BMI≥17
- Moderate: BMI=16–16.99
- Severe: BMI=15–15.99
- Extreme: BMI<15

Risk Factors

Studies have shown that certain factors may increase a person's risk for anorexia nervosa:

- **Temperament.** People who have *anxiety disorders* or show obsessive traits in childhood.
- **Environment.** Living in a culture in which being thin is valued. People who work in fields that promote thinness, such as models, dancers, and athletes, are at higher risk.
- **Genetics.** People with a first-degree blood relative (parent, sibling) who had anorexia nervosa.

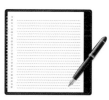

Helena's Story

Helena was a 16-year-old girl who lived at home with her parents and younger sister. Throughout her teenage years, she had been a normal or healthy weight, but she worried a great deal about her body weight and shape. She often compared her body weight with that of other girls and women she met or saw—and then judged herself as too heavy.

Often, Helena checked her body weight by looking in the mirror. She would pinch the skin on her sides and notice that her thighs touched each other. At about age 14 she began to diet, first off and on, and then all the time. At 15, she decided to become a vegetarian and began to cut out many foods from her diet. She was 5'6" and weighed 125 pounds at age 15, but by her 16th birthday she had dropped to 110 pounds.

Rather than being relieved by this weight loss, she kept seeing herself as too heavy. She weighed herself throughout the day. She spent most of her time worrying about her weight. Time spent on her weight concerns took the place of other activities she used to enjoy, such as schoolwork and having fun with friends. She spent more time alone. And she kept losing weight.

Her parents became more alarmed about her weight loss and behavior. They talked about this between themselves and started watching and checking her eating behavior at meals. They urged her to eat more often, without success. She kept losing weight, and 6 months later she weighed 98 pounds.

Helena appeared very thin. She often was withdrawn, hard to talk to, and distracted. She seemed weak—but did heavy exercise twice each day. She preferred to stand or pace rather than to sit and relax. Because of their concerns, her parents took Helena to see the family doctor for an evaluation.

Helena was diagnosed with *anorexia nervosa, restricting type.* Her low food intake, low weight (BMI of 15.8), frequent exercise, and constant concern about her body weight despite being very thin are hallmarks of the diagnosis.

Bulimia Nervosa

People with *bulimia nervosa* binge eat often. At these times, they consume large amounts of food in secret, often high in calories, sugars, carbohydrates, and fat. They can eat very quickly, sometimes gulping down food without even tasting it. Binges may end only when another person disrupts them, or they have stomach pain from the stomach being stretched beyond capacity.

People with bulimia nervosa can be slightly underweight, healthy weight, overweight, or, rarely, obese. They often diet and do intense exercise to keep their weight down but are never as underweight as people with anorexia nervosa.

During an eating binge, the person feels out of control. After a binge, people with bulimia purge by constant exercise, throwing up, or using a laxative, often because of stomach pains, shame about their extreme eating, and the fear of weight gain. This cycle is repeated at least several times a week, or in extreme cases, several times a day. The constant bingeing and purging can damage the digestive system. Frequent vomiting can also cause swelling of the cheeks and tooth decay.

People with this disorder manage to almost always hide their binges and purges. Because they don't become severely thin, family members and friends may not notice these behaviors. The chance of getting better increases the sooner bulimia nervosa is detected and treated.

Bulimia nervosa affects 0.5%–1.5% of teenage girls and young adult women in the United States. The disorder is much more common in girls and women than in boys and men.

Other mental disorders can occur with bulimia nervosa. These most often include *bipolar, depressive,* and *anxiety disorders.*

 Bulimia Nervosa

Bulimia nervosa is diagnosed when a person has:
- Repeated episodes of binge eating with both of the following:
    - Eating in a discrete period of time (such as within 2 hours) a larger amount of food than what most people would eat in that same time.
    - A lack of control over eating during this episode (feeling unable to stop eating or control how much to eat).
- Frequent use of unhealthy purge behaviors to prevent gaining weight, such as self-induced vomiting, laxative or diuretic abuse, fasting, or extreme exercise.

- Both binge-eating and purging behaviors that occur at least once a week for 3 months.
- Extreme concern with body weight and shape.

These symptoms need to occur outside an episode of *anorexia nervosa* for a diagnosis. The number of episodes per week of unhealthy purge behavior suggests how severe the disorder is. Problems with work, school, family, or friendships can increase the rating:
- Mild: 1–3 purging episodes per week
- Moderate: 4–7 purging episodes per week
- Severe: 8–13 purging episodes per week
- Extreme: 14 or more purging episodes per week

Risk Factors

A few factors may play a role in the development of bulimia nervosa:

- **Temperament.** Weight concerns, low self-esteem, depressive symptoms, *social anxiety disorder*, or childhood *generalized anxiety disorder* may be risk factors.
- **Environment.** A strong belief that being thin is ideal increases the risk for weight concerns and thus the risk for bulimia nervosa. Childhood sexual or physical abuse increases risk for the disorder. A series of stressful life events can also increase risk.
- **Genetics.** Childhood obesity and early puberty raise the risk. Having a first-degree blood relative (parent or sibling) with an eating disorder may also increase risk.

Binge-Eating Disorder

People with *binge-eating disorder* often eat unusually large amounts of food. This overeating is often done in secret. Unlike bulimia nervosa, the binge episodes are not paired with purging through vomiting or other means.

A person of any weight size—from healthy weight to obese—can have binge-eating disorder. Studies have shown that people with the disorder consume more calories and have more problems in daily function and overall quality of life than those who are obese.

Binge-eating disorder affects two to three times more women than men. Each year in the United States, about 1.6% of women and 0.8% of men are diagnosed. The disorder is found across races and ethnic groups equally in the United States.

People with binge-eating disorder may also be diagnosed with *major depressive disorder* and *alcohol use disorder*.

 Binge-Eating Disorder

Binge-eating disorder is diagnosed when a person binge eats at least once a week for 3 months and has the following symptoms:

- Repeated episodes of binge eating that is characterized by both of the following:
    - Eating in a discrete period of time (such as within 2 hours) a larger amount of food than what most people would eat in that same time.
    - A lack of control over eating during this episode (unable to stop eating or control how much to eat).
- Binge-eating episodes that involve at least three of the following:
    - Eating much faster than normal.
    - Eating until feeling uncomfortably full.
    - Eating large amounts of food although not feeling hungry.
    - Eating alone because of being ashamed by the amount consumed.
    - Feeling disgusted, depressed, or very guilty afterward.

The binge eating must occur outside periods of *bulimia nervosa* or *anorexia nervosa* and be a source of distress. The number of episodes per week of binge eating suggests how severe the disorder is. Problems with work, school, family, or friendships because of the disorder can increase the rating:

- Mild: 1–3 binge-eating episodes per week
- Moderate: 4–7 binge-eating episodes per week
- Severe: 8–13 binge-eating episodes per week
- Extreme: 14 or more binge-eating episodes per week

Risk Factors

Binge-eating disorder appears to run in families, which signals a possible genetic link.

Treatment

Eating disorders can lead to serious health trouble, such as malnutrition and heart problems. Proper medical and mental health care can be lifesaving. With treatment, people with these disorders can learn healthy eating habits, restore their weight to a healthy range, and control binge and purge episodes.

Any plan for treating anorexia nervosa, bulimia nervosa, or binge-eating disorder must include a thorough assessment of the person's medical condition. This involves a physical exam, lab tests, and often X-rays to check for osteoporosis (thinning of bones common in eating disorder patients).

While the main goals of treating the various eating disorders differ slightly, the treatments are similar. With anorexia nervosa, the first step is to restore a healthy weight. For people with bulimia nervosa, stopping the binge-purge cycle is key. And for people with binge-eating disorder, it is vital that binge episodes stop.

Restoring weight, curbing binge and purge episodes, and psychotherapy are the mainstays of treatment. Cognitive-behavior therapy can help the person address disturbed thoughts, feelings, and behaviors related to the eating disorder. Group and family-based therapy may help the person resolve any relationship problems or conflicts that may have caused the unhealthy eating behavior.

Medications such as antidepressants, antipsychotics, and mood stabilizers are sometimes used. These can help relieve depression, anxiety, or unstable moods that can impede treatment.

Nutritional counseling can help manage diet and eating habits. With nutritional counseling, a dietitian and other health care providers can explain how nutrition affects the body and how to return to healthy eating patterns of three meals each day. These measures help rebuild physical well-being and healthy eating habits.

A Healthy Mind and Body

Getting healthy again, both mentally and physically, is the number one goal of overcoming an eating disorder. Along with the treatment plan set by the mental health care provider and treatment team, these steps can help:

- **Set and conquer small goals.** Whether it's eating three meals a day that include all food groups or trying a new activity, changing behavior is a good start.
- **Build a support network.** Join a support group with others who are trying to heal. The National Association of Anorexia Nervosa and Associated Disorders (www.anad.org) and the National Eating Disorders Association (www.nationaleatingdisorders.org) provide a di-

rectory of groups around the country, as well as online forums. These organizations also offer toll-free help lines.

- **Practice embracing a positive body image.** People with eating disorders find that a top-ten list of things they like about themselves—that aren't related to weight or looks—helps. They read the list often. Looking at themselves as a whole person, not just as a body or only one body part, is key to recovery.

Other Eating Disorders

Pica, rumination disorder, and *avoidant/restrictive food intake disorder* involve disturbed feeding behaviors. These often first occur in childhood and can also occur in teens and adults.

Pica

Pica is the eating of nonfood items on a regular basis. Objects that people with pica eat include paint chips, paper, chalk, hair, talcum powder, starch, dirt, and ice. These items have no nutrients. They can be harmful if they are toxic, harm the person's stomach or bowels, or pose other medical risks. The disorder can occur in children, teens, and adults, including pregnant women. In some cases, a lack of certain nutrients, such as iron, can trigger the behavior. The disorder is diagnosed by the presence of the following:

- Constant eating of nonfood items with no nutritional value for at least 1 month.
- Eating nonfood items does not fit the person's stage in life (for instance, young children under 3 may attempt to eat or put in their mouths a variety of nonfood objects, but this is not standard for teens or adults).
- The eating behavior is not part of the person's cultural practice.

The eating behavior can occur with other conditions, such as *intellectual disability* and *autism spectrum disorder*.

Rumination Disorder

Rumination disorder occurs when a person *regurgitates* often (brings food up from the stomach into the mouth) and rechews the food. This occurs without gagging or disgust. It is frequent and occurs at least several times per week, often daily.

Rumination disorder can occur in people of all ages. Risk factors include lack of social contact, neglect, stressful life events, and problems in the parent-child relationship. People who have *intellectual disability* may be more at risk. When it occurs in infants, it tends to start between ages 3 and 12 months. Teens and adults may attempt to disguise the regurgitation behavior by placing a hand over their mouth or coughing. The regurgitation and rumination behavior appears to have a self-soothing function. It can lead to problems with growth, learning, and severe malnutrition if it persists. The disorder is diagnosed when the following occur:

- Repeated regurgitation of food to rechew, re-swallow, or spit out several times per week, often daily, for at least 1 month.
- The repeated regurgitation is not due to a gastrointestinal or other medical condition.

The behavior does not occur as a symptom of another eating disorder. The symptoms can occur with another mental disorder, such as *intellectual disability* or another childhood disorder.

Avoidant/Restrictive Food Intake Disorder

Avoidant/restrictive food intake disorder is a condition in which people avoid or restrict food intake and fail to meet needs for proper nutrition and energy. It is more common in children than adults and in boys with *autism spectrum disorder*. People with the disorder do not seem to like eating or food. They may have problems digesting certain food, avoid foods of certain colors and textures, or not tolerate the smell of other people's food. The disorder is diagnosed when the:

- Eating or feeding problem, such as a lack of interest in eating, causes a failure to take in proper calories or nutrition, signaled by at least one of the following:
  - Marked weight loss (or in children, failure to reach height or weight for age).
  - Marked nutritional deficits.
  - Dependence on a feeding tube or oral nutrition supplements.
  - A disruption of social function (such as avoiding work lunches or social events with family and friends where food is present).

The problem is not due to lack of food or because of cultural practice. The symptoms do not occur as part of another *eating disorder.* Symptoms are also not due to another mental disorder or medical condition. The disorder can occur with other mental disorders, such as *anx-*

iety disorders, obsessive-compulsive disorder, autism spectrum disorder, attention-deficit/hyperactivity disorder, and *intellectual disability.*

Key Points

- *Eating disorders* can lead to major health trouble, such as malnutrition and heart problems. Proper medical and mental health care are lifesaving for people with these disorders.
- Nutritional counseling can help manage diet and eating habits. A dietitian and other health care providers can explain how nutrition affects the body and how to return to healthy eating patterns of three meals each day. These measures help rebuild physical well-being and healthy eating habits.
- Restoring weight, curbing binge and purge episodes, and psychotherapy are the mainstays of treatment. Cognitive-behavior therapy is often used to help address the disturbed thoughts, feelings, and behaviors related to the eating disorder. Group and family-based therapy may help the person resolve any relationship problems or conflicts that may have caused the unhealthy eating behavior.
- Medications such as antidepressants, antipsychotics, and mood stabilizers are sometimes used. These can help relieve depression, anxiety, or unstable moods that can impede treatment.
- Along with the treatment plan set by the mental health care provider and treatment team, the following steps can help combat eating disorders: setting and meeting small goals, building a support network, and embracing a positive body image and self-image.

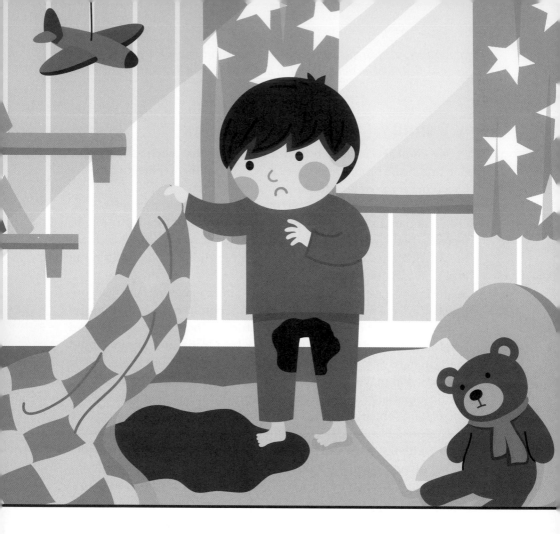

Enuresis

Encopresis

For a complete list of DSM-5-TR disorders, see Appendix A.

CHAPTER 11

Elimination Disorders

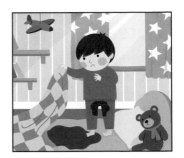

People with *elimination disorders* pass their urine or stools into bedding, clothing, or other inappropriate places. These problems with urinating (passing urine from the bladder) are called *enuresis*, and problems with defecating (passing stools from the bowels) are called *encopresis*. Both disorders can occur during the day or at night. A person can have one or both disorders at the same time. These disorders are most often first diagnosed in children, after the age when a child is expected to be toilet trained. The disorders occur less often in teens and adults.

The causes of these disorders are not always known. Medical conditions or medications can affect bowel or bladder function and cause these problems. Thus, seeing a doctor is key to rule out medical causes. When the medical issue is resolved, often so is the elimination disorder.

These disorders are included in DSM-5-TR because they also can result from problems with toilet training or stress, such as the start of school or the birth of a sibling. Although most often these behaviors are not done on purpose, sometimes they are. This points to an emotional or psychological reason for the behavior. No matter the reason, these disorders cause great distress to children and parents.

These disorders often resolve on their own without treatment as the child grows. If people with these disorders feel shame, embarrassment, or guilt from the disorder or are dealing with other stresses and worries in their life that could be making it worse, psychotherapy ("talk therapy") can help. Psychotherapy can also address emotional reasons for the behavior if it is done on purpose. One form of psychotherapy is *behavior therapy,* which works with parents and child to teach methods to change behaviors and learn new skills. Parents and the child can learn new habits that they can work on together. Parents' support, love, and calm attitude as new skills are practiced will greatly help the child learn to control their bladder or bowel and use the toilet.

Enuresis

Enuresis involves urinating into bedding, clothing, and other inappropriate places. Enuresis may be caused or worsened by heavy fluid intake (drinking), particularly before bedtime.

Children who have never been able to control urination during the day or night have *primary enuresis.* Those who begin to wet their beds after at least 1 year of normal bladder control have *secondary enuresis.* The most common type of enuresis involves urinating in the bed during the night (bed-wetting). The second type occurs during the day (urinary incontinence, or daytime wetting). Most often the urinating is by accident and out of the child's control. However, in rare cases it is done on purpose. Stress is a risk factor for this disorder.

Enuresis is common in children. Daytime wetting affects 3%–9% of children age 7 years, and bed-wetting occurs in 5%–10% of children age 5 years. Bed-wetting at night is twice as common in boys than in girls, and daytime wetting is more common in girls than in boys. Urinary tract infections are linked with daytime wetting, especially in girls. The disorder is most common among children ages 5–8 years. There is an increased risk for the disorder if either parent also had this problem when younger. The disorder tends to resolve in most children by the time they are teens. In 1% of cases, the disorder lasts into adulthood.

The condition is diagnosed only in those age 5 years and up. In younger children it is not considered a disorder because it can be part of normal development.

 Enuresis

Enuresis is diagnosed when the person, at least age 5 years:

- Urinates repeatedly into bed or clothes, whether by accident or on purpose.
- Does so for at least twice a week for 3 months in a row.

- Has trouble with daily life in going to work or school or taking part in social activities because of the behavior.

Enuresis is not diagnosed if the problem is caused by a medication (such as a diuretic) or another medical condition, such as a problem with bladder anatomy or a bladder infection.

Treatment

Children with nighttime enuresis often outgrow the problem on their own. After a doctor has ruled out any physical cause of the bed-wetting, parents are counseled on changing bedtime habits to reduce the amount of fluid the child drinks at night and to make sure the child uses the bathroom regularly during the day and evening.

If the problem lasts, bed-wetting alarms that wake the child or parent when the child starts to urinate also can train the child to get up and use the bathroom during the night. The child will need a parent's help. It may take 2–12 weeks to see gradual results, from fewer accidents, to smaller accidents, to complete dryness. Use of the alarm (often referred to as the *bell-and-pad method*) can be stopped after 14 days in a row of dryness. (For more tips, see box at the end of this chapter.)

Adults with urinary incontinence also are treated with bladder retraining exercises. They are asked to keep a "bladder diary" to record how much and how often during the day they urinate. The doctor then uses the diary to find a pattern and to suggest specific times for the person to control their bladder and use the bathroom. For women with urinary incontinence, *Kegel exercises* strengthen certain muscles in the vagina that control the flow of urine and can also help improve bladder control.

Children and adults who have enuresis may be prescribed medication to help calm the bladder. For children, behavior therapy (such as the bell-and-pad method) is just as useful and leads to less risk of relapse and side effects.

Encopresis

Encopresis involves repeatedly defecating (passing stools) in inappropriate places (such as in underwear or on the floor) after the age when bowel control is normally expected. It is also called fecal incontinence.

The most common reason for encopresis is chronic constipation, which can be caused by stress, not drinking enough water (stools become too hard to pass), and pain caused by a sore near the anus. Poor diet (such as too much sugar or fatty, fried foods) and lack of exercise can also worsen constipation. If a person is not fully passing stool, overflow incontinence can occur and result in leakage. Risk factors for encopresis include early childhood abuse or neglect, anxiety, depression, being bullied, poor school performance, and low income.

Over 4% of children ages 4–6 years have encopresis, and it is more common in boys than in girls. In most cases, encopresis is not done on purpose but is out of the person's control, usually because of constipation. It may result from anxiety that leads the person to avoid defecating. This results in overflow when the amount of stool can no longer be retained. When encopresis is clearly done on purpose, it may be related to *oppositional defiant disorder* or *conduct disorder* (see Chapter 15, "Disruptive and Conduct Disorders").

The condition is diagnosed only in those age 4 years and up. In younger children, it is not considered a disorder because it can be part of normal development.

 Encopresis

Encopresis is diagnosed when the person, at least age 4 years:

- Repeatedly passes stools in inappropriate places, whether by accident or on purpose.

- Does so for at least once a month for 3 months in a row.

- Has trouble with daily life in going to work or school or taking part in social activities because of the behavior.

Encopresis is not diagnosed if the problem is caused by a medication (such as a laxative) or another medical condition.

Treatment

Because encopresis is often due to constipation, treating the medical cause may resolve the problem. Preventing any constipation and teaching good toilet-training habits are the goals of treating encopresis (for more tips, see box).

Changing the child's diet to include foods high in fiber (fruits, vegetables, and whole grain foods) and making sure the child is drinking enough water during the day can help. If this doesn't relieve the constipation, stool softeners or suppositories can help. These also may be used under the guidance of a doctor or mental health care provider to build a regular pattern of bowel habits. A mental health care provider also may help to address any emotional issues that may be causing the problem.

Young or physically small children will often sit on the toilet with their feet dangling. This position makes it hard for them to relax enough or to use the muscles needed for a bowel movement. A footstool can be placed under their feet while they are sitting on the toilet. This sturdy support for their feet can help the child have the seating position needed to have a bowel movement.

Quick Tips for Parents

These basic techniques from behavior therapy can help parents whose child has enuresis or encopresis.

- When accidents happen, maintain a neutral and matter-of-fact, problem-solving attitude. This helps the child not to be afraid of reporting accidents—or not to try hiding the accident until it is discovered.
- The child who had the accident can help with the cleanup of soiled bedding and clothing in age-appropriate ways, such as putting soiled clothes in the washing machine, cleaning themselves as best they can, or helping to put clean sheets on the bed. These tasks are performed by the child to take part in getting better, not to punish the child.
- Parents need to be supportive and patient. Reward small steps taken to improve and slight progress made (such as fewer accidents or smaller accidents).
- Solving the problem together can help the parent and child learn new skills and increase their bond.

Key Points

- *Elimination disorders* can occur during the day or at night. They often are not done on purpose and are accidents. These disorders are more common in children, and they are diagnosed after the age when a child is expected to be toilet trained.
- These disorders can be very upsetting to both children and their parents. Keeping a neutral, supportive attitude when accidents happen lowers the child's stress about the accident. Solving the problem together includes the child's help in cleaning up accidents in ways that suit their age.
- Medical conditions or medications can affect bowel or bladder function and cause these disorders. When these conditions are treated (or certain medications stopped or replaced under a doctor's guidance), the elimination disorder can resolve. Seeing a doctor to rule out

medical causes for the problem is key. If not caused by medical conditions or medications, these disorders often end on their own without treatment as the child grows.

- Treatments for *enuresis* include drinking less fluid at night, regular bathroom use during the day and evening, bed-wetting alarms if the problem lasts, and medications. Adults can take medication, learn bladder retraining exercises, keep a bladder diary, and strengthen muscles to help bladder control.
- Treatments for *encopresis* include limiting sugar and fried, fatty foods; eating more fiber (vegetables, fruit, whole grains); drinking water during the day; getting more exercise; using stool softeners or suppositories; and placing a footstool under the child's feet while they are sitting on the toilet to achieve the posture needed.

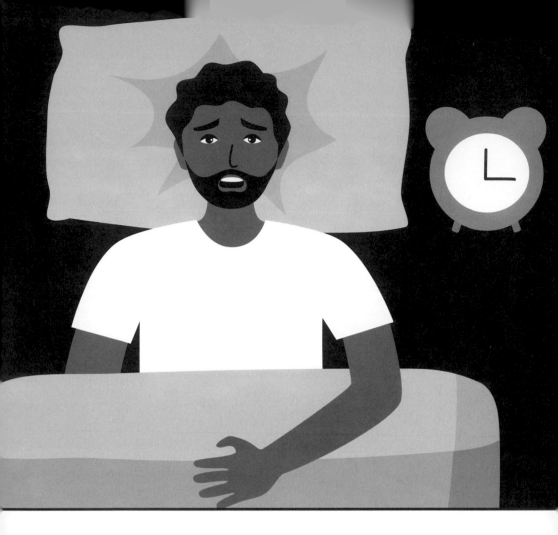

Insomnia Disorder
Narcolepsy
Breathing-Related Sleep Disorders
    Obstructive Sleep Apnea Hypopnea
    Central Sleep Apnea
    Sleep-Related Hypoventilation
Parasomnias
    Non–Rapid Eye Movement Sleep Arousal Disorders
    Nightmare Disorder
    Rapid Eye Movement Sleep Behavior Disorder
Other Sleep-Wake Disorders
    Hypersomnolence Disorder
    Circadian Rhythm Sleep-Wake Disorders
    Restless Legs Syndrome

For a complete list of DSM-5-TR disorders, see Appendix A.

CHAPTER 12

Sleep-Wake Disorders

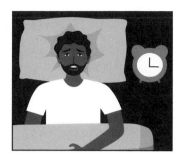

The purpose of sleep is a mystery, yet it fills about one-third of our lives. Ongoing sleep problems can make it hard to function well at school or work. They can cause people to lose needed sleep each day, to feel very sleepy and tired during the day, or to feel tired despite longer hours of sleep. Regular and consistent sleep can make a big difference in quality of life, day-to-day function, and mood. It is no wonder that sleep complaints are among the most common that people report to their doctors.

To feel fully rested and refreshed, most healthy adults need from 7 to 9 hours of uninterrupted sleep each night, although some people need more and some less to feel rested. Teens need about 8 to 10 hours. Without these needed hours of sleep, the body doesn't have enough hours to repair and restore itself for the next day. The longer a person has been awake, the more quickly they tend to fall asleep.

Sleep-wake disorders disrupt the quality, timing, and amount of sleep. These disorders are linked with a wide range of physical and emotional problems, such as fatigue, depression, concentration problems, irritability, and obesity. On any given night, one in three people has a problem falling or staying asleep.

This chapter details the sleep-wake disorders of *insomnia disorder, narcolepsy, breathing-related sleep disorders* (*obstructive sleep apnea hypopnea, central sleep apnea,* and *sleep-related hypoventilation*), and *parasom-*

nias (*non–rapid eye movement sleep arousal disorders, nightmare disorder, and rapid eye movement sleep behavior disorder*). Also described briefly are *hypersomnolence disorder, circadian rhythm sleep-wake disorders,* and *restless legs syndrome.*

How Are Sleep Disorders Diagnosed?

To diagnose sleep problems, the doctor will review medical history and use of medications. Certain medical conditions and medications are known to affect sleep.

People with sleep problems should keep a sleep log to track the following daily, for 1–2 weeks:

- Bedtime
- Amount of time (best guess) before they fall asleep
- Wake time(s)
- Number of awakenings
- Daytime naps (when and for how long)
- Any use of drugs or medications

The person's bed partner may be able to describe the person's snoring, breathing difficulties, leg jerks, or other body movements that might help the doctor diagnose a sleep disorder.

If the sleep disorder is severe or greatly impairs home and work function, getting a sleep study at a sleep disorders clinic is needed. Several tests can help identify the problem, but the most common is *polysomnography.* This test traces electrical activity in the brain and eye muscles during sleep, as well as other major body functions. The results can help to diagnose a range of sleep-wake disorders, such as *narcolepsy, breathing-related sleep disorders,* and *rapid eye movement sleep behavior disorder.*

Knowing about the normal stages of sleep can explain how different disorders cause problems in the night. Sleep stages in adults are divided into *rapid eye movement* (REM) and *non-REM* (NREM) sleep. These sleep stages switch back and forth in a cycle that lasts 70–120 minutes. In normal sleep, three to six NREM/REM cycles occur nightly.

- When people fall asleep, they enter NREM sleep that takes up most (75%) of the night. During this stage, body functions are restored, breathing becomes slower, muscles are relaxed, body temperature drops, and tissue growth occurs. The deepest level of sleep occurs during NREM sleep.
- The first stage of REM sleep occurs about 90 minutes after falling asleep and lasts 5–10 minutes. During REM sleep, the brain is active and the eyes dart back and forth. REM sleep repeats about every 90 minutes,

with each REM period getting longer later in the night. During the night, REM periods become closer together.

Without the full cycle of both REM and NREM sleep stages, the body may not feel fully restored. These changes from sleep to wakefulness are controlled by messages from the brain. Receiving a diagnosis and treatment, changing sleep habits and settings, and making lifestyle changes can return these sleep stages to more normal patterns. See the box at the end of this chapter for tips on building good sleep and lifestyle habits that can improve and prevent sleep disorders.

Insomnia Disorder

People with *insomnia disorder* are often unable to fall asleep or stay asleep. They do not get enough sleep or do not feel restored (with energy) or refreshed when they wake. As a result, they may have low energy and feel tired, worried, or depressed. It is the most common sleep problem of all the sleep disorders.

About 30% of adults report insomnia symptoms in any given year. Sometimes insomnia can happen during stressful events, such as loss of a loved one, loss of a job, or relationship problems. Looking forward to a happy event such as a wedding or vacation also can disrupt a person's sleep. Sleep schedules that vary can cause insomnia in children and teens, as well as adults.

Insomnia can be situational (also known as acute), episodic, persistent, or recurrent (chronic).

- *Situational insomnia* lasts a few days or weeks and is often brought on by life events or changes to sleep schedules or settings.
- *Episodic insomnia* occurs for at least 1 month but less than 3 months.
- *Persistent insomnia* occurs when the sleep problems last 3 months or longer after the life event or changes to sleep schedules or settings.
- *Recurrent insomnia* is when two or more insomnia episodes recur at least twice within 1 year. People with recurrent (chronic) insomnia often have trouble sleeping for a few nights, followed by a few nights of good sleep, before the trouble returns.

Insomnia is more common in women, people in middle age, and older adults. Women often have symptoms during pregnancy, as well as menopause. Insomnia can also occur with other medical conditions, such as diabetes, heart disease, arthritis, cancer, traumatic brain injury, and chronic pain conditions. Among people who suffer from insomnia, 40%–50% also have *alcohol use disorder* or another mental disorder.

Persistent insomnia is a risk factor for *bipolar, depressive,* and *anxiety disorders.* People with the condition often begin to rely on medications to help with sleep or use caffeine to stay awake during the day. This practice also can lead to a *substance use disorder.*

 Insomnia Disorder

The disorder is diagnosed when:

- A person does not get enough sleep or good sleep because of at least one of the following symptoms:
  - Problems falling asleep (children may have trouble falling asleep without the help of parent or caregiver).
  - Problems staying asleep (waking up often or problems going back to sleep after being awake).
  - Waking early in the morning and being unable to go back to sleep.
- The sleep problem causes much distress or hinders social, work, school, behavior, or other major functions.
- The problem occurs at least 3 nights a week.
- The problem lasts for at least 3 months.

The insomnia is not due to another sleep-wake disorder, such as *narcolepsy* or a *parasomnia*. It is not due to a drug, alcohol, or medication. Another mental disorder or medical condition is not the main cause of the insomnia.

Risk Factors

The following factors may make people more prone to insomnia. A life event, such as illness, separation, or chronic stress, can trigger a sleep problem in people with these traits:

- **Temperament.** People who tend to be anxious or worried are more prone to insomnia, as well as people who have difficulty expressing their emotions.
- **Environment.** Noise, light, a room that is too warm or cold, and a high altitude can increase risk for insomnia.
- **Genetics.** Having a first-degree blood relative (parent or sibling) with the condition.

Warren's Story

Warren, a 30-year-old graduate student, saw a doctor to discuss his problems staying asleep. The trouble began 4 months prior when he started to wake up at 3:00 A.M. every morning, no matter when he went to bed, and he was unable to fall back to sleep. As a result he felt "out of it" during the day. This led him to feel more worried about how he was going to finish his thesis when he was unable to focus due to extreme fatigue. At first, he did not recall waking up with any concern on his mind. As the problem lasted, he found himself dreading the next day and wondering how he would teach his classes or focus on his writing if he was only getting a few hours of sleep. Some mornings he lay awake in the dark next to his fiancée, who was sleeping soundly. On other mornings he would cut his losses, rise from bed, and go very early to his office on campus.

After a month of poor sleep, Warren went to the student health services clinic, where he received his medical care. (He had asthma, for which he sometimes used an inhaler.) He was prescribed a sleep medication, which did not help. Falling asleep was not his problem, Warren explained. Meanwhile, he followed some advice he read online. Although he often relied on coffee during the day, he never drank it after 2:00 P.M. An avid tennis player, he chose to play only in the early morning. He did have a glass or two of wine every night at dinner with his fiancée, however. "By dinner, I start to worry about whether I'll be able to sleep," he said, "and to be honest, the wine helps."

Warren did not appear tired but told the doctor, "I made a point to see you in the morning, before I hit the wall." He did not look sad or on edge and was not sure if he had ever felt depressed. But he was certain of nagging, low-level anxiety. "This sleep problem has taken over," he explained. "I'm stressed about my work, and my fiancée and I have been arguing. But it's all because I'm so tired."

Warren was diagnosed with *insomnia disorder*. His sleep problem began during a period of high stress. His worries about not sleeping may have made the problem worse. Warren had also begun to self-medicate with caffeine to stay alert during the day and with wine to calm down in the evening.

Also noted is a past medical history of asthma, for which Warren sometimes uses an inhaler. Because the inhaler medication may be stimulating, knowing when and how much he uses would be helpful.

Treatment

There are many methods used to treat insomnia and most people find relief—although it may take a bit of time for some. Treatment often combines both behavior therapy and medication.

With behavior therapy, one of the first steps may be to create a sleep environment that promotes sleep, as well as practicing good sleep hygiene (see box at the end of this chapter). Relaxation techniques, such as yoga and meditation, can also be very helpful in getting the body to sleep.

Prescription sleeping pills, such as one of the benzodiazepines or a sedating antidepressant, may be very helpful, but these should only be taken for short-term use. Some over-the-counter sleeping aids may also be effective, such as doxylamine or melatonin, but these also should be taken only for a short time. Those with insomnia disorder should talk to their doctor (whether primary care or mental health care provider) about these medications and their use.

Narcolepsy

People with *narcolepsy* have an extreme need to sleep during the day, with frequent daytime naps or sleep attacks that are hard to stop. They also may have *cataplexy*—a sudden loss of muscle tone triggered by emotions such as laughter or surprise. Cataplexy can affect the neck, jaw, arms, legs, or whole body, resulting in falls.

Narcolepsy can make people fall asleep while talking, while at work or school, while driving, or at other inappropriate times. The sleep attacks can last from seconds to minutes. People with the disorder often wake up through the night, for brief or long amounts of time. Right before falling asleep or just before waking up, they may also have *hallucinations* (seeing, smelling, or hearing things that are not there) or *sleep paralysis* (a brief loss of muscle tone, being unable to move or speak). Vivid dreams and nightmares are also common, as is *REM sleep behavior disorder* (described later in this chapter).

Social life can suffer as people with the disorder try to control their emotions to prevent symptoms. They may avoid social contact because they are embarrassed by their symptoms. Because the disorder impairs the ability to pay attention, it causes problems with school, work, driving, and other activities that require focused attention. When treated, people with the disorder can drive for short distances, but they should not drive or operate machines for a living because of safety concerns.

Symptoms of narcolepsy often start in childhood, teen years, or young adulthood. It rarely first appears in older adults. The disorder is also linked to obesity and early puberty. Young children who suddenly develop symptoms often have rapid weight gain. People with *bipolar, depressive,* and other *sleep disorders* (such as *sleepwalking, REM sleep behavior disorder, obstructive sleep apnea,* and *restless legs syndrome*) may also suffer from narcolepsy.

Narcolepsy

Narcolepsy is diagnosed when people have:

- Periods of a strong urge to sleep, followed by a short nap (sleep attack). These naps happen at least three times per week over the past 3 months.
- The presence of at least one of the following:
  - Episodes of cataplexy (either one of the following) that occur at least a few times per month:
    - In people whose symptoms have lasted for a long time, a brief and sudden loss of muscle tone while awake that makes them unable to move and is triggered by emotions such as laughter or joking.
    - In children or people whose symptoms have lasted for 6 months or less, sudden grimaces or episodes with an open jaw and thrusting tongue, without any clear emotional triggers.
  - Lab tests showing a low amount of hypocretin (a chemical in the brain that controls wakefulness).
  - Nighttime sleep study results showing that REM sleep occurs more quickly than in normal sleep cycles.

Risk Factors

The following factors may make people more prone to narcolepsy:

- **Temperament.** Those with narcolepsy often notice that they need more sleep than other family members.
- **Environment.** Certain types of flu or strep throat, immune system problems, head trauma, and sudden changes in sleep-wake patterns, such as job changes or stress, may be triggers.
- **Genetics.** People with a first-degree blood relative (parent or sibling) with narcolepsy are at a higher risk of also developing the condition.

Treatment

Treatment of narcolepsy often combines both behavior therapy and medication. These may relieve the symptoms enough for many people with the condition to once again have almost-normal sleep habits.

Behavior therapy may include making lifestyle changes, such as taking several short naps (10–15 minutes) during the day and sticking to a regular schedule for sleep, exercise, and meals. Avoiding heavy meals and alcohol, which can disturb or induce sleep, is also suggested.

Stimulants, such as methylphenidate, are often used to treat sleep attacks and can help with staying alert. Modafinil is an effective alternative to the stimulants and is well tolerated. Tricyclic antidepressants are sometimes prescribed to treat cataplexy or sleep paralysis but have little impact on sleep attacks. Sodium oxybate can be used to treat cataplexy.

Breathing-Related Sleep Disorders

Breathing-related sleep disorders cause problems in a person's normal breathing that disturb sleep. These often lead to more serious health and social concerns. Seeking treatment quickly for these disorders can prevent serious health problems. This group of disorders includes *obstructive sleep apnea hypopnea, central sleep apnea,* and *sleep-related hypoventilation.* The most common of these disorders is obstructive sleep apnea hypopnea.

Obstructive Sleep Apnea Hypopnea

Obstructive sleep apnea hypopnea—or sleep apnea—causes breathing to briefly stop during sleep. *Apnea* refers to a total pause in breathing, and *hypopnea* refers to reduced breathing for at least 10 seconds (in children, two missed breaths). The pause or reduction in breathing occurs when the muscles in the back of the throat do not keep the airway open. This can happen hundreds of times throughout the night.

Sleep apnea is the most common breathing-related sleep disorder, affecting more than 22 million American adults. Most people who have sleep apnea, however, don't know it because it only happens while they are asleep. A family member or other person sharing the bedroom might be the first to notice the symptoms. Sleep apnea is more common in men, people ages 40–60, older adults, and people who are overweight. Weight loss can resolve the problem.

At least 1% to 4% of children also suffer from sleep apnea. The disorder tends to peak in children ages 3–8 years, when enlarged tonsils may cause the problem. Sleep apnea can resolve as the child grows. At any age, problems with sleep or complaints about being sleepy during the day are important to see a doctor about. Sleep problems have a vital impact on health. In children, delayed growth and behavior and learning problems can result from sleep apnea. Children with the disorder may have problems breathing while asleep, a dry mouth, morning headaches, problems swallowing, bed-wetting, and problems with speech.

For all people with the condition, sleep apnea can cause disturbed sleep and low oxygen levels. The most common symptoms in adults include snoring, dry mouth, sleepiness during the day, heartburn, morning headaches, and loss of sex drive. Sleep apnea is linked with an increased risk of death, high blood pressure, heart disease, heart failure, stroke, diabetes, and depression.

Obstructive Sleep Apnea Hypopnea

The condition is diagnosed when a person has either one of the following:

- A sleep study shows at least five obstructive apneas or hypopneas per hour of sleep and either of the following sleep symptoms:

  - Snoring, snorting/gasping, or breathing pauses during nighttime sleep.

  - Daytime sleepiness, fatigue, or unrefreshing sleep, despite enough time to sleep, that is not due to another mental disorder or medical condition.

- A sleep study shows at least 15 obstructive apneas and/or hypopneas per hour of sleep regardless of other symptoms.

Carlos's Story

Carlos, a 57-year-old man, came in for reevaluation of his antidepressant medication. He described several months of worsening fatigue, daytime sleepiness, and generally "not feeling good." He lacked the energy to do his usual activities, but he still enjoyed them when he took part in them. He had some trouble staying focused on his work in computers and was worried that he would lose his job. A selective serotonin reuptake inhibitor (SSRI) antidepressant had been prescribed 2 years earlier, and symptoms improved somewhat. Carlos insisted he was still taking the medication.

He said he didn't feel stressed. Along with *depression,* he also had high blood pressure, diabetes, and heart disease. He complained of heartburn as well as erectile dysfunction, for which he had not seen a doctor.

Carlos was married and had two grown children. He did not smoke or drink alcohol but did drink several servings of coffee each day to help stay alert.

The exam showed he was 5 feet 10 inches tall, weighed 235 pounds, and had a body mass index (BMI) of 34.

More questions revealed that Carlos not only had trouble staying awake at work, but sometimes nodded off while driving. He slept for 8–10 hours nightly but woke up often, made nightly trips to the bathroom (nocturia), and often woke with a choking sensation and sometimes with a headache. He had snored since childhood, but he added, "All the men in my family are snorers." Before his wife chose to sleep in their guest bedroom, she said he snored very loudly and sometimes stopped breathing and gasped for air.

Carlos was sent for a sleep study, which showed he had 25 events of apnea per hour. He was diagnosed with *obstructive sleep apnea hypopnea.* His history of loud snoring and episodes of choking and gasping suggested that apnea was likely the problem.

Carlos has many of the risk factors for obstructive sleep apnea hypopnea. For example, he is over age 50 and obese, and has a family history of "all the men" being snorers. Snoring is a specific sign of sleep apnea, especially when the snoring is very loud, occurs more than 3 days per week, and is accompanied by episodes of choking and gasping.

Risk Factors

Many genetic and physical factors increase the risk of sleep apnea, such as having a first-degree blood relative (parent or sibling) with the condition, obesity, a small jaw, or a large overbite. Men are at higher risk than women because of the design of their airway structure. Menopause or pregnancy can increase risk in women.

Treatment

Treatment for sleep apnea helps people to breathe normally during sleep and relieves symptoms such as loud snoring and daytime sleepiness.

- Lifestyle changes are a major part of treating apnea. Because many people with sleep apnea are overweight or obese, weight loss can help in many cases.
- People also find that sleeping on their side instead of their back helps keep the throat open, and can reduce the symptoms of sleep apnea.
- Seeing a doctor for any medical or medication problems that might be causing the sleep apnea can also resolve the sleep problem.
- A custom-made mouthpiece can be used to adjust the lower jaw and tongue to keep the airways open during sleep.
- For those with moderate to severe apnea, a *continuous positive airway pressure (CPAP)* device is prescribed. A CPAP machine consists of a face mask that gently blows air into the person's throat to keep airways open during sleep.

- In rare and severe cases, surgery can help to keep the airway open during sleep.

Central Sleep Apnea

Central sleep apnea is a disorder in which the brain fails to correctly control breathing during sleep. This causes people to make no effort to breathe for brief periods. The condition is a rare type of sleep apnea.

Central sleep apnea is more common in people with certain medical conditions, such as heart failure, stroke, or kidney failure. People with these health problems usually develop a type of disturbed breathing pattern known as *Cheyne-Stokes breathing*. Breathing increases and decreases, sometimes quickly, like a tidal wave, with periods of sleep apnea and waking. Hyperventilation (fast, deep, rapid breaths) and hypoventilation (shallow and few breaths) occur.

Central sleep apnea is more common in men over age 60. It is also more common in people who use long-acting opioids (painkillers), with about 24% of such opioid users having the condition.

 Central Sleep Apnea

The condition is diagnosed when:

- A sleep study shows at least five central apneas per hour of sleep.
- The disorder is not due to another current sleep disorder.

Risk Factors

Many genetic and health factors increase the risk of central sleep apnea, such as heart failure, older age, acid reflux, being male, kidney failure, stroke, and taking long-acting opioid medication.

Treatment

Treating the underlying condition that is causing central sleep apnea can help relieve and manage symptoms. If opioid medications are causing the apnea, the doctor may lower the dose or change the medicine. Devices used during sleep to aid breathing also may be used. These include CPAP (described above for obstructive sleep apnea hypopnea), bilevel positive airway pressure (BiPAP), and adaptive servo-ventilation (ASV). These devices provide pressured air in different ways. BiPAP and ASV can deliver a breath if one hasn't been taken for a certain number of seconds. Some types of central sleep apnea are treated with medicines that promote breathing. Oxygen treatment may help ensure the lungs get enough oxygen while sleeping.

Sleep-Related Hypoventilation

Sleep-related hypoventilation is a rare condition marked by shallow breathing with either high carbon dioxide or low oxygen levels only during sleep. It can occur on its own or with medical conditions, medication use, or *substance use disorders*. Daytime sleepiness, frequent waking during sleep, morning headaches, and complaints of insomnia are common. The disorder is slow to progress and can occur at any age, even in infants. It can result in heart failure and problems in brain, blood, and heart function.

 Sleep-Related Hypoventilation

The condition is diagnosed when:

- A sleep study shows decreased breathing with high carbon dioxide or low oxygen levels.
- The disorder is not due to another current sleep disorder.

Risk Factors

The following factors increase the risk of developing the condition:

- **Environment.** People who take central nervous system depressants to treat anxiety or insomnia, such as benzodiazepines, opiates, or alcohol.
- **Genetics and biology.** Other medical conditions, such as obesity, breathing disorders (such as chronic obstructive pulmonary disease [COPD]), hypothyroidism, neuromuscular or chest wall disorders, or spinal cord injury.

Treatment

Treating the underlying condition that is causing sleep-related hypoventilation can help relieve and manage symptoms. When the other condition improves or worsens, it can likewise improve or worsen sleep-related hypoventilation. Treatments also can include oxygen treatment and CPAP.

Parasomnias

Parasomnias are disorders that involve abnormal behaviors and experiences, such as frequent nightmares, that happen during sleep or as someone begins to awake. *Non–rapid eye movement (NREM) sleep arousal disorders* and *rapid eye movement (REM) sleep behavior disorder* are the most common.

When episodes of parasomnias are frequent and cause much distress, medications are usually prescribed for treatment. In most cases, benzodiazepine tranquilizers or antidepressant medications can be very helpful in stopping the episodes.

Non–Rapid Eye Movement Sleep Arousal Disorders

The most common type of *NREM sleep arousal disorders* are *sleepwalking* and *sleep terrors*. These disorders involve partial waking during the night, and the person's eyes may be open when these events occur. The person is confused when wakened or can be hard to wake. There is little or no recall of what occurred. Many people have both sleepwalking and sleep terrors. Rare episodes of sleepwalking or sleep terrors do not count as symptoms of NREM sleep arousal disorders.

Early stages of sleepwalking may involve just sitting up in bed, looking about, or picking at the blanket or sheet. For the disorder, these behaviors progress to more complex movement and repeated episodes. People with a sleepwalking disorder get up from bed and walk about. They may leave the room, use the bathroom, or talk with someone, but they are not aware or awake when this happens. Most episodes last from 1–10 minutes but may last up to a full hour.

During a sleep terror, people will suddenly sit up in bed, screaming or crying, with a scared look on their face. They show signs of great fear, such as sweating and rapid breathing. It is difficult to comfort or wake them. They seem to have an extreme sense of dread and danger, and an urge to escape. They return to sleep after this event. There may be several episodes of terrors throughout the night, but it is more common to have only one episode in the night. For the disorder, sleep terrors are repeated experiences rather than a rare event.

It is common for sleepwalking or sleep terrors to occur just once or rarely repeat (after a long while if it happened before). Between 10% and 30% of children have sleepwalked at least once, and 5% sleepwalk more often. Between 7% and 30% of adults around the world sleepwalk at some point during their lifetime, and between 2% and 4% sleepwalk in any given year. Sleep terror episodes (not the disorder) are more common in young children under age 3 (20%–40%) than in adults (2%).

 NREM Sleep Arousal Disorders

The disorder is diagnosed when the following occur:

- Repeated episodes of incomplete awakening from sleep, usually during the first third of the sleep hours, along with one of the following:
  - **Sleepwalking:** Repeated episodes of rising from bed during sleep and walking about. While sleepwalking, the person has a blank, staring face; does not respond to others trying to talk to them; and can be hard to wake.
  - **Sleep terrors:** Repeated episodes of extreme nightmares that wake a person from sleep, most often with a panicked scream. There may be intense fear, rapid breathing, and sweating during each episode. The person does not respond to others who try to give comfort during the episode.
- None or little of the dream is recalled.
- The person does not recall that sleepwalking or sleep terrors occurred.
- The episodes cause much distress or disrupt social life, work, or daily functions.

The problem is not due to the effects of a substance such as drugs or medication. It is not due to another mental disorder or medical condition.

Risk Factors

These factors increase the risk of sleepwalking or sleep terrors:

- **Environment.** Use of sedatives (medicines that cause sleep or rest), lack of sleep, change of sleep schedule, fatigue, fever, and physical or emotional stress.
- **Genetics.** Up to 80% of people who sleepwalk have a family history of sleepwalking or sleep terrors. Children whose mother and father both sleepwalk are up to 60% more likely to also have the problem. And those with a first-degree blood relative (parent or sibling) who sleepwalks or has sleep terrors are up to 10 times more likely to have sleep terrors as well.

Nightmare Disorder

Nightmares are vivid, detailed dreams that cause worry or fear. They seem real when they occur. Attempts to avoid danger are a common theme, and feelings of worry or fear may persist after waking. Nightmares occur during REM sleep. They involve quick waking after the dream and good recall of the dream content.

Episodes of nightmares increase through childhood into teenage years. Between 1% and 4% of parents report that their preschool-age children "often" or "always" have nightmares. Nightmares often begin between ages 3 and 6 years but become more frequent and severe in the teens and early adult years. About 5% of children ages 5–15 years report nightmares. About 6% of adults have nightmares at least once a month, and 1% to 2% have them frequently. Parents who soothe their children after nightmares may protect them against chronic nightmares.

 Nightmare Disorder

The disorder is diagnosed when:

- Repeated instances of long, unhappy, and well-remembered dreams that often involve trying to avoid physical harm and safety threats. These happen during the second half of sleep hours.
- The person wakes from a dream and quickly is alert.
- The episodes cause much distress or interfere with social life, work, or other major daily functions.

The problem is not due to the effects of a substance such as drugs or medication. It is not due to another mental disorder or medical condition. The nightmares can occur less than once a week, more than once a week, or each night. They can happen for 1 month or less, more than 1 month, or 6 months or more.

Risk Factors

In middle-aged adults, low income; symptoms of depression, anxiety, and insomnia; and frequent heavy alcohol use are linked with nightmare disorder. Other factors increase the risk of nightmares:

- **Environment.** Lack of sleep, jet lag, and changing the times for sleeping and waking can upset REM sleep stages and increase risk.
- **Genetics.** A family history of nightmares.

Rapid Eye Movement Sleep Behavior Disorder

People with *REM sleep behavior disorder* act out their dreams during sleep. They may perform strong and violent acts in dreams of being attacked or escaping harm. The violent behavior includes loud, profane screams or movement, such as falling, jumping, punching, thrusting, hitting, or kicking. These movements may harm the person or bed partner, and about 55% of those with the disorder have had an injury from these movements. The person's eyes may be closed during these episodes. When awakened, the person is quickly alert and may be able to recall the upsetting dream.

The disorder is more common in men over age 50, but it can occur in women and younger people. It may be more common in people who take medications for a mental disorder. The disorder has been found in 30% of those with *narcolepsy*.

 REM Sleep Behavior Disorder

The disorder is diagnosed when:

- Repeated episodes of waking during sleep occur, with talking and/or complex movement.
- These behaviors arise during REM sleep and often happen more than 90 minutes after sleep begins, tend to occur later in the sleep cycle, and rarely happen during daytime naps.
- The person wakes fully alert, and not confused or disoriented.
- Either of the following exists:
  - REM sleep without relaxed muscles on sleep study recording.
  - A history of possible REM sleep behavior disorder and a diagnosis of a disease with abnormal levels of synuclein protein (a type of protein in the brain), such as *Parkinson's disease* or *Lewy body disease.*
- The behaviors cause much distress or interfere with social life, work, or other major daily functions.

The problem is not due to the effects of a substance such as drugs or medication. It is not due to another mental disorder or medical condition. Special regard is given to how often symptoms occur, the potential for harm, and the degree of distress in other household members.

Risk Factors

REM sleep behavior disorder is often a side effect of many antidepressant medications.

Other Sleep-Wake Disorders

These other sleep-wake disorders also cause distress and disrupt social, work, or other major daily functions. They require treatment and are discussed briefly below: *hypersomnolence disorder, circadian rhythm sleep-wake disorders,* and *restless legs syndrome.*

Hypersomnolence Disorder

Hypersomnolence is a condition that causes people to sleep for long periods during the day or night. Most people with the condition sleep 9 or more hours each night but do not feel refreshed or energized when they awake. In the United States, about 5%–10% of people who complain of being sleepy during the day and get examined at a sleep clinic are later diagnosed with *hypersomnolence disorder.* The same treatments for *narcolepsy* also improve symptoms of this disorder.

The condition is diagnosed when:

- Extreme sleepiness occurs with 7 or more hours of sleep, with at least one of the following symptoms:
  - Frequent periods of sleep or sleep attacks within the same day.
  - Sleeping for more than 9 hours per day without feeling refreshed.
  - Trouble fully waking up.
- The problem happens at least three times per week for at least 3 months.

The problem is not due to the effects of drugs or medication. It is not due to another sleep disorder, mental disorder, or medical condition, although these can also be present. Hypersomnolence disorder may require a special evaluation, and a number of medical disorders may need to be ruled out as the cause.

Circadian Rhythm Sleep-Wake Disorders

Circadian rhythm sleep-wake disorders occur with changes to the normal sleep-wake routine, such as with shift work. *Circadian rhythm* is a 24-hour cycle often referred to as the "body clock." This internal body clock is affected by factors such as sunrise and time zones. When the body's circadian rhythm is disrupted (for instance, by jet lag), sleeping patterns can be affected. Treatment involves resetting the sleep-wake schedule by fixing environmental cues and the use of light therapy. Behavior approaches also help (see the box at the end of this chapter).

These disorders are diagnosed when:

- A constant or frequent pattern of disturbed sleep occurs when a person's normal sleep-wake schedule is changed.
- The disturbed sleep leads to extreme sleepiness, insomnia, or both.

Restless Legs Syndrome

Restless legs syndrome causes uncomfortable feelings in the legs, often in the evenings, while sitting or lying down. It makes people feel like getting up and moving around, which eases the discomfort. The uncomfortable feelings are often described as creeping, crawling, tingling, or burning. As with the other sleep disorders, this condition can interrupt the sleep of the person's bed partner. The disorder can delay falling asleep. For some people, a lack of iron may cause the problem. Treatment may include benzodiazepines and medicines that increase levels of dopamine (a chemical in the brain)—for instance, pramipexole.

The condition is diagnosed when:

- A person has an urge to move the legs in response to uncomfortable sensations, characterized by all of the following happening at least three times a week for at least 3 months:
  - The urge to move the legs begins or worsens during periods of rest or inactivity.
  - The urge to move the legs is partly or totally relieved by movement.
  - The urge to move the legs is worse at night or only happens at night.

The problem is not due to the effects of alcohol, drugs, or medication. It is not due to another mental disorder or medical condition, such as arthritis or leg swelling.

Practice Good Sleep Hygiene

While many factors can disrupt sleep, these steps can help provide a better night's rest:

- **Make your bedroom comfortable.** Have a quiet setting that is dark and cool and a bed with cozy bedding and pillows. Remove the distractions of computers, televisions, phones, and other electronic devices. Use the bed for sleeping and sex only. Paying bills or going over work issues will link sleep with stress.
- **Get regular exercise.** Brisk exercise, such as cycling or swimming, at least three times a week is best. Any form of exercise can help as long as it does not occur close to sleep time.
- **Maintain sleep times.** Get as much sleep as you need, not too much or too little.
- **Limit worry.** Schedule a regular worry time earlier in the day to think about issues in your life. Write down concerns and possible solutions so they don't prevent you from sleeping.
- **Set a routine.** Stick to a regular pattern of sleep and wake hours—wake up and go to bed every day at the same time and avoid daytime naps even on weekends.
- **Stay away from stimulants and alcohol.** Cut off substances such as caffeine, nicotine, and alcohol at least a few hours before bedtime.
- **Find a relaxing bedtime routine.** A regular ritual of a warm bath or listening to soft music can mentally prepare the body and mind for sleep.
- **Create a soothing sleep environment.** Keep the lights turned down. Use earplugs or a sound machine that produces soothing or neutral sounds.

Key Points

- *Sleep-wake disorders* disrupt the quality, timing, and amount of sleep. These disorders can cause a wide range of physical and emotional problems, such as fatigue, depression, concentration problems, irritability, and obesity. On any given night, one in three people has a problem falling or staying asleep.
- Certain medical conditions and medications are known to affect sleep. To diagnose sleep problems, the doctor will review medical history and use of medications.
- People with sleep problems should keep a sleep log to track the following items daily for 1–2 weeks for their doctor: bedtime, amount of time (best guess) before they fall asleep, wake time(s), number of awakenings, daytime naps, and any use of drugs or medications. The person's bed partner may be able to describe the person's snor-

ing, breathing difficulties, leg jerks, or other body movements that might help the doctor diagnose a sleep disorder.

- If the sleep disorder is severe or greatly impairs home and work function, getting a sleep study at a sleep disorders clinic is needed. Several tests can help identify the problem, but the most common is polysomnography. This test traces electrical activity in the brain and eye muscles during sleep, as well as other major body functions.
- Seeking a diagnosis and treatment, changing sleep habits and settings if needed, and making lifestyle changes can greatly improve sleep. The following tips can help: make your bedroom comfortable and use it only for sleep and sex; get regular exercise as long as it does not occur close to sleep time; schedule a "worry time" during the day; stick to a regular pattern of sleep and wake hours; stay away from caffeine, nicotine, and alcohol at least a few hours before bedtime; find a relaxing bedtime routine; and create a soothing sleep environment.

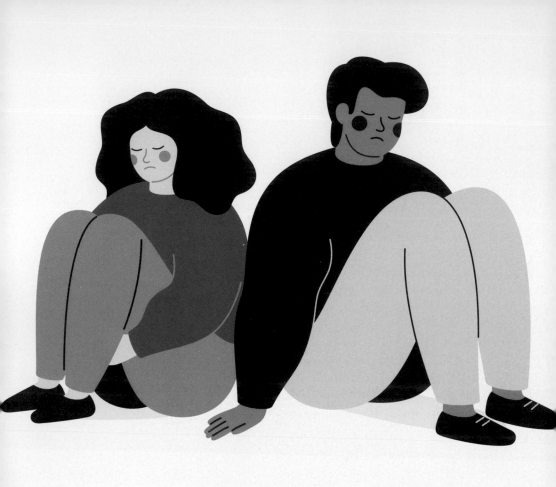

Substance/Medication-Induced Sexual Dysfunction

Erectile Disorder

Premature (Early) Ejaculation

Female Orgasmic Disorder

Other Sexual Dysfunctions

    Delayed Ejaculation

    Genito-Pelvic Pain/Penetration Disorder

    Female Sexual Interest/Arousal Disorder

    Male Hypoactive Sexual Desire Disorder

For a complete list of DSM-5-TR disorders, see Appendix A.

CHAPTER 13

Sexual Dysfunctions

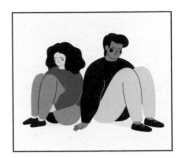

Sexual intimacy with another person can provide intense joy—and it can also produce distress.

Sexual dysfunctions disrupt the ability to respond to sexual activity or to enjoy sex. Sexual dysfunctions occur across a range of sexual response stages (see box). Learning the reasons for the problem is key to how these disorders are diagnosed and treated. For instance, aging brings a normal decrease in sexual response. Because the sexual response involves the body, mind, and emotions, often more than one factor is involved:

- *Partner factors,* such as a partner's sexual or health problems, or lack of desire.
- *Relationship factors,* such as not talking openly about feelings, likes, and dislikes; not feeling close; having levels of desire that differ.
- *Individual factors,* such as aging, poor body image, low self-esteem, *depression, anxiety,* stress (such as from job loss, divorce, loss of a loved one), inhibitions with sexual activity, past sexual or emotional abuse.
- *Cultural or religious factors,* such as laws or rules against sexual activity or pleasure.
- *Medical factors,* such as injury, diabetes, thyroid problems, and heart disease.

> ## Stages of Human Sexual Response
>
> Four stages of human sexual response help describe sexual function:
> - **Desire** is the key factor that begins sexual response.
> - **Sexual excitement** causes biological changes in the man (erection) and woman (vaginal lubrication).
> - **Orgasm** produces ejaculation in men and vaginal contractions in women.
> - **Resolution** involves a state of well-being and relaxing as sexual organs return to their normal, nonexcited state.

The disorders described in this chapter can affect men, women, transgender persons, and those who may not identify with any gender. For *male hypoactive sexual desire disorder* and *female sexual interest/arousal disorder,* the symptoms and feelings of these disorders are not limited to the person's specific sex or gender. Disorders linked to reproductive anatomy (such as *erectile disorder, premature ejaculation, delayed ejaculation,* and *genito-pelvic pain/penetration disorder*) are based on the person's current body and not on the person's sex assigned at birth. Much more research is needed to understand experiences of sexual dysfunction among gender diverse people.

It is normal for sexual problems to occur from time to time, and a diagnosis of a sexual dysfunction involves problems that last for at least 6 months (except for substance/medication-induced sexual dysfunction, which can occur shortly after a drug, alcohol, or medication is taken). Sexual dysfunctions include the following: *substance/medication-induced sexual dysfunction, erectile disorder, premature (early) ejaculation, female orgasmic disorder, delayed ejaculation, genito-pelvic pain/penetration disorder, female sexual interest/arousal disorder,* and *male hypoactive sexual desire disorder.* They can be mild, moderate, or severe, and are described based on when they begin or occur:

- *Lifelong* sexual problems are present since the first sexual experience.
- *Acquired* problems begin after a time of normal sexual activity.
- *Generalized* problems occur with any partner or sexual act.
- *Situational* problems occur with only certain types of stimulation, situations, or partners.

Substance/Medication-Induced Sexual Dysfunction

Sexual problems can occur from using certain kinds of substances, such as alcohol, opioids (narcotic painkillers such as codeine and oxycodone), sedatives or hypnotics (sleep medications), amphetamines, cocaine, and other stimulants. Some medications that may have sexual side effects include antidepressants, antipsychotics, estrogens, steroids, and medications for heart, stomach, and high blood pressure problems.

Sexual problems can occur when people start or stop taking a medication or substance or when their dosage is increased. Sexual problems that seem to occur with medication may cause some people to stop the medicine right away, but this can lead to harmful health problems. Report sexual problems that may result from medication to the doctor, who can help find a better medicine and advise on how to stop a medicine that may cause sexual problems.

People who use drugs often have problems with sexual desire, keeping erections, and reaching orgasm. About 60% to 70% of heroin users have these problems, but the numbers are lower for those who abuse amphetamines or cocaine. Men who drink and smoke on a regular basis often have trouble getting or keeping an erection.

Sexual problems caused by antidepressants can start fairly soon after the first dose. The most common problems relate to reaching orgasm in women and keeping an erection or ejaculating in men. For example, selective serotonin reuptake inhibitors (SSRIs) can have sexual side effects, such as loss of sexual desire and ejaculation problems in men. Other antidepressants, such as bupropion and mirtazapine, are less likely to cause these problems.

About one-half of the people taking antipsychotic medications have sexual side effects. These include problems with sexual desire, erection, dryness (in women), ejaculation, or having orgasm.

 ## Substance/Medication-Induced Sexual Dysfunction

The condition is diagnosed when there is:

- A major problem in sexual function.

- Information based on the person's history, lab tests, and physical exam show that

  - The problem began during or soon after starting or stopping the use of a medication.

  - There is a medication or substance used that can cause sexual problems.

- Great distress about the problem.

A substance/medication-induced sexual dysfunction is *not* diagnosed when any of the following occur: the sexual dysfunction was present before the substance or medication use began; the sexual dysfunction lasts more than 1 month after the person stops using the substance or medication; and the sexual dysfunction occurs only during a *delirium* (see Chapter 17, "Dementia and Other Memory Problems").

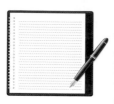

Daniel's Story

Daniel, a 55-year-old married accountant, saw a psychiatrist for a second opinion about his ongoing *major depression*. He had not improved after trying two antidepressants (fluoxetine and then sertraline) at high doses for 3 months. He had not taken medications for about a month after the sertraline did not work.

Daniel was severely depressed, with poor concentration, early morning waking, decreased sex drive, and loss of interest in normal activities. He didn't abuse any substances, drank little, and did not smoke.

Daniel was treated with the antidepressant clomipramine and the antianxiety medication buspirone. After 5 weeks, he said he felt much better. He was sleeping and eating well and taking part in activities with greater enthusiasm. For the first time in many months, he felt a return of his sexual interest.

After not having sexual intercourse in months, Daniel tried to have sex several times. He was distressed to find that he couldn't keep an erection during intercourse. He was also unable to ejaculate during masturbation. These problems lasted for a month. He recalled having had slightly delayed ejaculation while taking fluoxetine. He did not recall sexual problems while using sertraline.

Daniel was diagnosed with *medication-induced sexual dysfunction* and *depression*. His erection and ejaculation problems appear to have begun directly after starting clomipramine. The antidepressant is known to cause problems with sexual function, most often erectile dysfunction. Clomipramine's sexual side effects also include delayed or inhibited ejaculation.

Treatment

The first approach to treating substance/medication-induced sexual dysfunction is to find out which substance or medication is causing the problem and to see whether it can be stopped. In some cases, the condition being treated also may cause the problem. The dosage for some medications must be slowly reduced to avoid adverse effects or health problems. The doctor can then suggest other medication that can replace the agent causing the problem and provide guidance on switching and starting new medications. SSRI antidepressants often can be replaced with a different kind of antidepressant that is less likely to cause sexual problems. Alcohol, heroin, and cocaine are some drugs that can cause sexual dysfunctions. If a drug of abuse is involved, learning about the problems caused by the drug and seeking treatment for substance abuse are important.

Erectile Disorder

Erectile disorder (impotence) involves a man's repeated failure to get or keep an erection during sex with his partner. The disorder may be caused by many factors, including health problems (such as diabetes and heart disease), certain medications, and alcohol or cigarette smoking.

Generalized erectile disorder occurs with all types of stimulation, in any setting, and with all partners. Situational erectile disorder only occurs with certain types of stimulation, settings, or partners. Many men with the condition have low self-esteem, feelings of guilt, self-blame, anger, a sense of failure, and concern about disappointing their partner. Low confidence may lead them to fear or avoid sexual encounters.

Erectile disorder affects less than 10% of men under age 40. Symptoms of erectile disorder increase as a man ages—often after age 50. About 13% to 21% of men between ages 40 and 80 have the disorder, and it affects between 50% and 75% of men age 70 and older.

Erectile disorder occurs in men with other sexual disorders, such as *premature (early) ejaculation,* as well as *anxiety* and *depressive disorders*. It is also common in men with urinary tract problems related to an enlarged prostate gland.

 Erectile Disorder

The disorder is diagnosed when:

- At least one of the following symptoms happens almost every time (at least 75% of the time) during sexual activity:

    - Problems getting an erection during sexual acts.

    - Problems keeping an erection until a sexual act is finished.

    - Erections are much less rigid or hard than in the past.

- Symptoms have lasted for at least 6 months.

The symptoms cause the man much distress. They are not due to a nonsexual mental disorder, stress in the relationship or in other areas of life, another medical condition, or drug, alcohol, or medication use.

Risk Factors

Erectile problems may be more common in men with *depressive disorders, posttraumatic stress disorder,* and diabetes. Smoking, older age, heart disease, and lack of exercise each increase risk. Stress and anxiety also can play a part in erectile problems.

Treatment

Treatment of erectile disorder may involve medication, psychotherapy, and lifestyle changes. Men with erectile disorder may be prescribed medication that causes an erection by increasing blood flow to the penis: avanafil, sildenafil, vardenafil, or tadalafil. With therapy, couples are taught how to give sexual pleasure without having intercourse. Without the pressure to have an erection, a man often is soon able to have an erection and have intercourse. Lifestyle changes (see box at end of this chapter) also may help. In some cases, men may benefit from the use of penile implants or vacuum pumps.

Premature (Early) Ejaculation

Men with *premature (early) ejaculation* ejaculate before or within 1 minute after vaginal penetration and before the man wishes it. Those with the disorder often feel a sense of lack of control over ejaculation and concern about being able to delay ejaculation in future attempts.

Up to 30% of men around the world report a concern for ejaculating too quickly. Premature ejaculation may increase with age. The disorder affects about 1%–3% of men. The guideline of ejaculation in 1 minute or less may apply to men of all sexual orientations.

 Premature (Early) Ejaculation

The condition is diagnosed when:

- Ejaculation happens during sexual activity with a partner within about 1 minute after vaginal penetration or before the person wishes it.

- The problem has occurred for at least 6 months and happens during almost all sexual activity (75%–100% of the time).

The symptoms cause the man much distress. They are not due to a nonsexual mental disorder, stress in the relationship or in other areas of life, another medical condition, or drug, alcohol, or medication use.

Risk Factors

Factors that may increase risk for premature ejaculation include the following:

- **Temperament.** Premature ejaculation is more common in men with anxiety disorders, especially *social anxiety disorder*.
- **Genetics and biology.** Lifelong premature ejaculation may be inherited. Acquired premature ejaculation can occur with thyroid disease or drug withdrawal.

Treatment

Treatment of premature ejaculation may include medication or behavior therapy. An SSRI antidepressant (fluoxetine, paroxetine, or sertraline) is often prescribed because a common side effect is delayed ejaculation. Another option is a topical anesthetic cream that contains lidocaine. It lessens sensation to the penis and helps delay ejaculation.

In behavior therapy, the man's partner learns to stimulate his penis until he signals that ejaculation is near. The partner stops stimulation and then restarts once the man's level of arousal is lowered. Over time, the man gains greater control over ejaculation. Another popular method is the "squeeze technique," in which a man's partner is instructed to squeeze the end of the man's penis for several seconds when he feels the urge to ejaculate, until the urge passes. With practice, the man learns how to delay ejaculation.

Female Orgasmic Disorder

Women who have *female orgasmic disorder* have trouble reaching orgasm after sexual arousal and stimulation. Women with the disorder also may have problems with sexual interest or arousal. The disorder can be linked to physical causes, such as medications or surgery, or psychological stress, such as marital or family conflict.

About 8%–72% of women who have not reached menopause report problems with having an orgasm, varying across age, culture, and how long the problem has lasted. A women's first time having an orgasm can happen anytime from before puberty until well into adult years. About 10% of women around the world report that they have never experienced an orgasm.

Female Orgasmic Disorder

The condition is diagnosed when:

- One of the following symptoms happens almost all the time during sexual activity (75%–100% of the time):
    - Delayed, infrequent, or no orgasm.
    - Reduced orgasmic sensations.
- Symptoms have lasted for at least 6 months.

These symptoms cause the woman much distress. They are not due to a nonsexual mental disorder, severe stress in the relationship (such as partner violence), another medical condition, or drug, alcohol, or medication use.

Risk Factors

These factors can increase a woman's risk for female orgasmic disorder:

- **Temperament.** A wide range of factors, such as *anxiety* or concerns about getting pregnant, can disrupt a woman's ability to have orgasm.
- **Environment.** Problems with relationships, physical health, and mental health are strongly linked to orgasm problems in women. Cultural beliefs about strict gender roles and religious laws against sexual pleasure or activity also play a role.
- **Genetics and biology.** Medical conditions and medications can cause women's orgasm problems. Medical conditions include multiple sclerosis, pelvic nerve damage, and spinal cord injury. Medications such as the SSRIs can delay or prevent orgasm.

Treatment

Treating female orgasmic disorder may include training the woman to have an orgasm through masturbation. Other methods include *sensate focus* (a method of touching skin, being aware of what is pleasing, and not touching sex organs or genitals until later sessions), clitoral stimulation, and Kegel exercises (these involve tightening and relaxing the muscles around the vagina). Once women have orgasm through self-stimulation, they can teach their partners the most pleasurable ways to stimulate them. Therapy also involves teaching the couple exercises to improve intimacy and communication.

Other Sexual Dysfunctions

Symptoms for these other sexual dysfunctions also cause much distress and must last for at least 6 months for a diagnosis. They are not due to severe stress in the relationship (this includes partner violence) or drug or alcohol use. These other disorders are *delayed ejaculation, genito-pelvic pain/penetration disorder, female sexual interest/arousal disorder,* and *male hypoactive sexual desire disorder.* The mental health care provider should ensure that no medications, other mental disorders, or other medical conditions are causing the symptoms.

Delayed Ejaculation

Delayed ejaculation occurs when a man takes a long time to reach sexual climax and ejaculate during sex with his partner. Some men are unable to ejaculate at all, despite a desire to do so.

There is no exact definition of *delayed* and what is a reasonable time for a man to reach climax. Men and their partners may report prolonged thrusting to achieve orgasm, to the point of fatigue, pain, or injury, at which point they cease their effort. Some partners may report feeling less sexually attractive because their partner cannot easily ejaculate with them, but can do so if masturbating. Men older than age 50 are at increased risk because of changes with aging. About 1%–5% of men in the United States have the disorder.

The condition is diagnosed when a man experiences one of the following during almost every sexual encounter with his partner:

- Unwanted, long delay in ejaculation.
- No or rare ejaculation.

Treatment can include meditation, relaxation, and psychotherapy. Cognitive-behavior therapy may include asking the man to refrain for a time from all sexual acts leading to orgasm. Sexual exercises with a partner that involve masturbation or vibrators may be used.

Genito-Pelvic Pain/Penetration Disorder

Women with *genito-pelvic pain/penetration disorder* have pain with sexual intercourse or at other times of vaginal penetration, such as during a gynecology exam or when inserting a tampon. The intense pain is often described as "burning," "cutting," "shooting," or "throbbing."

Women who have this type of pain often become fearful of intercourse or penetration. They may begin to avoid sexual or intimate acts.

Risk factors include early puberty, vaginal infections, and prior sexual or physical abuse. Having a *bipolar, depressive,* or *anxiety disorder* before genito-pelvic pain symptoms occur can increase risk for the disorder. Although the number of women who have genito-pelvic pain/penetration disorder is unknown, about 10%–28% of U.S. women report ongoing pain during intercourse.

The disorder is diagnosed when a woman has frequent problems with at least one of the following:

- Vaginal penetration during intercourse.
- Vulvovaginal or pelvic pain during vaginal intercourse or other attempts at penetration.
- Fear of vulvovaginal or pelvic pain before, during, or after penetration.
- Tensing or tightening of the pelvic muscles during attempts at vaginal penetration.

Treatment options include cognitive-behavior therapy (group or one-on-one) and sex therapy (such as sex education, sensate focus, and Kegel exercises that strengthen the pelvic floor). Physical therapies to help dilate the vagina also may be helpful. Surgery to remove sensitive tissue causing painful intercourse has been used with success. Treatment should be tailored to the woman and involve health care providers across different fields (such as mental health and gynecology).

Female Sexual Interest/Arousal Disorder

Women with *female sexual interest/arousal disorder* have low or absent desire for sex for 6 months or more. Having a level of desire lower than a partner's is not enough for diagnosis. Rather, it is the woman's own distress about the problem that prompts the diagnosis. Short-term changes in arousal or interest because of life events are common and do not represent a dysfunction.

Women with the disorder may no longer get pleasure during sex. They often will describe themselves as feeling numb. Causes may include past physical and sexual abuse, fear of pregnancy, performance anxiety, body image problems, and marital discord. Diabetes and thyroid problems may increase risk. About 30% of women report chronic low desire for sex, and about 7% of women report both chronic low desire and their own distress about this.

The disorder is diagnosed when a woman has low or no interest in sexual activity as shown by at least three of the following:

- No or low interest in sexual activity.
- No or few sexual thoughts or fantasies.
- Stops or reduces initiating sexual activity and often is not open to a partner's attempts to start.
- No or low sexual excitement or pleasure during almost all sexual activity.
- No or low interest in sex in response to any sexual cues (such as written, verbal, visual).
- No or low genital or other body sensations during almost all sexual activity.

Treatment includes a number of options, which can be combined. These involve sex education, sensate focus exercises, and stopping intercourse for a time. Couples therapy may be helpful in building an emotional connection between the couple to address any discord. Cognitive-behavior therapy can help address any thoughts that are not helpful or true that the woman may have about herself and sex. It has been shown to increase women's sexual pleasure and satisfaction.

Male Hypoactive Sexual Desire Disorder

Male hypoactive sexual desire disorder occurs when a man has little or no interest in sexual fantasies or acts for 6 months or more. Having a level of desire lower than a partner's is not enough for diagnosis. How long the symptoms have lasted is key to the diagnosis, as well as the man's distress about his low desire.

Risk factors include mood and anxiety symptoms, alcohol use, and job stress. About 6% of men worldwide report low interest in sex lasting for 6 months or more, but less than 2% report distress about their low sexual desire.

Treatment includes psychotherapy or couples therapy based on the nature of the problem. If testosterone is below normal levels, testosterone replacement therapy with a daily patch or gel may be prescribed, with evaluation and education about side effects. Weight loss (if needed) and changing sexual activities to increase levels of desire also may help.

Key Points

- Sexual intimacy involves the whole person and can bring great joy. *Sexual dysfunctions* disrupt the ability to respond to sexual activity or to enjoy sex.
- These problems occur for many reasons, which can impact how the disorder is diagnosed and treated. Often, more than one factor causes a sexual dysfunction. These include health problems, medications, poor body image or low self-esteem, and relationship issues (such as lack of trust or communication).
- Treatment for sexual dysfunctions considers all the factors that can cause these problems and that are unique to each person and their partner. There may be medications that can be taken or changed, medical conditions to be treated, techniques to learn, and behaviors to help build trust and communication.
- Drugs, alcohol, and tobacco can impair sexual response. Alcohol is a depressant that can blunt response to sex. Smoking slows blood flow to the sexual organs, which decreases sexual arousal. Quitting or cutting back on these substances can improve sex.
- Others ways to improve sexual health include getting regular exercise (boosts stamina, mood, and self-esteem), coping with stress (so it won't distract from sex), and sharing feelings and preferences (to build closeness and learn what pleases the other).

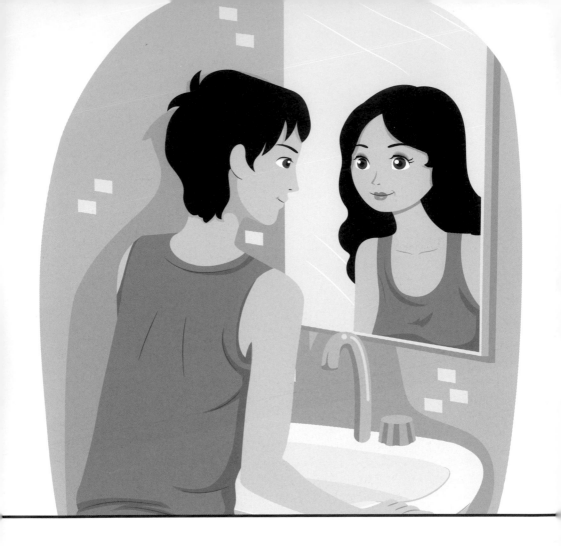

Gender Dysphoria in Children

Gender Dysphoria in Teens and Adults

For a complete list of DSM-5-TR disorders, see Appendix A.

CHAPTER 14

Gender Dysphoria

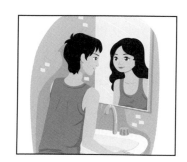

For some people, their gender is never something to question nor a source of conflict for their sense of identity. Other people strongly identify themselves as a member of a gender different from the sex they were assigned at birth, whether that be as a girl/woman, boy/man, *gender nonbinary* (that is, neither only girl/woman nor only boy/man, and may be between or beyond genders), or another identity. Some experience great distress that their gender features do not match the way they think and feel about themselves. This distress and sense of conflict is called *gender dysphoria.* The gender that fits with the way they feel is called their *experienced gender,* and the gender they were born with is called their *assigned gender.*

Gender dysphoria is a symptom or experience, as described above. It is also the key feature of the DSM-5-TR disorder *gender dysphoria.* Gender dysphoria is diagnosed when the person's assigned gender and experienced gender mismatch for at least 6 months and result in problems with social, school, or other key aspects of function in addition to their distress.

Gender dysphoria may start in childhood or later. It can sometimes start with the unwanted changes of puberty in the teen years. For some, gender dysphoria arises in adulthood. Dysphoria starting in childhood may end or worsen with the changes of puberty.

In children, the disorder is defined by the presence of firm statements that they are or desire to be the other sex. Their behavior reflects such statements. *Gender nonconforming behavior* (patterns of behavior that differ from those often expected with the assigned gender) tends to start between ages 2 and 4 years—the age that most children begin to develop gender-specific behaviors and interests.

- Young children assigned female at birth may say they wish to be a boy and prefer boys' clothing and hairstyles, boy playmates, and rough-and-tumble play and sports. Many such children are labeled "tomboys" at this age. Such behaviors are quite common and are often not gender dysphoria. To have a diagnosis of gender dysphoria, the child must have the firm thought that they are truly a boy and will become upset when told that they must behave as a girl.
- Young children assigned male at birth may wish to be a girl, prefer dressing in girls' clothing, and engage in playing house and playing with dolls. They often avoid rough play and sports. Some may pretend not to have a penis and insist on sitting down to urinate. These behaviors are fairly common in children assigned male at birth and do not always mean that the child has gender dysphoria.

As teens and adults, those with gender dysphoria experience distress based more on the conflict between their experienced gender and their assigned gender. Teens and adults with gender dysphoria may be more upset by their primary and secondary sex characteristics (see box) than are children with gender dysphoria.

- When puberty brings body changes, girls with gender dysphoria may wear baggy clothing or bind their breasts to hide them. Boys may shave their body hair at the first sign of hair growth. Such behaviors relieve their distress, which lessens when their looks match the way they feel about themselves.
- Adults with gender dysphoria may want to get rid of the physical features of their sex assigned at birth and adopt the behavior, clothing, and manners of the other sex. They may try to reduce their symptoms of dysphoria by living in the role of their experienced gender as much as possible in their work, looks, and social lives.

If social support is lacking, emotional and behavioral problems may arise in children with gender dysphoria—such as depression, anxiety, and disruptive or impulsive behavior. As children become teens, teasing or conflicts with their peers may increase and lead to more problems. Teens and adults are at increased risk to have *anxiety* and *depressive disorders*, as well as suicidal thoughts or behavior.

Sex Features: Growth Brings Changes

People with gender dysphoria may be distressed by one or both types of sex features as they grow from children to adults:

- **Primary sex features** are organs for reproduction present at birth (such as a uterus or penis).
- **Secondary sex features** appear in puberty (such as body hair or breasts).

 ## Gender Dysphoria

Gender dysphoria is diagnosed as a disorder when the following symptoms have occurred for at least 6 months.

Gender Dysphoria in Children

- A clear mismatch between one's expressed gender and assigned gender as shown by the first trait on the list and at least five more of the following:

    - Strong desire to be, or insistence that one is, the other gender.

    - In boys, a strong preference for cross-dressing in women's clothing. In girls, a strong preference for wearing only masculine clothing and strong resistance to wearing anything that is feminine.

    - Strong preference for cross-gender roles in make-believe or fantasy play.

    - Strong preference for toys, games, or activities that are often used or done by the other gender.

    - Strong preference for playmates of the other gender.

    - In boys, a strong rejection of masculine toys or games and avoidance of rough-and-tumble play. In girls, a strong rejection of feminine toys, games, or activities.

    - Strong dislike of one's sexual anatomy.

    - Strong desire for the primary sex features (sex organs) and/or secondary sex features (breasts, facial hair) to match one's experienced gender.

Gender Dysphoria

- The condition causes much distress and impairs social, school, or other key aspects of function.

Gender Dysphoria in Teens and Adults

- A clear mismatch between one's expressed gender and assigned gender as shown by at least two of the following:
  - A clear mismatch between one's expressed gender and primary or secondary sex features.
  - Strong desire to be rid of one's primary and/or secondary sex features because of a strong disagreement with one's expressed gender.
  - Strong desire for the primary and/or secondary sex features of the other gender.
  - Strong desire to be the other gender.
  - Strong desire to be treated as the other gender.
  - Strong conviction that one has the typical feelings and reactions of the other gender.
- The condition causes much distress and impairs social, work, or other key aspects of function.

Risk Factors

The following factors have been linked with gender dysphoria:

- **Temperament.** At early preschool age, those who often behave out of character in their culture from the gender they were assigned at birth may be more likely to develop gender dysphoria.
- **Environment.** Those with gender dysphoria who were assigned male at birth are more likely to have older brothers.

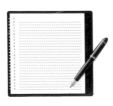

Christine's Story

Christine is a 25-year-old salesperson. She was assigned male at birth and raised as a boy. As long as she could remember, she had been teased and called a "sissy" by neighborhood boys. She had generally preferred the company of girls throughout childhood. During her teen years, she had many female friends but thought of herself then as a gay male and dated a few other gay teens. She recalled trying her best to "fit in" but noted that she had always felt like an outsider.

Understanding Mental Disorders

At age 19, during a romantic relationship with a man, she become aware of an intense desire to be a woman. That relationship ended, but Christine's desire to be a woman evolved into a strong sense that she had been born as the wrong gender. She tried to figure out whether this sense had existed earlier, but all she could recall was sometimes wishing she were a girl to fit in more comfortably with her friends.

By age 20, Christine was very unhappy about being seen as a man. She viewed her genitals as "disgusting" and a "mistake of nature." Her family and some of her friends had not supported her growing sense about herself, and she recalled feeling increasingly hopeless. She sometimes had suicidal thoughts and had attempted suicide once by overdose at age 21.

Beginning at age 22, Christine lived as a female, including changing her name and wearing only women's clothes. She struggled to access appropriate health services and faced multiple barriers to obtaining appropriate treatments—but at the age of 24, Christine was evaluated by two psychiatrists skilled in transgender health. They agreed with her perspective, and she started gender-affirming hormone therapy.

As her transition progressed, she began to feel more comfortable in the female role and pleased with having secondary sexual characteristics that were more consistent with her experienced gender. She explored her sexuality during this time, dating both gay and straight men. Her anxiety lessened. However, being transgender, she felt vulnerable to many types of aggression, including potential partner violence.

The following year, at age 25, Christine had the gender on her driver's license and passport changed from male to female and had gender-affirming surgeries. These included vaginoplasty (creation of a vagina) and breast augmentation. She was pleased with the results of the surgeries, and reported feeling as "more comfortable in her skin" than she had ever been. Despite not feeling accepted by her family of origin or by some of her old friends, she found warm support from other friends and colleagues at work. Although she has many friends who are gender nonbinary/gender nonconforming, Christine identifies as a heterosexual female.

Treatment

Some people can feel happy with their lives and manage their gender dysphoria by living in their experienced gender without having gender-affirming surgeries or hormones. Other people may dress and live at times as their experienced gender but not feel any distress about a mismatch between their body and identity. Neither of these people have gender dysphoria. One clue that treatment is needed is the presence of great distress and frequent unhappiness.

Psychotherapy can help those with gender dysphoria by offering support and helping the person consider treatment options. It can benefit those who do not choose gender-affirming surgery or hormones to cope with any issues gender dysphoria may cause. In addition to mental health care, gender-affirming treatments may involve hormones and surgery to better match physical characteristics with experienced gender, also called *medical transition.*

Gender dysphoria requires care not only for the person who experiences it, but also for the rest of the family to adjust and try to understand how the person is feeling. Family and friends may have a hard time accepting what is happening and what it means to experience gender dysphoria. Family education can lessen the person's distress and the risk for other mental disorders that may result from gender dysphoria, such as *anxiety* and *depressive disorders.*

Many children go through phases of behavior as they are learning who they are. They may at times show gender nonconforming behavior without identifying as or wanting to be a gender different from that assigned at birth. Often it is helpful simply to give support and encourage them to choose activities, toys, and clothes that they enjoy the most. If there are signs of ongoing distress or problems at school because of these gender diverse behaviors, such as refusing to use the restroom for their assigned gender, then it is helpful to seek out a mental health care professional who is experienced in assessing and treating gender concerns.

Children may do best if they can live in environments and build relationships that do not exclude or shame their gender nonconformity. This includes being able to pursue activities, interests, and relationships that come naturally to them.

The physical changes of puberty may trigger the first expressions of gender dysphoria or worsen prior symptoms of gender dysphoria. In either case, the distress may respond to hormone treatment to stop for a time the upsetting advance of puberty. Next, after a period of psychotherapy to explore the person's gender dysphoria and treatment options, different sex hormones that promote the individual's experienced gender may be started.

For a male transition to female, hormones are often prescribed for a time before any gender-affirming surgery. Different types of hormones reduce growth of beard and body hair and cause breast development and other bodily changes to create a more feminine appearance. Once the breasts have developed as much as possible with hormone treatment, the person may consider surgical breast enlargement. Permanent procedures for the genitals, as well as facial surgeries, may follow if desired.

For a female transition to male, hormones may be given to increase muscle mass and deepen the voice. Some persons may choose to have

surgery to remove breast tissue, uterus, and ovaries, and construct a male chest. Surgeries are now available to construct male external genitals.

For someone with nonbinary experienced gender and wishes, medical treatments that enhance female or male features may desired.

Key Points

- People with the diagnosis of *gender dysphoria* strongly identify as a member of a gender other than their gender assigned at birth. They have great distress that their sex assigned at birth does not match the way they think and feel about themselves.
- Gender dysphoria may start in childhood or may start later in the teen or adult years. Children may at times show gender nonconforming behavior without identifying as or wanting to be a gender different from that assigned at birth. One clue that treatment is needed is the presence of great distress and frequent unhappiness about their gender.
- Psychotherapy can help those who have gender dysphoria. It can offer support and assist those who are thinking about treatment options. Treatment for gender dysphoria includes therapy for the family to adjust and know how the person is feeling. Family education may also reduce the risk of other mental disorders that may result from gender dysphoria, such as *anxiety* and *depressive disorders*.
- Some people with gender dysphoria in the adolescent and adult years will choose to have gender affirming hormones and surgery.
- Whether or not gender affirming hormones and surgery are chosen, people can change their appearance and begin living fully in the role of a different gender. Some people can feel happy with their lives and manage the gender dysphoria by living in their experienced gender without having gender affirming surgeries or hormone treatments.

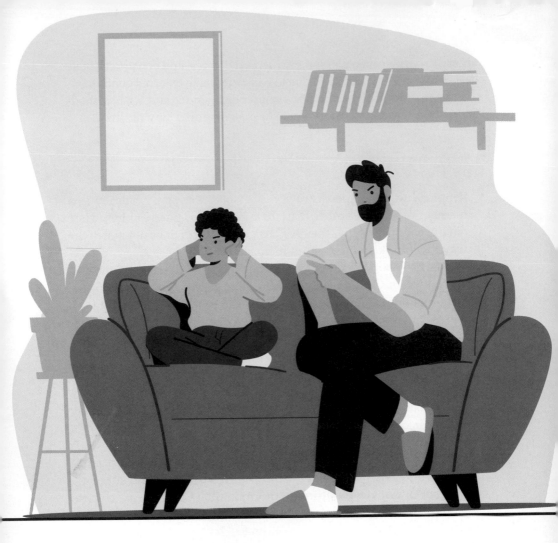

Oppositional Defiant Disorder
Intermittent Explosive Disorder
Conduct Disorder
Other Disruptive and Conduct Disorders
　　　Pyromania
　　　Kleptomania

For a complete list of DSM-5-TR disorders, see Appendix A.

CHAPTER 15

Disruptive and Conduct Disorders

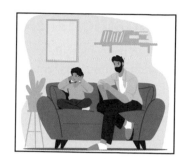

All children and teens sometimes misbehave. Stress may cause them to act out, such as when there is the birth of a sibling, a divorce, or a death in the family. *Disruptive and conduct disorders* are more severe problems that last a longer time than normal acting out. People with these disorders have a hard time controlling their angry feelings and may display hostile behaviors. These disorders can cause them to be aggressive toward other people or property, to break rules and laws, and to disobey or rebel against authority figures.

The disorders discussed in this chapter are *oppositional defiant disorder, intermittent explosive disorder, conduct disorder, pyromania,* and *kleptomania.* All these disorders tend to begin in childhood or teenage years, and many are more common in boys than girls. Conduct disorder, for instance, is one of the most frequent mental disorders seen in teenage boys.

These conditions are often called *externalizing disorders* because the behaviors get attention and are "out there" for all to see. Distress is expressed by acting it out through angry behaviors that impact others. In contrast, people with *internalizing disorders*—such as *depressive* and *anxiety disorders*—keep distress inward and self-directed. These disorders are less likely to cause conflict with others.

Many factors can increase the risk for these disorders. These include harsh or inconsistent parenting, being neglected by parents, frequent changes in caregivers, physical or sexual abuse, lack of supervision, and having a parent involved with crime or an addiction to drugs or alcohol. These disorders can occur with other mental disorders, such as a *depressive, bipolar,* or *substance use disorder,* or *attention-deficit/hyperactivity disorder* (ADHD).

Oppositional Defiant Disorder

Children or teens with *oppositional defiant disorder* display difficult behaviors such as tantrums, arguing, and angry or disruptive acts. They may often argue with their parents, refuse to comply with adult requests or rules (such as cleaning their rooms or meeting curfews), and be angry and resentful toward others. These behaviors go beyond normal misbehavior when they last for at least 6 months and disrupt home or school life.

For the diagnosis, these behaviors must be seen during contact with others who are not siblings. Symptoms often are displayed with adults or peers whom the child or teen knows well. The behaviors may not be shown during a visit with a doctor or a mental health care provider.

Symptoms of oppositional defiant disorder often reflect a pattern of problems in relating with others. People with this disorder tend not to see themselves as angry, oppositional (combative), or defiant. Instead, they often justify their behavior as a response to unfair demands or events. The first symptoms tend to appear during the preschool years and rarely later than the early teens.

Parent management training has proved useful for oppositional defiant disorder and also may help improve *conduct disorder* symptoms, discussed later in the chapter. This method equips parents with behavior management techniques to improve how they respond when their child disobeys and obeys. It can help build the parent-child relationship and teaches ways to give clear instructions and results for behavior. Practice at home is key.

 Oppositional Defiant Disorder

The disorder is diagnosed when the following occurs:

- There is a pattern of angry or irritable moods, arguing or defiant behavior, or spite or revenge lasting at least 6 months as shown by at least four symptoms from any of the following types. The behavior is shown during contact with at least one person who is not a sibling:

Angry or Irritable Mood

- Often loses temper.
- Often touchy or easily annoyed.
- Often angry and resentful.

Arguing or Defiant Behavior

- Often argues with authority figures (or in children and teens, with adults).
- Often defies or refuses to follow the rules or requests from authority figures.
- Often annoys others on purpose.
- Often blames others for their own mistakes or misbehavior.

Spite or Revenge

- Has been spiteful or sought revenge at least twice within the past 6 months.

The behavior causes distress for the person or others in close daily life (such as family, peers, coworkers), or has a negative impact on the person's social, school, work, or other key aspects of function. The behaviors are not due to any *psychotic, substance use, depressive,* or *bipolar disorder.*

Intermittent Explosive Disorder

People with *intermittent explosive disorder* respond with quick, angry, forceful outbursts that are out of proportion to the situation. For instance, an outburst could occur in response to a mild criticism from a loved one or friend. The outbursts often last for less than 30 minutes and can be in the form of temper tantrums, arguments, fights, or assault.

These symptoms can persist for many years. At risk are people with a history of physical and emotional trauma during the first 20 years of life. The disorder is more common in people younger than age 35–40 years than in those older than age 50. It is more common in those with a high school education or less.

Cognitive-behavior therapy is a helpful treatment for intermittent explosive disorder. It involves training in relaxation and coping skills, as well as changing thought patterns tied to anger and aggression.

Some medications also have been found to be helpful. These include the selective serotonin reuptake inhibitor (SSRI) antidepressants and mood stabilizers. (See Chapter 20, "Treatment Essentials," for more information on these medications.)

Intermittent Explosive Disorder

The disorder is diagnosed when the following occurs:

- Frequent outbursts show a failure to control aggressive (angry, hostile, forceful) impulses as shown by either of the following:
  - Verbal aggression (such as temper tantrums, rants, arguments) or physical aggression toward property, animals, or other people. Either occurs about twice a week for 3 months. The physical aggression does not damage property or injure others.
  - Three outbursts that involve property damage, physical assault, or both. The physical assault causes physical harm to animals or other people. These acts have occurred within 1 year.
- The force of the outbursts is beyond the extent of what might have provoked the person or any stress the person has.
- The frequent aggressive outbursts are impulsive (not planned) and are not done to achieve a certain goal, such as money, power, or fear.
- The frequent aggressive outbursts cause much distress for the person, disrupt work function or relationships, or have legal or financial costs (such as arrests and fines).
- The person is at least 6 years old.

The frequent aggressive outbursts are not due to a medical condition or drug, alcohol, or medication use. Other mental disorders in which assault or aggressive behaviors are symptoms need to be ruled out. These include *bipolar disorder, psychotic disorders,* and *antisocial* or *borderline personality disorder.* A sudden behavior change along with such outbursts in someone who seems healthy may suggest a brain disorder or head trauma, which also needs to be ruled out.

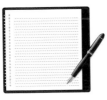 ## Sam's Story

Sam, a 32-year-old landscape architect, sought help from a mental health care provider to gain better control of his anger. His wife, who came with him to the appointment, said that Sam always had a temper. However, now he was angry so often that she worried that he would become violent with her or their two young children.

Their most recent quarrel began when Sam came home after a "hard day at work" to find that dinner was not on the table. When he entered the kitchen and saw his wife reading the paper, he exploded and launched into a rant about how "bad" a wife she was. When his wife tried to explain her own long day, Sam cursed at her and broke glasses and a kitchen chair. Frightened, Sam's wife ran out of the kitchen, gathered up their toddlers, and left for her mother's house a few miles away. The next day, she told Sam that he would need to get help right away or prepare for a divorce. She had reached the limit of what she could take.

Sam said his "blow-ups" began in childhood but did not become a problem for him until age 13. At about that time, he started having frequent fights with classmates that would at times result in visits to the principal's office. In between fights, he was a social and solid student.

Sam guessed that he had about four verbal outbursts a week in recent years, often in response to frustration, unexpected demands, or perceived insults. He also described violent acts about every 2 months. For instance, he threw a computer across the room when it started "acting up," he kicked a hole in a wall when one of his children would not stop crying, and he destroyed his mobile phone during an argument with his mother. He denied physical fights since his teens, although he came close to hitting a neighbor, a number of strangers, and the employees at his landscaping firm. His company had high turnover because of his quick temper. The idea that he might physically hurt someone scared Sam "to the core."

Sam described his angry episodes as short, reaching a peak within seconds, and rarely lasting more than a few minutes. Between episodes, he described feeling "fine." He was worried about his behavior and was sorry about his outbursts and actions toward his wife. Sam drank socially, but neither he nor his wife linked his outbursts to the alcohol.

Sam noted at least two other close family members with major "anger issues." His father was emotionally abusive and demanding, and his older sister had problems with her temper. Sam said her three divorces were caused by her emotionally abusive behavior.

Sam was diagnosed with *intermittent explosive disorder*. Treatment for Sam is a crucial issue not only for his marriage but also to stop the cycle of violence for his children.

Conduct Disorder

Conduct disorder describes a pattern of frequent behavior in children or teens that disregards the rights of others or involves breaking of rules or laws at home, school, and work. This can include using weapons, bullying, breaking into people's homes, and physical cruelty to people or animals. People with conduct disorders infringe on the rights of others. They may wrongly think others have a hostile intent against them and feel they are acting justly in response to perceived threats. They are likely to deny their behavior or downplay the degree of harm they caused.

Problems can start as early as the preschool years, but the first serious signs often appear during middle childhood through middle teenage years. For boys, the common signs are fighting, stealing, vandalism, and school discipline problems. Girls more often lie, skip school, or run away, and may become sexually active earlier than their peers. The disorder rarely begins after age 16.

If the conduct problems start no later than age 15 and last into age 18 (and beyond), the problems are then diagnosed as *antisocial personality disorder*. The symptoms of antisocial personality disorder include deceit, hurting or mistreating others without any regret, and disregard for the rights of others (see Chapter 18, "Personality Disorders," for more detail). Conduct disorder is seen as the childhood warning sign for antisocial personality disorder—but it is important to know that a young person with conduct disorder does not always go on to have antisocial personality disorder. Early diagnosis and treatment are key to helping learn healthy ways of thinking and acting and how to control angry feelings.

Helpful treatments for conduct disorders include parent management training (as described for *oppositional defiant disorder*) and functional family therapy (FFT). Either option lasts for about 12 weeks. FFT tackles unhealthy family beliefs about the problem, builds relationships and positive parenting skills, and helps plan use of community resources to prevent relapse.

Conduct Disorder

Conduct disorder is diagnosed when the following occurs:

- A frequent and steady pattern of behavior that infringes on the basic rights of others or breaks social rules or laws, as shown by at least 3 of the 15 behaviors below in the past 12 months, with at least 1 behavior in the past 6 months:

Aggression Toward People and Animals

- Often bullies, threatens, or intimidates others.
- Often starts physical fights.
- Has used a weapon that could cause serious physical harm to others, such as a bat, knife, brick, or gun.
- Has been physically cruel to people.
- Has been physically cruel to animals.
- Confronts and steals from a victim, such as mugging, purse snatching, armed robbery.
- Has forced someone into a sexual act.

Destruction of Property

- Has set fires with the intent of causing great damage.
- Has destroyed other people's property on purpose.

Deceit or Theft

- Has broken into someone's house, building, or car.
- Often lies to obtain goods or favors, or to avoid duties (cons others).
- Has stolen items without confronting a victim (such as shoplifting, but without breaking and entering).

Serious Violations of Rules

- Often stays out at night despite parental rules against this.
- Has run away overnight at least twice from a parent's home, or once without coming back for a lengthy time.
- Often skips school, starting before age 13.

The behavior greatly impairs social, school, or work function. For the diagnosis to apply to someone age 18 years or older, the person must *not* meet the guidelines and standards for *antisocial personality disorder.* Some people with conduct disorder may show a lack of remorse or guilt for their actions, lack of concern for others' feelings, or lack of concern about their school or work duties and function. The disorder can be mild, moderate, or severe, based on the number of symptoms and degree of harm caused.

Thomas's Story

Thomas was a 12-year-old boy who angrily agreed to see a mental health care provider after getting arrested for breaking into a grocery store. His mother said she was "worn out," adding that it was hard to raise a boy who "doesn't follow the rules."

As a young child, Thomas was often aggressive, bullying other children, and taking their things. When confronted about his actions by his mother, stepfather, or a teacher, he would curse, punch, and show no concern for getting punished.

Thomas, his mother, and his teachers agreed that he was a loner and not well liked by his peers. There was no history of sexual or physical abuse.

The year before his arrest, Thomas had been caught stealing from school lockers (a cell phone, a jacket, a laptop computer). He also stole a classmate's wallet and was suspended after many physical fights with classmates. Thomas had no regret for his acts, blamed others for his stealing and fights, and did not care about others' feelings. When his parents or teachers scolded him about his behavior, he would say, "What are you going to do, shoot me?" Because of this pattern of behavior, Thomas was diagnosed with *conduct disorder.*

Treatment

Getting early treatment for any of these disorders will more quickly lessen distress and the impact of problems in the child's or teen's life. The sooner treatment begins, the better the chances of improved symptoms and behavior. Treatment can be a challenge, however. Children and teens may resist therapy, not cooperate, and display fear and distrust of adults. Learning new attitudes and behavior patterns takes time and patience for all involved.

Behavior therapy and psychotherapy—either one-on-one or in a group or family setting—can help children and teens express and control their anger. Therapy is aimed at helping young people be aware of their behavior and its effect on others. Parent training teaches skills to learn how best to support good behavior and relate with the child or teen (see box "Tips for Parents"). For children and teens who also have ADHD or a *depressive* or *bipolar disorder,* medications for these disorders may reduce the disruptive behaviors by bringing relief to some of the feelings that worsen them.

Other Disruptive and Conduct Disorders

These disorders are marked by poor impulse control for certain behaviors that relieve inner tension. They include *pyromania* (fire setting) and *kleptomania* (stealing objects). These disorders are not due to *conduct disorder,* a manic episode (as in *bipolar I disorder*), a hallucination or delusion (as in a *psychotic disorder*), or *antisocial personality disorder.* Those who have pyromania or kleptomania may also have a *substance use, depressive,* or *bipolar disorder.*

Pyromania

Pyromania is the repeated setting of fires on purpose for pleasure or satisfaction. People with the disorder often have an unusual interest in or fascination with fire. They may set off false alarms, spend time at the local fire department, and often watch fires in their neighborhoods. Fire-setting behavior is more common in teenage boys, often in those with poor social skills and learning problems. Although the age that pyromania begins is unknown, more than 40% of those arrested for arson in the United States are younger than age 18. Those who are 18 and younger with the disorder may also have *conduct disorder, ADHD,* or *adjustment disorder.*

Pyromania is diagnosed when the person displays the following:

- Fires are set on purpose more than once.
- Tension or excitement before the act.
- Fascination with, curiosity about, or attraction to fire.
- Pleasure, gratification, or relief when setting fires or watching their aftermath.

The fire setting is not done for financial gain, to express social or political views, to conceal a crime, to improve the person's living condition, or as a result of impaired judgment, a *delusion*, or *hallucination*.

Cognitive-behavior therapy that includes conflict- and problem-solving skills, as well as parent education, is useful in stopping the behavior and its causes. Fire-safety education and guided visits to burn units also have been shown to be helpful.

Kleptomania

People with *kleptomania* do not resist their urge to steal objects that are not needed for personal use or for their monetary value. They know the act is wrong and senseless, but are not able to control the impulse. They often are afraid of getting caught stealing and may feel depressed or guilty about the thefts. Women are three times more likely to have kleptomania than men, and the disorder often begins in teenage years.

Kleptomania is diagnosed when the following occur:

- Frequent failure to resist the impulse to steal objects that are not needed for personal use or that have little value.
- Increased tension right before stealing.
- Pleasure, gratification, or relief while stealing.

Treatment for kleptomania may include the medication naltrexone, which can reduce the impulse and pleasure of stealing. Psychotherapies include *exposure and response prevention therapy* (which includes the practice of thinking of stealing but not doing it), *covert sensitization* (which involves thinking of stealing and picturing a strong negative result, such as vomiting), and *cognitive-behavior therapy* (which involves changing thoughts that stealing will relieve distress). Sometimes medication is prescribed, especially if the person also has *major depressive disorder* or an *anxiety disorder*.

Key Points

- *Disruptive and conduct disorders* cross the line from normal misbehavior that occurs from time to time in children or teens or that is due to stressful life events. These are more severe problems in which people often do not control their angry feelings and display hostile behaviors. They may also act on impulse in ways that damage property or inflict financial cost on others.
- All these disorders tend to begin in childhood or teenage years, and many are more common in boys. Some of these disorders last into adult years or are first diagnosed then. These disorders may reflect distress that is expressed by acting it out through angry behaviors that impact others.
- Many factors can increase the risk for these disorders. These include harsh or inconsistent parenting, neglect, frequent changes in caregivers, physical or sexual abuse, lack of supervision, having a parent involved with crime or an addiction to drugs or alcohol, and other mental disorders, such as a *depressive* or *bipolar disorder*, or *attention-deficit/hyperactivity disorder* (ADHD).
- Getting early treatment for these disorders will more quickly lessen distress and the impact of the problems in the child's or teen's life. The sooner treatment begins, the better the chances of improved symptoms.

- Behavior therapy and psychotherapy—either one-on-one or in a group—can help children and teens express and control their anger. Therapy is aimed at helping young people realize and understand the effect their behavior has on others. Parent training teaches skills to learn how best to support good behavior and relate with the child or teen. For children and teens who also have depression or ADHD, medications for these disorders may reduce the disruptive behaviors by bringing relief to some of the feelings that worsen them.

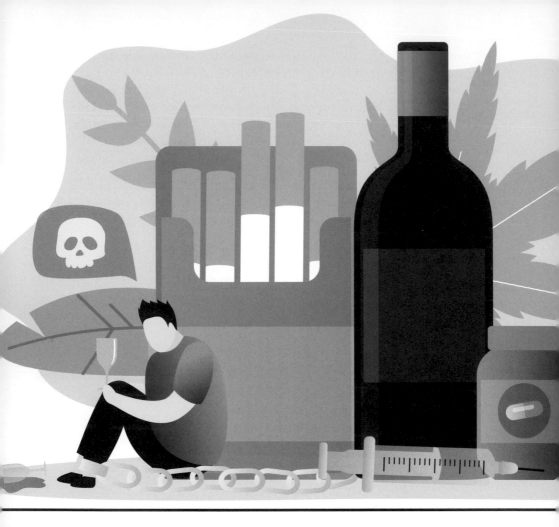

Substance Use Disorder

Substance Intoxication

Substance Withdrawal

Substance/Medication-Induced Mental Disorder

Gambling Disorder

For a complete list of DSM-5-TR disorders, see Appendix A.

CHAPTER 16

Addictive Disorders

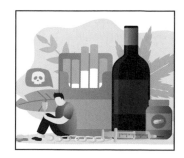

Drinking, other drug use, and gambling are often woven into the culture as social or fun pursuits. Alcohol, drugs, and gambling seem to quickly affect a portion of the brain called the *reward system*. This leads to intense pleasure (or a "high") and a craving to repeat what led to those feelings. A craving for the substance or behavior can send a message to both the brain and body that they must have the substance or these feelings of pleasure. What seemed harmless at first may become harmful. People with an *addictive disorder* have an intense focus on using a certain substance (such as alcohol or drugs) or taking part in a certain activity (such as gambling) to the point that it takes over their life.

Those with addictive disorders spend a great deal of time and effort trying to obtain the substance to use or the money to gamble. This begins to outweigh the value of other people and duties in their lives. The addictive disorder may cause them to have problems with fulfilling their roles at work, school, and home (such as finishing assignments and caring for children). Those with the most serious addictive disorders sometimes break the law to satisfy their craving or urges. Some addictive drugs are illegal or obtained through illegal channels. People with the addictive disorder may be aware of the problems caused by their substance use or gambling but cannot stop on their own, even when they want to. The addictive disorder causes concern and distress for those in their lives.

Table 1. Ten classes of substances	
Substance class	Examples
Alcohol	Beer, wine
Caffeine	Coffee, cola, energy drinks
Cannabis (marijuana)	Joints, blunts, bongs, vaping products, edibles (foods or drinks)
Hallucinogens	Phencyclidine (PCP), LSD (acid), salvia
Inhalants (breathed in through the nose or mouth)	Paint thinners, glue, aerosol spray
Opioids	Heroin, painkillers such as codeine and oxycodone
Sedatives, hypnotics ("sleeping pills"), and anxiolytics (medicines for anxiety, such as tranquilizers)	Barbiturates (such as Nembutal), benzodiazepines (such as Valium and Xanax), benzodiazepine hypnotics (such as Rohypnol or "roofies")
Stimulants	Cocaine, amphetamines ("uppers" such as methamphetamine or "meth")
Tobacco (nicotine)	Cigarettes, vaping products
Other (or unknown)	Prescription medicines, over-the-counter medicines

The addictive disorders included in this chapter are those caused by misuse of substances. These are ordered across 10 different substance classes as shown in Table 1. Addictive disorders include *substance use disorder, substance intoxication, substance withdrawal*, and *substance/medication-induced mental disorders. Gambling disorder* is included in DSM-5-TR as an addictive disorder (rather than as an impulse-control disorder).

The good news is that people can recover from an addictive disorder. The first step on the road to recovery is to know there is a problem. Often this process is hindered by denial of the problem or a lack of knowledge about substance misuse and addictive behavior. In these cases, an intervention with concerned friends and family can prompt treatment.

An *intervention* is a careful, structured, planned meeting with the person with an addictive disorder and their family, friends, and others concerned. Seeking advice and support from a mental health care provider before and after the meeting is crucial. The mental health care professional can also lead or direct the intervention. These people gather to talk with the person about the addictive behavior, express their concern, give examples of the behavior and the problems that result, and outline a clear treatment plan. One person leads the planning and guides the meeting. (See Appendix C, "Helpful Resources" for support groups that may be of help.)

When Someone You Care About Has a Drinking, Drug, or Gambling Problem

People with an addictive disorder are swept up in their behavior and cannot see as clearly as those who do not have the problem. They need people who care about them to get involved in healthy ways and be honest with them. Here are some key ways to engage with the person:

- Preaching, blaming, and scolding won't help.
- Don't try to address the problem when the person is high, intoxicated, or engaged in gambling.
- Don't join in the activity or setting where the addictive behavior occurs.
- Give feedback that is direct and focused on a certain behavior (such as, "You promised you would be there for our son's baseball game. When you didn't show up, I was worried—then upset when I learned you were at the bar drinking all night. Our son was sad you weren't there.").
- Learn as much as you can about the problem and its effects. Find resources for recovery and support in your area (see Appendix C, "Helpful Resources" for support groups). Seek help from a mental health care provider.
- Addictive behaviors cause painful problems with home, school, work, relationships, and finances—as well as brain and body effects. Pain causes those with these behaviors to seek help. If you remove a painful result of their addictive behavior, you remove a main reason for seeking change. Do not cover up the problem, give them money, make excuses for them, shield them from the results of their behavior, feel responsible for their addictive behavior, or feel guilty for their behavior.
- Don't give up on showing care, concern, and emotional support. People with addictive disorders need help to get better. Recovery is often a process without a quick fix.
- Realize that you cannot force people with addictive disorders to stop. You can urge them to get help. Support them when they choose to get help and during the process of change.
- If the addictive behavior impacts children, take steps to ensure that children are safe from harm and neglect.
- Seek help for yourself. Protect your finances, emotions, and health. Don't try to manage the problem of someone else's addictive disorder on your own. Being alone can increase fear and loss of hope.

Source. Adapted from Missouri Department of Mental Health; National Council on Alcoholism and Drug Dependence.

Substance Use Disorder

People can develop a *substance use disorder* with any of the drugs listed in Table 1 earlier in this chapter, except caffeine. Substance use disorder with caffeine is not a current diagnosis and is being studied. (People can have *caffeine intoxication* or *caffeine withdrawal*, as shown in Table 2 later in this chapter.) People with a substance use disorder have a mix of disturbed thinking, behavior, and body functions, and they keep using the substance when they know that problems will result.

The substances listed in Table 1 can cause harmful changes in how the brain functions. These changes can last well after the intoxication is over. *Intoxication* is recent use of the drug that can cause intense pleasure, calm, and increased senses—or a high, as well as problems with function and behavior. (Intoxication symptoms differ for each drug and are described in the "Substance Intoxication and Withdrawal" section of this chapter.)

Changes to the brain and body are more severe in those with heavy or frequent drug use. The changes in the brain's wiring are what cause people to have intense cravings for the drug and make it hard to stop using the drug. The craving may be so strong that the person cannot think of anything else. Craving can be strongest in settings where the drug has been used before. Increased craving can be a warning sign for a relapse after recovery.

People with substance use disorders may spend a lot of time trying to obtain the substance, use the substance, or recover from its effects. In severe substance use disorders, the person's entire life may revolve around the substance.

Over time, people with substance use disorder can develop a *tolerance* for the substance. When this happens, they need a larger amount to feel high. Tolerance differs from person to person. It depends a great deal on the type of substance and a person's gender and weight.

Each drug shares the same checklist of symptoms for substance use disorder. The symptoms are grouped by the effects of substance use: impaired control, social problems, risky use, and drug effects. People have a substance use disorder when the problem lasts at least 1 year. The degree of how severe the problem is depends on how many symptoms they have.

Substance Use Disorder

A problem of substance use leading to great impairment or distress, as shown by at least two of the following within 1 year:

Impaired Control

- The substance is often taken in larger amounts or over a longer period than was planned.
- There is a constant desire or failed attempts to cut down or control substance use.
- A great deal of time is spent trying to get the substance, use the substance, or recover from its effects.
- There is a craving, or a strong urge, to use the substance.

Social Problems

- Regular substance use causes failure to complete major tasks at work, school, or home.
- Continued substance use despite having constant or regular social or personal problems caused or made worse by the effects of the substance.
- Important social, work, or leisure activities are given up or cut back because of the substance use.

Risky Use

- The substance is often used in settings where it is unsafe.
- The substance keeps being used despite the known problems caused or made worse by the substance. These problems can be physical (linked to the body) or psychological (how someone thinks and feels), or both.

Drug Effects

- Tolerance as defined by either of the following:
  - A need for larger amounts of the substance to get intoxicated or high.
  - The same amount of the substance gives fewer effects.
- Withdrawal, as evident by either of the following:
  - Symptoms of withdrawal (symptoms differ for each substance; see Table 2 later in this chapter). These symptoms occur when the amounts of the substance in the body decline with stopping or less use.
  - The substance is taken to avoid or relieve withdrawal symptoms.

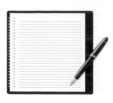

Keith's Story

Keith, a 45-year-old plumber, was referred for a psychiatric evaluation after his family met with him to express their concern about his heavy drinking. Since making the appointment 3 days earlier, Keith denied having a drink.

For 20 years after high school, Keith drank 3–5 beers per evening, five times per week. Over the last 7 years, Keith drank almost daily, with an average of 6 beers on weeknights and 12 beers on weekends and holidays. His wife repeatedly voiced her concern that he was "drinking too much." Despite his efforts to limit his alcohol intake, Keith spent much of the weekend drinking, sometimes missing family get-togethers, and often passed out while watching TV in the evening. He remained productive at work and never called in sick. Keith was able to stop drinking twice for 1 month in the past 4 years. Both times, he said he had gone "cold turkey" in response to his wife's concerns. He denied having had symptoms of alcohol withdrawal either time.

Keith had been married for 18 years and had one 17-year-old daughter. He was a high school graduate with 2 years of community college. He owned a successful plumbing company and had never seen a psychiatrist.

Keith was diagnosed with *alcohol use disorder.* His lack of success in cutting down, overall time spent intoxicated or recovering from being intoxicated, missed family events, and frequent alcohol use despite problems all fit the criteria for the disorder.

Stan's Story

Stan, a married 46-year-old pastor, was referred to the psychiatry outpatient department by his primary care doctor for depressive symptoms and misuse of opioids (painkillers) for his chronic right knee pain.

Stan injured his right knee playing basketball 17 months earlier. His mother gave him several tablets of hydrocodone-acetaminophen that she had for back pain, and he found this helpful. When he ran out of the pills and his pain continued, he went to the emergency room. He was told he had a mild sprain. He was given a 1-month supply of hydrocodone-acetaminophen. He took the pills as prescribed for 1 month, and his pain went away.

After stopping the pills, however, Stan began to have pain again in his knee. He saw an orthopedist (a doctor who treats bone and muscle problems), who ordered imaging scans and determined there was no major damage. He was given another 1-month supply of hydrocodone-acetaminophen. This time, however, he needed to take more than prescribed in order to ease the pain. He also felt sad and "achy" when he did not take the medication, and said he had a "craving" for more opioids. He returned to the orthopedist, who referred him to a pain specialist.

Stan was too embarrassed to go to the pain specialist. He believed that his faith and strength should help him defeat the pain. He found that he could not live without the pain medication, because of the pain and muscle aches when he stopped the medication. He also began to enjoy the high and had intense craving. He began to frequent emergency rooms to get more opioids, often lying about the timing and nature of his right knee pain, and even stole pills from his mother on two occasions. He became fixed on trying to find more opioids, and his work and home life suffered. After a while, he told his primary care doctor about his opioid use and sadness, and that doctor referred him to the outpatient psychiatry clinic.

During the evaluation, Stan reported that his mood was "lousy." He denied symptoms of paranoia or hallucinations, or having any thoughts of harming himself or others.

Stan was diagnosed with *opioid use disorder*. The number of people who abuse prescription opioids ranks second among substance use disorders. Stan's use led to out-of-control opioid use that had a negative impact on his life.

Substance Intoxication and Withdrawal

When people use the substances listed in Table 2, they can have substance intoxication or withdrawal. *Intoxication* occurs when the substance use was recent. *Withdrawal* occurs when the person stops or uses less of the substance.

Table 2. Symptoms of intoxication and withdrawal		
Substance class	Intoxication symptoms	Withdrawal symptoms
Alcohol	Slurred speech, incoordination, unsteady walk, quick eye movements	Sweating or fast pulse, increased hand tremors, trouble sleeping, nausea or vomiting, hallucinations, anxiety
Caffeine	Restlessness, nervousness, excitement, trouble sleeping, flushed face, upset stomach, increased urination	Headache, fatigue or drowsiness, quickly annoyed or angry, sad mood, trouble staying focused
Cannabis	Red eyes, increased appetite, dry mouth, fast heart rate	Quickly annoyed or angry, nervousness, trouble sleeping, decreased appetite, restlessness

Substance class	Intoxication symptoms	Withdrawal symptoms
Hallucinogens	*With phencyclidine (PCP):* quick eye movements up and down or side to side, fast heart rate, loss of muscle coordination *With other hallucinogens:* large pupils, fast heart rate, sweating, blurred vision, tremors	None
Inhalants	Feeling dizzy, quick eye movements, incoordination, slurred speech, unsteady walk, slow reflexes, blurred vision	None
Opioids	Small or large pupils, drowsiness or coma, slurred speech, impaired attention or memory	Sad mood, nausea or vomiting, muscle aches, large pupils
Sedatives	Slurred speech, incoordination, unsteady walk, quick eye movements, impaired attention or memory	Sweating or fast pulse, hand tremors, trouble sleeping, nausea or vomiting, hallucinations, anxiety, seizures
Stimulants	Fast or slow heart rate, large pupils, higher or lower blood pressure, sweating or chills, nausea or vomiting	Fatigue, trouble sleeping, vivid nightmares, increased appetite
Tobacco	None	Quickly annoyed or angry, trouble keeping thoughts focused, increased appetite, restlessness, sad mood, trouble sleeping

Table 2. Symptoms of intoxication and withdrawal *(continued)*

When people are intoxicated, they show behavioral, physical, or psychological changes shortly after the substance is taken. Substance intoxication most often causes people to have problems with perception, staying awake, thinking, judgment, body movement, and personal behavior. They may become aggressive or moody.

How people use a substance plays a part in how quickly it is absorbed into the bloodstream and how strongly they become intoxicated. For instance, smoking, snorting, or shooting a drug intravenously (into the vein) causes a more intense intoxication. These methods are also more likely to lead people to use the substance more often. Also, the substance can continue to have effects even after tests no longer detect the substance in the body.

 Substance Intoxication

Substance intoxication occurs when:
- Recent use of the substance has occurred.
- Major problems appear with behavior, body function, and thinking or feeling during or shortly after the substance is taken, due to the effect on the central nervous system.
- Certain symptoms appear after the substance is taken (see Table 2).
- Symptoms are not due to another medical condition or mental disorder.

When people stop using a substance—or use less of it—substance withdrawal can also occur. Withdrawal symptoms can cause problems with social, work, or other tasks. Most people who have substance withdrawal have the urge to start using the substance again to relieve the withdrawal symptoms. If people use medications as directed by their doctor, any withdrawal symptoms that result from a reduced dose are not signs of a substance use disorder. They should contact their doctor if they are concerned about withdrawal symptoms.

 Substance Withdrawal

Substance withdrawal occurs when:
- The person stops or reduces use of the substance.
- Certain symptoms appear after the substance use is stopped or reduced (see Table 2).
- These symptoms cause great distress or problems with social, work, or other key, daily tasks.
- Symptoms are not due to another medical condition or mental disorder.

Drug Use and Risks Among U.S. Teens and Young Adults

Did you know...

- In 2021, 54% of 12th graders in the United States said they used alcohol in the past month, and 20% said they used marijuana.
- Caffeine can mask the effects of alcohol in the person taking it and to those who can see and speak with the person. Combined, caffeine and alcohol increase risk of harm to health, as well as risk for car accidents and other injuries.
- In 2021, marijuana was the most commonly used illegal drug across all ages in the United States.
- Although many people think marijuana use is harmless, it can have negative and long-term effects, even after marijuana use is stopped:
    - The brain is actively developing until around age 25. Marijuana use may harm the developing brain. It can cause permanent IQ loss when people start using it at a young age.
    - Marijuana use impairs driving. It causes slower reactions, lane weaving, decreased coordination, and difficulty reacting to signals and sounds on the road.
    - Marijuana use during pregnancy may cause premature birth, stillbirth, and problems with brain development. Chemicals from marijuana can be passed from a mother to her baby through breast milk.
    - Marijuana use can also lead to long-term problems with memory and has been linked with increased risk for psychosis.
- In 2020, nearly 21% of people age 12 and older have used nicotine (such as in cigarettes or through vaping) in the past month. Of these, 63% of teens ages 12–17 vaped nicotine in the past month. Vaping harms the lungs of both users and bystanders.
- There is a high risk of death from misuse of prescription opioids, illicit opioids (such as heroin), and synthetic opioids (such as fentanyl).
    - Fentanyl is deadly. The amount of fentanyl that can fit on the tip of a pencil can kill someone.
    - Fentanyl and other deadly drugs can be made to look like candy or medicine, such as methylphenidate for *attention-deficit/hyperactivity disorder*.
- No pill purchased on social media is safe. If a doctor did not prescribe your medicine, do not take it.

Source. Centers for Disease Control and Prevention; National Institute on Drug Abuse; Substance Abuse and Mental Health Services Administration; United States Drug Enforcement Administration.

Compared to others in the general population, young people ages 18–25 have the highest rates of alcohol use disorder and another substance use disorder. Those between ages 12–17 who use alcohol and cigarettes are at high risk to use other drugs. Intoxication is often the first substance-related disorder to occur and often begins during the teen years. Withdrawal can happen at any age as long as the substance has been taken for a long time on a frequent basis.

People can have a wide range of symptoms when intoxicated or in withdrawal. Examples of intoxication and withdrawal symptoms for certain substance classes are shown in Table 2.

Substance/Medication-Induced Mental Disorders

Sometimes, the use of drugs and medications can bring on symptoms of certain mental disorders. These mental disorders often stop within days or weeks after the drug or medication was last used. For instance, *alcohol-induced depressive disorder* is a *depressive disorder* caused by alcohol.

Of the drugs in Table 1, tobacco causes the fewest mental disorders. Withdrawal from tobacco (quitting smoking) can cause sleep disorders (such as trouble sleeping).

The other drugs in Table 1 can cause more severe mental disorders. For example, intoxication from drugs that cause sedation (sleepiness)—such as sedatives, hypnotics, or alcohol—can lead to a *substance-induced psychotic, bipolar, depressive,* or *sleep disorder* or a *substance-induced sexual dysfunction.* Withdrawal from these same drugs can lead to *substance-induced anxiety disorders* and *sexual dysfunctions.* Substances that cause stimulation (wakefulness)—such as cocaine and amphetamines—can cause *substance-induced psychotic, bipolar, depressive, sleep,* and *anxiety disorders* and *sexual dysfunctions.*

Some people are more prone than others to develop a substance-induced mental disorder from using drugs. The risk of developing one of these disorders increases with frequent use and larger amounts taken. Some drugs can have a rapid, severe, and harmful impact on the brain and body even if used just once in a small amount.

 ### Substance/Medication-Induced Mental Disorder

The following are common features of this disorder:
- The disorder shows the same distinct symptoms of a certain mental disorder.
- There is proof from the person's health history, physical exam, or lab tests of both of the following:

- The disorder began during or within 1 month of intoxication or withdrawal from the substance or from taking a medication.
- The substance or medication can cause the mental disorder.

- The disorder is *not* due to a separate mental disorder (such as one that is not substance/medication-induced). Proof of a separate mental disorder could include the following:

  - The disorder symptoms started before the severe intoxication, withdrawal, or exposure to the substance or medication began.
  - The full mental disorder lasted for an ample amount of time (such as at least 1 month) after the severe withdrawal, intoxication, or exposure to the substance or medication ended.

- The disorder is not part of a *delirium* (confusion and reduced attention caused by a substance, medication, or medical condition).
- The disorder causes much distress and problems with social, work, or other daily functions.

Gambling Disorder

Gambling involves risking something of value in hopes of getting something of greater value. Gambling has occurred in almost every part of the world throughout time. People in many cultures gamble (or place bets) on games and sporting events. Many gamble for fun and leisure and never have problems with it. But for some people, gambling becomes an addictive behavior that they find hard to resist. When that happens, it can lead to major problems that include family and marital discord (such as fighting over money or time away spent gambling), financial crises (such as losing savings, not paying bills), and trouble at work (being late, missing work).

People with *gambling disorder* get the same effect from gambling as someone with an alcohol or other substance use disorder gets from having a drink or using a drug. The gambling changes their mood and they keep up the habit, trying to achieve that same effect. They may feel a sense of power, control, and confidence when gambling. People with a gambling disorder then begin to crave gambling like people with a substance use disorder who begin to crave a substance. People who gamble also may abuse alcohol or other drugs.

People with a gambling disorder often get into a cycle of placing larger bets after they lose money on a bet. They then try to win back what they lost, which leads to an urgent need to keep gambling. This is called "chasing losses."

Those with a gambling disorder may see money as the source of and answer to their problems. They may begin to lie to family members and others to conceal how much they gamble. They may slip into illegal behavior (such as forgery and theft) to obtain more money to keep gambling. They also may ask others to loan them money for gambling, to pay back debts, or to help in a financial crisis.

Among those ages 18 to 21, the disorder is more common in young men than in young women. Young men tend to bet on active pursuits for the thrill, such as card games or sports betting, often with family or friends. Internet gambling among young men in this age group has been linked with more financial risk and is more often done while alone. Older people tend to bet using slot machines and playing bingo. Gambling disorder in later life is more common among women, and the disorder can become more serious more quickly in this group. Women may gamble as an unhealthy approach to relieve feeling angry or sad.

Gambling can increase during times of stress. There may be times of heavy gambling that cause severe problems in life, followed by times when the person is able to control the gambling behavior. Some people with gambling disorder decide to fully stop on their own, but others will benefit from the help of a mental health care provider. Some others may think they are recovered and do not know their risk. After they gamble a few times without problems, they may assume they are immune and continue to gamble—only to return to a gambling disorder.

 Gambling Disorder

The disorder is diagnosed when:
- Frequent gambling leads to problems and distress, as shown when someone has at least four of the following symptoms in 1 year:

  - Needs to gamble with increasing amounts of money to get excited.
  - Is restless or quickly annoyed or angry when trying to cut down or stop gambling.
  - Has tried but cannot control, cut back, or stop gambling.
  - Has constant thoughts about gambling (for instance, thinks about past gambling times, plans the next venture, thinks about ways to get more money to gamble).
  - Often gambles when feeling stressed (helpless, guilty, depressed).
  - After losing money gambling, often returns another day in an effort to win back money lost (chasing losses).

- Lies to conceal the extent of the gambling habit.
- Has placed at risk or lost a close relationship, job, or major school or career prospect because of gambling.
- Relies on others to provide money to make up for money lost through gambling.

- The gambling behavior is not due to a *manic episode* (spells of high energy and mood that can occur in *bipolar disorder*).

How severe the gambling disorder is depends on how many symptoms a person has. A person can have a mild, moderate, or severe gambling disorder. Those with 4–5 symptoms on the list above have a mild gambling disorder. People with 6–7 symptoms have a moderate disorder, and those with the most severe form have 8 or all of the symptoms.

Risk Factors

The following factors increase people's risk of gambling disorder:

- **Temperament.** People who begin gambling in childhood or early teenage years have an increased risk for the disorder. *Antisocial personality, depressive, bipolar* and *substance use disorders* have been linked with gambling disorder.
- **Genetics and biology.** The disorder runs in families. This could be due to both genetics and environment (being exposed to gambling at home).

Treatment

An addictive disorder is a lifelong or chronic illness like heart disease, high cholesterol, or high blood pressure. Although people with an addictive disorder are at risk of relapse, they can live full, healthy lives with treatment and support. *Relapse* occurs when someone has stopped use for a while and is getting back to daily life and doing well—but then resumes the addictive behavior, even just once. This return to drugs or gambling can pull the person back into the addictive disorder. Relapse is not failure and can strengthen efforts for recovery. Learning to be aware of triggers for relapse can prevent it (see box, "Tips to Help Recovery"). Because an addictive disorder affects many aspects of a person's life, combined forms of treatment are often used. For most, a mix of medication and individual or group therapy works best.

Tips to Help Recovery

The following tips have been adapted from the Web site **"Rethinking Drinking"** by the National Institute on Alcohol Abuse and Alcoholism (http://rethinkingdrinking.niaaa.nih.gov). These tips for problem drinking can apply to other addictive disorders and can help prevent relapse once recovery has begun. The main goals are to stay in control, learn and use refusal skills, and build a new life without addictive behavior.

- **Avoid triggers.** What triggers your urge toward your addictive behavior? If certain people or places make you drink, use a drug, or gamble even when you don't want to, try to avoid them. If certain activities, times of day, or feelings trigger the urge, plan something else to do instead.
- **Plan to handle urges.** When you cannot avoid a trigger and an urge hits, try these options:
  - Remind yourself of your reasons for changing (it can help to carry them in writing or store them in an electronic message you can access quickly, such as on a mobile phone).
  - Talk things through with someone you trust.
  - Get involved with a healthy, distracting activity, such as physical exercise or a hobby that doesn't involve the addictive behavior.
  - Instead of fighting the feeling, accept it and ride it out without giving in, knowing that it will soon crest like a wave and pass.
- **Be prepared to say "no."** You're likely to be offered a drink, a drug, or a chance to gamble at times when you don't want to or with old friends who joined you in your addictive behavior. Have a polite, firm "no, thanks" ready. Review what might occur and script your response. The faster you can say "no" to these offers, the less likely you are to give in. If you hesitate, it allows you time to think of excuses to go along. In some cases, it may be best to avoid the setting or the people who cannot take "no" for an answer.
- **Rebuild your life without the addictive behavior.** This may involve the following:
  - Let family and friends know about the problem and share information with them about the addictive behavior. Enlist their support and let them know what helps you in the process of change and recovery.
  - Develop new interests and social groups.
  - Find rewarding ways to spend your time that don't involve the addictive behavior.
  - Ask for help from others.
  - Decline taking on new demands, such as complex projects or new duties.

- Consider joining a support group (see Appendix C, "Helpful Resources"). People in recovery who attend groups on a regular basis do better than those who do not. Groups can vary widely, so shop around for one that's comfortable. You'll get more out of it if you become involved by having a sponsor and reaching out to other members for help.
- **Don't give up.** Changing unhealthy behaviors such as drinking too much can take a lot of effort. Setbacks are common, but you learn more each time. Each try brings you closer to your goal. Whatever course you choose, give it a fair trial. If one approach doesn't work, try something else. If a setback happens, get back on track as quickly as possible. In the long run, your chances for success are good. Research shows that most people who drink heavily can cut back a great deal or quit.

Medications can help control drug cravings and relieve severe symptoms of *withdrawal* (how the body and brain respond when the substance or gambling is stopped or decreased). These medications include naltrexone and benzodiazepines, among others (see Appendix B, "Medications"). Withdrawal symptoms differ for each drug and are described in the "Substance Intoxication and Withdrawal" section of this chapter.

Therapy can help those with addictive disorders learn about their behavior and why they use the drug or gamble. It can help them learn to stop, rebuild their life without addictive behavior, build higher self-esteem, and cope with stress. Other treatments may be given in hospitals, outpatient programs, and community settings that provide a controlled, drug-free environment.

Self-help groups can provide support for those with an addictive disorder. These programs often follow the 12 steps of treatment based on Alcoholics Anonymous. Sister organizations focus on those who abuse other substances (Cocaine Anonymous, Narcotics Anonymous), gambling (Gamblers Anonymous), and family members (Al-Anon, Gam-Anon, Nar-Anon Family Groups). These groups all provide a support system to those affected by an addictive disorder and help reinforce messages learned in treatment.

Key Points

- Certain drugs—and gambling—seem to quickly affect a portion of the brain called the *reward system*. This leads to intense pleasure (or a "high") and a craving to repeat that pleasure. Those with *addictive disorders* spend a great deal of time and effort trying to obtain the substance to use or the money to gamble. This begins to outweigh the value of other people and duties in their lives.

- Addictive disorders cause painful problems with home, school, work, relationships, finances, brain, and body. At the same time, the pain of an addictive disorder causes people to seek help. People with an addictive disorder must choose to get better. They cannot be forced to change. People with addictive disorders often cannot stop on their own, even when they want to. They must get proper help.
- Treatment can involve medications to help control drug cravings and relieve severe symptoms of withdrawal. Therapy can help those with an addictive disorder learn about their behavior and why they engage in it, rebuild life without the addictive behavior, build higher self-esteem, develop new and healthy coping skills, and cope with stress. Self-help or support groups play a major role in recovery for people with addictive disorders. They also provide valued guidance and support for their loved ones.
- For those with an addictive disorder and their loved ones, learning as much as they can about the problem and its effects is important. Loved ones and those with an addictive disorder should seek help from others. It is best for loved ones not to cover up the addictive behavior, make excuses for the addictive behavior, or take responsibility for it.
- *Relapse* occurs when someone has stopped the addictive behavior for a while and is getting back to daily life and doing well—but then resumes the behavior. The following tips help to prevent relapse: learn what triggers the addictive behavior, avoid those triggers, plan to handle urges for the addictive behavior, be prepared to say "no" to offers to engage in the behavior, and replace the behavior with other rewarding activities and relationships.

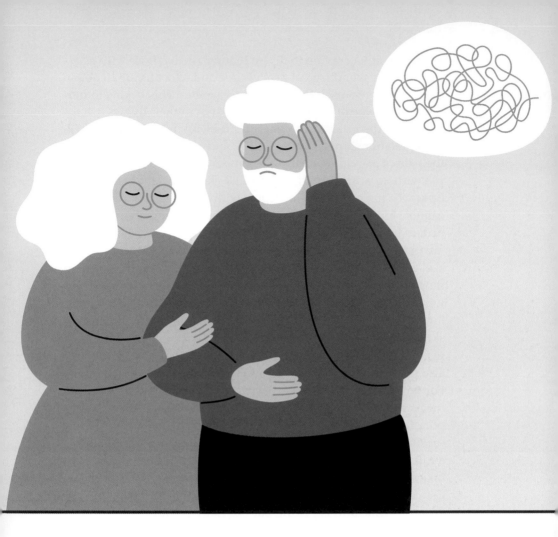

Delirium

Neurocognitive Disorder Due to Alzheimer's Disease

Neurocognitive Disorder Due to Traumatic Brain Injury

Neurocognitive Disorder Due to Parkinson's Disease

Frontotemporal Neurocognitive Disorder

Neurocognitive Disorder With Lewy Bodies

Vascular Neurocognitive Disorder

Other Dementia and Memory Problems

    Neurocognitive Disorder Due to HIV Infection

    Neurocognitive Disorder Due to Prion Disease

    Neurocognitive Disorder Due to Huntington's Disease

For a complete list of DSM-5-TR disorders, see Appendix A.

CHAPTER 17

Dementia and Other Memory Problems

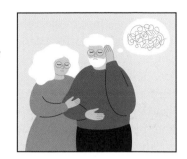

People with *dementia* have a decline in mental function that is severe enough to disrupt their daily life. The decline lessens their ability to think, remember, and plan. Dementia is not a disease itself, but a group of symptoms, such as memory loss and personality change. These symptoms may be caused by different disorders, so there are different types of dementia based on the cause.

Emotional problems, such as stress, anxiety, or depression, can make a person more forgetful—which might be mistaken for dementia. For instance, someone who has recently retired or who is coping with the death of a loved one may feel sad, lonely, worried, or bored. Trying to deal with these life changes leaves some people confused or forgetful. These memory problems are often short-term and go away when the feelings fade. If these feelings and memory problems persist, seek help from a doctor or other mental health care provider.

Some memory problems are linked to health issues that may be treated. These include medication side effects, lack of vitamin B_1 (thiamine) or vitamin B_3 (niacin), and *alcohol use disorder*. Some thyroid, kidney, or liver disorders also can lead to memory loss. A doctor should treat medical conditions like these as soon as possible. Some of these conditions may lead to dementia, and others do not. Early diagnosis and treatment can help limit and manage memory symptoms.

Alzheimer's disease is one of the most common causes of dementia. Dementia can also be caused by conditions such as a stroke, Parkinson's disease, or serious head injury. Dementia tends to worsen over time. How quickly symptoms worsen differs from person to person.

In DSM-5-TR, disorders that describe dementia and other disorders that affect brain function are called *neurocognitive disorders*. These disorders are caused by illness, disease, or injury. These disorders affect memory, thinking, and reasoning (see Table 1 for brain functions that doctors assess). Together, these abilities are referred to as *cognitive functions*. Not all neurocognitive disorders occur only in older people.

One of the neurocognitive disorders is *delirium*. This is a short-term state of decreased awareness and reduced attention. Delirium is not a dementia, although the two can overlap. Unlike the other neurocognitive disorders, delirium is a temporary state that usually resolves, whereas the other neurocognitive disorders persist.

All other neurocognitive disorders are named by the medical disease or injury causing the symptoms: *Alzheimer's disease, traumatic brain injury, Parkinson's disease, frontotemporal degeneration, Lewy body disease, vascular disease, HIV infection* (from AIDS), *prion disease*, and *Huntington's disease*. These neurocognitive disorders are diagnosed as either "major" or "mild" based on how severe symptoms are. When people say "dementia," *major neurocognitive disorder* is the diagnosis described in DSM-5-TR. The problems are not explained by delirium and are not the result of another mental disorder (such as *major depressive disorder* or *schizophrenia*). Other symptoms may appear with major or mild neurocognitive disorders, such as apathy (a lack of will or interest), agitation (such as resisting care, being unruly), psychosis, and anxiety.

What marks the disorder as major or mild is defined as follows:

Major Neurocognitive Disorder

- A major decline in at least one area of mental function—such as attention, ability to plan and make decisions, memory and learning, language, and motor skills. The decline is enough to cause concern from a loved one or a doctor, or is confirmed by testing.
- The major decline in mental skills impairs or disrupts the ability to do daily tasks. The person needs the help of others or must rely on others to perform these tasks, such as paying bills or keeping track of medications to take.

Mild Neurocognitive Disorder

- A slight decline in at least one area of a person's mental function— such as attention, ability to plan and make decisions, memory and

learning, language, and motor skills—that causes concern from the person, a loved one, or a doctor, or is confirmed by testing.
- The slight decline in mental skills permits doing daily tasks without help, such as paying bills or keeping track of medications to take. These tasks now take more mental effort to perform.

Table 1. Brain functions (neurocognitive domains) and disorder impact		
Domain (a type of thinking skill)	Examples of possible symptoms	
	Major neurocognitive disorder	Mild neurocognitive disorder
Complex attention (includes sustained attention, divided attention)	Needs simple, limited content to keep focus. Cannot keep attention when there are other distractions nearby (radio, TV, other people's background conversations). Has trouble holding new information in mind, such as what was just said or a phone number just given.	Normal tasks take longer than before. Thinking is easier without distractions, such as radio, TV, driving, and other people's background conversations.
Executive function (includes planning, decision making, working memory)	Needs to focus on one task at a time. Needs others to plan daily living tasks or make decisions.	Has more problems doing more than one task at once, or finishing a task after being interrupted by a visitor or phone call. May complain of being more tired from the extra effort needed to organize, plan, and make decisions.
Learning and memory (includes immediate, recent, and long-term memory)	Repeats self in conversation, often within same conversation. Cannot keep track of short list of items when shopping or of plans for the day. Needs frequent reminders to focus on task at hand.	Has problem recalling recent events and depends more on list making or calendar. May sometimes repeat self over a few weeks to the same person.

Table 1. Brain functions (neurocognitive domains) and disorder impact *(continued)*		
Domain (a type of thinking skill)	Examples of possible symptoms	
	Major neurocognitive disorder	Mild neurocognitive disorder
Language (includes naming objects, correct grammar, and understanding word definitions)	Has great problems naming objects and understanding simple requests. May not re-call names of close friends or family. Uses vague phrases such as "that thing" and "you know what I mean," and uses gen-eral pronouns instead of people's names.	Has problem finding the correct words they want to say. May avoid using names of people they do not see often.
Perceptual-motor (includes assembling items that require hand-eye coordina-tion, identifying faces, and imitating gestures)	Has great problems with tasks that were once easy (such as using tools, driving a car), or getting around in familiar areas.	Needs to rely more on maps or others for directions. Takes more effort to do tasks such as assembly, sewing, or knitting.
Social cognition (includes recognizing other people's emo-tions or mental states)	Behaves clearly out-side social norms. Shows no awareness of what's proper to wear or say in conversations. Disregards own safety. Has no awareness about these changes.	Slight changes in behavior or personality appear. Less able to read facial expressions or feel empathy.

Delirium

Delirium occurs when normal brain signals are not working. Delirium causes a decreased awareness and reduced attention that results from drugs of abuse, alcohol, medications, toxins, or a medical condition, such as an illness or infection. *Alcohol* or *drug intoxication* or *withdrawal* can cause symptoms. People with delirium have problems staying fo-cused or paying attention. Delirium can start quickly, often within hours or a few days. One way to understand delirium is to think about what it is like to be "out of it," not being fully awake, having an illness with a high fever, or waking up from anesthesia.

People with delirium have disturbed mental function that causes a decreased awareness of their environment, memory problems, and confused thinking. They may be easily distracted and unable to answer questions. They can be sleepy during the day and awake at night. People with delirium may have other symptoms, such as anxiety, fear, depression, irritability, and anger. They may also call out, scream, curse, or moan, especially at night. Delirium can occur in someone who also has dementia.

Any condition that requires a hospital stay, especially in intensive care, increases the risk of delirium. Between 18% and 35% of people admitted to the hospital develop delirium. In older people admitted to intensive care units, the rate is as high as 81%.

 Delirium

- Reduced attention and awareness. For instance, not able to stay focused on a topic or to change topics. Normal tasks take longer than before, and thinking is easier when other things don't compete for attention, such as the radio, TV, and other conversations.

- The problem develops over a short time (usually hours to a few days), tends to become more severe through the day, and worsens in the evening.

- A problem in mental function, such as memory loss, disorientation, language problems, and problems with judging shapes and sizes.

The first and third items above must not be due to another neurocognitive disorder. There must be evidence (for instance, from testing, physical exam, or report by self or others) of another medical condition, alcohol or drug intoxication or withdrawal, or exposure to a toxin or a medication that might have caused the symptoms. Delirium can last for hours, days, weeks, or months.

Risk Factors

The following factors may increase the risk of delirium: vision or hearing loss, increasing age, severe illness or infection, *depression*, history of stroke, alcohol use, and having a *major* or *mild neurocognitive disorder*. Older people are at higher risk than young adults.

Treatment

While most people with delirium have a full recovery with or without treatment, early diagnosis and treatment can shorten the length of the illness. Delirium can progress to coma, seizures, or death if the cause for the symptoms remains untreated. The first goal of treatment is to address the underlying cause, such as stopping the use of a certain medication or substance. For that reason, the doctor will need to assess all possible causes for the delirium through a medical "workup." This involves a range of medical tests. For instance, if an infection that has caused a delirium is treated, it also will allow the delirium to resolve.

Alzheimer's Disease

Alzheimer's disease is a condition that causes dementia by slowly killing nerve cells in the brain. It destroys memory and the ability to learn, reason, make judgments, communicate, and carry out daily tasks.

Alzheimer's disease is one of the most common forms of dementia, striking nearly 6 million Americans of all ages. This includes an estimated 5.8 million people age 65 and older and about 300,000 people younger than age 65 who have a younger-onset (or early-onset) form of the disease. The Centers for Disease Control and Prevention (CDC) lists Alzheimer's disease as the sixth leading cause of adult death in the United States.

Symptoms most often start after age 70. People with Alzheimer's disease first show mild symptoms of personality changes and memory loss that differ from normal changes that happen with age (see box). They may become upset or anxious more easily or withdraw from their usual hobbies and activities. They may not cope well with change. For instance, they can follow their same daily routes, but travel to a new place confuses them and they quickly become lost. Another early sign of the disease is changes in judgment or decision making. They may pay less attention to grooming or keeping themselves clean.

In the early stages of the illness, people are often at risk of *depression.* Their condition also may be worsened by reactions to medications or changes in living arrangements. Because Alzheimer's disease happens late in life, the loss of a spouse or other close family members may increase the suffering of people with Alzheimer's disease.

As memory loss worsens, people with Alzheimer's disease may ask the same questions over and over and forget the names of longtime friends. Social life becomes harder, and they may become more isolated. In the later stages of Alzheimer's disease, people with the illness begin to lose physical coordination and may need help with dressing, bathing, and even walking.

Is It Alzheimer's Disease or Just Normal Aging?

While some changes in memory, thinking, and reasoning skills may be early warning signs of *Alzheimer's disease,* many changes are just a normal part of getting older. If you notice any of these signs of Alzheimer's disease, see a doctor right away for an evaluation.

Signs of Alzheimer's disease	Normal age-related changes
Memory loss that disrupts daily life (forgetting recently learned information or important dates or events)	Sometimes forgetting names or appointments but can recall them later
Challenges in planning or solving problems (trouble following a familiar recipe or keeping track of monthly bills)	Sometimes making errors when balancing a checkbook
Problems completing familiar tasks at home, work, or leisure (managing a budget at work or knowing rules of a favorite game)	Sometimes needing help to use the settings on a microwave or to record a television show
Confused about time or place (losing track of the date or the season)	Forgetting the day of the week but can recall it later
Trouble making sense of visual images and spatial relationships (problems reading, judging distance, and knowing colors)	Vision changes from cataracts
New problems with words while writing or talking with others (repeating statements, calling items by the wrong name)	Sometimes having trouble finding the right word
Misplacing things and being unable to retrace steps to find them	Losing or misplacing things from time to time
Decreased or poor judgment	Making a bad decision once in a while, such as not taking the car for an oil change
No longer or seldom taking part in work or social functions	Sometimes feeling weary of work, family, and social duties
Changes in mood and personality (becoming confused, suspicious, depressed, fearful, or anxious)	Having certain ways of doing things and getting annoyed when a routine is changed

Source. Alzheimer's Association.

Dementia and Other Memory Problems

Most people with Alzheimer's disease are older adults. They may suffer from a number of medical conditions that can make diagnosing the disease more complicated. These other medical conditions also play a role in the person's overall health and how quickly Alzheimer's disease may progress.

 ### Neurocognitive Disorder Due to Alzheimer's Disease

- Symptoms of either major or mild neurocognitive disorder are present.
- The disease begins with few or no symptoms, and memory or thinking slowly become impaired.
- There may be signs of Alzheimer's disease from family history or genetic testing.
- All three of the following are present:
  - Proof of decline in memory, learning, and at least one other mental process (such as attention or language) based on health history or testing.
  - Increasing, gradual decline in mental processes.
  - No proof of another disease that may cause the mental decline.
- The disorder is not due to the effects of alcohol, drugs, or medication.

Risk Factors

Factors that play a role in the development of Alzheimer's disease include smoking, *depression*, and getting little physical exercise, as well as the following:

- **Environment.** Low education level and little social contact with others are linked with the disorder. Traumatic brain injury (serious head injury) may increase the risk.
- **Biology.** High blood pressure, heart disease, obesity, hearing loss, and diabetes increase risk. Age is the greatest known risk factor for the disease, with a higher risk after age 75 years.
- **Genetics.** The disease also runs in families—having a first-degree blood relative (parent or sibling) with the disease increases a person's risk. A gene variation called apolipoprotein E4 may increase the risk of developing Alzheimer's disease. In African Americans, a gene that transports protein, *ABCA7*, has been linked with the disease.

Roger's Story

Roger, a 71-year-old man, was referred to a psychiatrist by his primary care doctor for symptoms of depression that had not responded to medication. Roger's wife reported that he had begun to change at age 68, about a year after his retirement. He had stopped playing golf and cards, which he had enjoyed for decades. He no longer looked forward to going out of the house, and he refused to socialize. Instead, he sat on the couch all day and watched TV or napped. His wife said he was sleeping 10–12 hours a day instead of his normal 7 hours.

His wife had become worried that retirement had left Roger depressed, and she had mentioned her concerns to their primary care doctor. Their doctor agreed and prescribed an antidepressant. Roger's symptoms did not improve on the medication, and the doctor then referred him for a psychiatric evaluation.

Roger's past psychiatric history was noted because one of his younger brothers had *major depression* that was treated with psychotherapy and antidepressant medication. His mother had developed *dementia* in her 70s.

Roger had graduated from college with a degree in business, had a successful career as a corporate manager, and retired at age 67. He and his wife had been married for 45 years, said there were no major marital problems, and had three children and four grandchildren, who were all in good health. Before this, he had been outgoing, energetic, and well organized.

Roger had high blood pressure and high cholesterol and was taking medication for these conditions. The exam showed he was alert and cooperative and had steady but slow speech. Roger had a limited range of emotional expression, denied feeling sad or guilty, but felt he had retired too early. He was aware that his wife was concerned and agreed that he had less energy and was less active than in the past. He blamed these changes on his retirement.

During the exam, Roger could name the year but not the month or day of the week for his appointment. He remembered one of three objects in 2 minutes, performed three of five subtractions correctly, named four common objects correctly, and repeated a complex sentence without error. He was able to draw the face of a clock and place the numbers correctly, but he was not able to correctly place the hands at 10 minutes after 2.

Roger was diagnosed with *Alzheimer's disease*. He had a 3-year history of gradual social withdrawal. He has a family history of depression in a brother and late-life dementia in his mother. The main symptoms were slowness, lack of concern about his decline, and increased sleep. The exam showed problems in memory, concentration, and math, as well as trouble with clock drawing.

Treatment

While there is no cure for Alzheimer's disease, there are two types of medications that may help lessen the memory symptoms for a short time. Cholinesterase inhibitors ("memory enhancers") often are prescribed in the early stages to treat symptoms such as memory loss, thinking, language, and judgment. About half the people who take the medication have a delay in their symptoms getting worse for about 6 to 12 months. Another medication, memantine, may help reduce the decline in memory, attention, reasoning, and ability to do simple tasks later in the disease. Antidepressants also may be used to treat mood symptoms or antipsychotic medications for hallucinations, agitation, and severe hostility.

Patients and families may benefit from the help of support groups and counseling. Families can also benefit from getting help with the care that is needed to maintain safety when a loved one has memory loss. Therapy can help family members learn ways to help their relative living with the disease to manage the illness. They also can learn coping skills to lessen the stress of caring for a loved one with Alzheimer's disease.

By taking advantage of group support and assistance in caregiving when needed, patients and their loved ones can prepare themselves for the disease and its progression. While the disease does not have a cure, quality of life can be greatly improved with support for patients and caregivers.

Tips for Caregivers

Taking care of a loved one with *Alzheimer's disease* or *other dementia* can be stressful. As a caregiver, follow these tips to take good care of yourself:

- **Know what resources are available.** Learn about the different levels of care your loved one will need depending on the stages of illness. Adult day programs, in-home assistance, and visiting nurses are just some of the services that can help you manage day-to-day tasks. Search for local resources in your area at www.alz.org or www.alzfdn.org.
- **Get help.** Don't try to do everything yourself. Ask family and friends for support. Helplines for caregivers are available 24/7, and local support groups for caregivers are also good sources for comfort (see Appendix C, "Helpful Resources," "Dementia and Other Memory Problems").
- **Practice relaxation techniques.** Meditation, breathing exercises, yoga, and visualization are just a few of the simple techniques that can help relieve stress.
- **Take time for yourself.** Although it may be hard to find time to do things just for you, it's important for your well-being to take time each week for an activity you enjoy or to stay connected to friends and family. Be sure to include time for exercise—even a brief walk—and healthy meals.

Traumatic Brain Injury

A *traumatic brain injury* (TBI) disrupts brain structure and/or function because of an impact to the head—or other rapid movement of the brain—that causes instant medical effects. These may include confusion, slowed thinking, loss of consciousness, or lost memory for events right before or after the injury. Falls, vehicle accidents, and being struck in the head cause most TBIs.

A neurocognitive disorder due to TBI causes lasting problems in brain function. These may involve problems with attention, balance, speech, learning, memory, planning, fatigue, irritability, and *depression*. More than 3 million people in the United States have a disability from TBI, which can affect their ability to work or do daily tasks of living. They may need ongoing care and services.

TBIs can be mild, moderate, or severe, depending on what is seen in brain imaging and whether and how long the person lost consciousness, had amnesia, and remained confused after the injury. Collisions and blows to the head that happen during contact sports are often a mild form of TBI. With mild TBIs, symptoms either go away in days to weeks or improve greatly within 3 to 12 months. Repeated mild TBIs may cause problems that last longer. Severe TBIs can cause seizures, emotional problems, weakness on one side of the body, vision problems, bleeding in the brain, and death.

In the United States, nearly 3 million TBIs occur each year, resulting in 2.5 million visits to hospital emergency rooms, 288,000 hospitalizations, and 56,000 deaths. Among these numbers, 837,000 TBIs occur in children each year. Men suffer more TBIs than women up until age 75, and after that age the rates are nearly the same because of falls.

The following problems can occur as a result of TBIs:

- Emotional problems, such as quick frustration, irritability, moodiness, tension, and anxiety.
- Personality changes, such as aggression, lack of motivation, and suspiciousness.
- Physical symptoms, such as headache, fatigue, sensitivity to light, sleep problems, and dizziness.
- Mental challenges, such as slower thinking, problems staying focused, and reduced ability to perform usual activities.

 ## Neurocognitive Disorder Due to Traumatic Brain Injury

- Symptoms of either major or mild neurocognitive disorder are present.
- There is evidence of a traumatic brain injury, with one or more of the following:

- Loss of consciousness.
- Posttraumatic amnesia (loss of memory after a traumatic event).
- Being disoriented and confused.
- Signs of neurological problems (such as seizures, loss of smell, or weakness on one side of the body).

- The disorder starts right after the brain injury or right after the person regains consciousness and lasts past the acute post-injury period.

Risk Factors

Alcohol and other *substance use disorders* increase the risk for a TBI. They also increase the risk for more adverse outcomes in mental function from the TBI, such as problems with memory, attention, and planning.

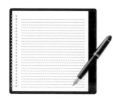

Olivia's Story

The parents of 19-year-old Olivia insisted she see a psychiatrist. "It's not me you want to see," Olivia proclaimed. "It's my insane parents who need your help." Olivia added, "Everything is going great in my life. I have plenty of friends, go out almost every night, and always have lots of fun."

Olivia agreed to have her parents join the session, and they told a different story. In tears, they disclosed that their daughter had become irritable, unproductive, and combative. In searching her room, they had found small amounts of marijuana, alprazolam (Xanax), cocaine, and prescription stimulants. The parents described major changes in Olivia's personality over the last few years. They also noted that Olivia's attitudes and behavior sharply differed from those of her family. Her sister went to a top university, and her younger brother excelled at a private high school. Her parents seemed to enjoy their careers as radiologists.

Her parents said that Olivia's sudden change began 4 years ago. At 15, she liked to study. She also had a lively sense of humor and a wide circle of "terrific friends." But "almost overnight," she began to shun her longtime friends in favor of "dropouts and malcontents" and began to get traffic tickets and school detentions. Her grades dropped from As to Ds. The parents were at a loss to explain the abrupt and dramatic change.

The change in school performance led the psychiatrist to ask Olivia to take a series of neuropsychological tests so the results could be compared with those of tests that she had taken when she had applied to a private high school several years ago. These involved two high school admissions tests that Olivia retook: the System for Assessment and Group Evaluation (SAGE), which tests a wide range of thinking skills, and the Differential Aptitude Tests (DAT), which focus on reasoning, spelling, and perception skills.

On the SAGE, her average scores dropped from the upper 10% for a 13-year-old to the bottom 20%. When Olivia took the DAT at age 13, she scored in the highest range for ninth graders across almost all measures. Upon repeating the test at age 19, she scored below the high school average in all measures.

A magnetic resonance imaging (MRI) brain scan displayed a clear "lesion" on the left side of the brain. This was a sign of prior injury to that area.

During more questions about the time in which she seemed to have changed, Olivia revealed that she had been in a traffic accident with her ex-boyfriend, Mark. Although Olivia did not recall much from this episode, she remembered that she hit her head and that she had bad headaches for many weeks thereafter. Because Olivia was not bleeding and there was no damage to the car, neither Mark nor Olivia reported the incident to anyone. With Olivia's permission, the psychiatrist contacted Mark, who remembered the incident well. "Olivia hit her head very, very hard on the dashboard of my car. She was not totally unconscious but very dazed. For about 3 hours, she spoke very slowly, complained that her head hurt badly, and was confused. For about 2 hours she didn't know where she was, what day it was, and when she had to get home. She also threw up twice. I was really scared, but Olivia didn't want me to worry her parents since they're so overprotective. And then she broke up with me, and we've hardly spoken since."

Olivia was diagnosed with *mild neurocognitive disorder due to traumatic brain injury* (TBI). The decision to retest Olivia's performance on high school aptitude and achievement examinations revealed the dramatic decline in her test scores. The questions about her history led to the discovery of the car accident that marked the start of Olivia's symptoms.

In the accident, Olivia suffered a TBI and had two of the four core symptoms for a TBI diagnosis: she was disoriented and confused for hours afterward, and she did not recall much about the accident (posttraumatic amnesia).

Treatment

Medical care should be sought as soon as possible for a brain injury. Treatment may require a short hospital stay or monitoring at home. Severe injuries need special hospital care that may take months. A medical workup will show how serious the injury is and if any treatment is needed (for example, to drain a subdural hematoma, which is a pool of blood within the skull that may occur after a head injury.) In Olivia's case, the symptoms from the TBI included both a change in personality and a change in thinking skills. Sometimes personality changes can include anxiety or depression symptoms that require treatment. Other times they can include being impulsive, being easily angered, making poor decisions, or tending to abuse drugs or alcohol. The type of treatment varies for each person and is based on the type of symptoms from the injury.

Parkinson's Disease

Parkinson's disease is a disorder of the nervous system that affects people's movement. It occurs when nerve cells in the brain stop making a chemical called dopamine, which helps control muscle movement. The disease progresses slowly and usually starts with a slight shaking or tremor in one hand. Over time, people with the disease may become stiff, move slowly, and have problems with balance and walking. They also may have confusion, slowed or quieter speech, and loss of thinking skills and facial expressions.

Each year in the United States, about 60,000 new cases of Parkinson's disease are diagnosed. About 1 million people in the United States currently have the condition. Symptoms of the disease often begin after age 50, and most often in the early 60s. Parkinson's disease occurs more often in men than in women. A dementia can develop in some people with Parkinson's disease.

When people have a neurocognitive disorder with Parkinson's disease, the loss of thinking skills often doesn't occur until years after the movement symptoms have been present. When thinking problems do begin, the main problems involve slow thinking and taking a long time to process new information or learn new things. Problems with memory, planning, and keeping focused attention may also occur.

 ### Neurocognitive Disorder Due to Parkinson's Disease

- Symptoms of either major or mild neurocognitive disorder are present.
- The problem occurs with a diagnosis of Parkinson's disease.
- The disease begins with few or no symptoms and progresses with gradual impairment.
- The disorder is not due to another medical condition or mental disorder.

Risk Factors

The following factors increase the risk of Parkinson's disease:

- **Environment.** Exposure to herbicides and pesticides.
- **Biology.** The risk of a neurocognitive disorder from Parkinson's disease includes older age at disease onset, growing severity of Parkinson's disease, and *rapid eye movement sleep behavior disorder*.

Treatment

There is no cure for Parkinson's disease, but treatment can help to reduce its symptoms. Treatment most often includes medication that helps replace the brain chemical dopamine that is lost with the disease.

These medications treat symptoms related to movement problems. One of the most effective is levodopa, which passes into the brain and transforms into dopamine. A class of medications known as dopamine agonists may also be given that mimic the actions that dopamine has in the brain. Dopamine agonists include pramipexole and ropinirole. These medicines help with the movement problems but do not help with the cognitive (thinking) problems with Parkinson's disease. Sometimes the medicines that help increase dopamine can cause side effects when people lose thinking skills from Parkinson's disease, and too much dopamine agonist medicine can cause hallucinations or confusion.

Although less common, surgery may be an option for some people to help ease symptoms. A procedure known as *deep brain stimulation* involves placing electrical stimulators on areas of the brain that control movement. This treatment is only used when medications do not work. The surgery may help with movement problems, but not with changes in thinking skills that happen later with Parkinson's disease. There is no treatment to relieve the cognitive symptoms of Parkinson's disease. Occupational therapy may help with tasks used in daily life (such as getting dressed) and learning how to avoid falls.

Frontotemporal Neurocognitive Disorder

Frontotemporal neurocognitive disorder is caused by cell damage in the brain's frontal lobes (area behind the forehead) or temporal lobes (area of the brain that is just above the ears). These parts of the brain control a person's planning, judgment, emotions, and speaking, and some types of movement.

The disorder can cause severe changes in personality. For instance, someone who once had flawless manners may become profane or vulgar in public. People with the behavioral symptoms of the disorder may lose their sense of social skills, so that they may do awkward things, such as stand too close to people or make rude comments that are out of character for their personality. Others may lose their skill with language, such as showing problems with naming objects, using correct grammar, or finding words to say what they mean.

Frontotemporal dementia occurs in 2 to 31 of every 100,000 people This type of dementia can be seen often in people younger than age 65 years.

The disorder occurs most often in those who are in their 50s. Only about 20%–25% of those with the disorder are diagnosed when they are older than age 65. Because of the younger age that symptoms appear, the disorder can disrupt work and family life in more ways than the dementias that start later in life.

 ## Frontotemporal Neurocognitive Disorder

- Symptoms of either major or mild neurocognitive disorder are present.
- The disease begins with few or no symptoms and progresses gradually.
- A decline in thinking skills centers mainly on behavior control or language, with few or no problems with memory, learning, motor, or visual skills.
- The disorder is not due to another disorder or disease, such as stroke, or the effects of a medication, drug, or alcohol.
- Either a behavioral type or a language type is present.

Behavioral Type

- At least three of the following behavioral symptoms:
  - Behavioral disinhibition (loss of social restraint).
  - Lack of emotion or interest.
  - Loss of sympathy or empathy.
  - Compulsive behavior.
  - Hyperorality (putting inappropriate objects in the mouth) and changes in diet, such as constant overeating or eating strange foods.
- Clear decline in social skills (such as decline in self-care, lack of interest in social interactions, less interest in personal responsibilities) and decline in ability to plan, organize, and make decisions.

Language Type

- Clear decline in language skills, such as the ability to make words easily, name objects, or read and write.

Risk Factors

About 40% of people with frontotemporal neurocognitive disorder have a family history of early-onset neurocognitive disorder. Certain gene mutations can increase the risk.

Treatment

There is no treatment for frontotemporal neurocognitive disorder. Because the problem often causes changes in behavior or personality, the most important treatment involves counseling and support for families and caregivers to understand the illness. Often people with the disorder need supervision and care from their families. When there are severe behavior changes that involve irritability or hostility, antidepressant or antipsychotic medications may help calm the person.

Lewy Body Disease

Neurocognitive disorder with Lewy bodies (NCDLB) is caused by abnormal microscopic deposits in the brain that damage brain cells over time. The disorder is named after neurologist Frederich H. Lewy, M.D., who discovered the abnormal brain deposits in the early 1900s.

The damage caused to brain cells leads to a gradual decline in thinking and reasoning. The disease also causes confusion and degrees of alertness that change greatly through the day or from one day to the next. People with the disorder may fall often or have spells of lost consciousness. They may have problems feeding themselves and using the toilet. Symptoms tend to begin between ages 50–89, and the most common age at onset is the mid-70s.

Some symptoms of NCDLB can look like the symptoms of Parkinson's disease. People with NCDLB have the same motor problems that are seen in Parkinson's disease, such as a very slow walking gait, slow speech, and loss of facial expression.

People with the disorder may have two major symptoms not found in other neurocognitive disorders: visual hallucinations (seeing things that are not there) and symptoms of *rapid eye movement (REM) sleep behavior disorder* (see Chapter 12, "Sleep-Wake Disorders," for details). Up to 50% of people with NCDLB also have severe reactions and side effects to antipsychotic medications, so a correct diagnosis of the condition is essential.

It is estimated that up to 10% of elderly people have NCDLB. The disorder is thought to be the third most common cause of dementia after *Alzheimer's disease* and *vascular dementia,* making up as much as 30% of dementia cases.

 Neurocognitive Disorder With Lewy Bodies

- Symptoms for either major or mild neurocognitive disorder are present.
- The disease begins with few or no symptoms and progresses gradually.
- There is a range of severity for this disorder. See a doctor if at least one of the following symptoms is present:
    - Fluctuating cognition with noticeable changes in attention and alertness.
    - Frequent visual hallucinations that are clear and detailed.
    - Symptoms of Parkinson's disease (such as muscle tremors or stiffness) and decline in thinking abilities (such as understanding, judgment, and memory).
    - Symptoms of REM sleep behavior disorder.
    - Severe side effects to antipsychotic medications.
- The disorder is not due to another disorder or disease, such as stroke, or the effects of a medication, drug, or alcohol.

Risk Factors

Several genes linked to the disorder increase the risk of developing NCDLB.

Treatment

There is no treatment for NCDLB. As a rule, people with NCDLB are very sensitive to side effects from all types of medicines. For this reason, doctors must take great care with prescribed medication. Changes in alertness with NCDLB can worsen greatly with medications. For instance, sometimes dopamine-increasing medicines are used to help treat symptoms of stiffness and motor slowness, but these medicines can have the unwanted effect of making visual hallucinations worse. Sometimes the cholinesterase inhibitors used to treat the memory and thinking symptoms of Alzheimer's disease are prescribed for people with NCDLB, but whether these medications are helpful is not certain. Careful prescribing to help with depression or sleep problems can be done with close watching for side effects.

Often the best help for NCDLB is to avoid things that may cause confusion. Keeping a home free of clutter and noise may help maintain focus and avoid distractions. Doing so may also lessen the risk for hallucinations. Setting routines can build structure into the day and keep tasks clear. Breaking down complex tasks into simple steps also helps.

Vascular Neurocognitive Disorder

Vascular neurocognitive disorder is caused by reduced blood flow to the brain because of a problem with the blood vessels that supply it. Parts of the brain become damaged and die from a lack of oxygen and nutrients.

The most common cause of the disorder is *cerebrovascular disease* (brain problems due to diseased blood vessels that supply the brain). This includes stroke and transient ischemic attacks (ministrokes). Changes in thinking skills sometimes follow these episodes. While thinking problems may begin mildly, they can worsen over time as a result of multiple minor strokes or other conditions that affect smaller blood vessels. Personality changes, mood changes, depression, and slowed movements may also occur.

In the United States, estimates for vascular neurocognitive disorder range from 1% of people ages 71–79 years to 4% of those ages 80–89. Within 3 months of having a stroke, 20%–30% of people are diagnosed with the disorder.

 Vascular Neurocognitive Disorder

- Symptoms of either major or mild neurocognitive disorder are present.
- The symptoms reflect a vascular problem, as shown by either of the following:
  - Start of cognitive problems is related to at least one cerebrovascular event (such as stroke).
  - Decline in mental skills is shown in memory, problem solving, reasoning, and planning.
- Evidence of cerebrovascular disease is shown in the person's health history, from physical exam, or from brain imaging.
- The disorder is not due to another brain disease or systemic disorder.

Risk Factors

The following factors increase the risk of the disorder:

- **Environment.** How well people overcome the effects of vascular brain injury depends on how well their brain forms new connections after portions of the brain have died. Keeping up education, physical exercise, social interaction, and mental activity throughout life helps.
- **Genetics and biology.** Factors that lead to cerebrovascular disease increase the risk, such as high blood pressure, diabetes, smoking, high cholesterol, and obesity.

Treatment

There is no treatment for vascular dementia. The most important "treatment" is to prevent it. A healthy diet, exercise, weight control, and reducing stress can lower blood pressure, blood sugar, and cholesterol levels. These lifestyle changes can greatly reduce the risk of vascular dementia and can reduce progress of the disease. Quitting smoking can also help. Sometimes the medicines used in *Alzheimer's disease* are prescribed for vascular dementia, but it is not certain if they offer any benefit.

Other Dementia and Memory Problems

The following neurocognitive disorders can result from HIV infection, prion disease, or Huntington's disease. For a diagnosis, symptoms of either major or mild neurocognitive disorder must be present. The neurocognitive disorder cannot result from another medical condition or mental disorder. There may be some medications that can treat the memory and thinking problems or mood symptoms for these disorders. The best care for all the dementias involves loved ones and care providers giving kindness, patience, respect, and dignity to those with these disorders.

Neurocognitive Disorder Due to HIV Infection

HIV disease infects the body's immune cells and some people with the infection develop dementia symptoms, such as memory loss and problems with planning, decision making, and learning new information. In the United States, about 25% of people infected with HIV have a mild neurocognitive disorder, and less than 5% have a major neurocognitive disorder due to HIV infection. Although more men have HIV infection than women, more women have a neurocognitive disorder due to the HIV infection.

To prevent or reduce neurocognitive symptoms of HIV, seeking treatment with medications that cross the blood-brain barrier is key. (The *blood-brain barrier* protects the brain; it restricts passage of certain substances in the blood from reaching the brain, such as certain medications.) Symptoms of a neurocognitive disorder due to HIV infection are as follows:

- There is proven infection with HIV.
- The neurocognitive disorder is not better explained by non-HIV conditions, such as brain disease.

Neurocognitive Disorder Due to Prion Disease

Prion disease describes a very rare group of diseases that affect humans and animals. *Prions* cause infection in nerve tissue, with rapid brain damage and major neurocognitive disorder in as little as 6 months. Prion disease most often occurs in those age 65 or older. The disease may begin with fatigue, anxiety, and problems with eating, sleeping, or keeping focus. After a few weeks, changes in vision, coordination, or walking occur, as well as jerking movements. The disease always causes death. Exposure to infected nerve tissue may cause the disease, but often it appears without a clear source of infection. One common type of prion disease is Creutzfeldt-Jakob disease, or "mad cow disease." Symptoms of a neurocognitive disorder due to prion disease are as follows:

- The disease begins with few or no symptoms and progresses rapidly.
- Motor features of prion disease, such as muscle jerks or lack of muscle coordination, are present.

Neurocognitive Disorder Due to Huntington's Disease

Huntington's disease is rare. It is inherited within families, so people often know that they are at risk for it. The disease causes people to have jerky movements that they cannot control. Problems progress with walking, speaking, swallowing, feeding themselves and chewing, and fine motor tasks such as writing. People with the disorder also have thinking problems and emotional changes that begin before the movement problems start. These may include irritability, anxiety, depression, impulsivity, lack of motivation, and problems with attention, planning, and organization.

Most people begin to develop the first signs and symptoms between ages 35 and 45. Symptoms of a neurocognitive disorder due to Huntington's disease are as follows:

- The disease begins with few or no symptoms and progresses gradually.
- There is clinically diagnosed Huntington's disease or a risk of the disease based on family history or genetic testing.

Key Points

- Everyone forgets from time to time, and minor memory problems are part of normal aging. They can also result from stress, grief, medication side effects, lack of vitamin B_1 (thiamine) or vitamin B_3 (niacin), drug or alcohol use, or medical problems. When the underlying cause is treated or the emotional event has passed, the memory problems often disappear.
- *Delirium* is a short-term state of decreased awareness and reduced attention that goes away, while the other neurocognitive disorders persist. Treatment helps pinpoint the cause of delirium and quickens the end of symptoms.
- *Dementia* describes a decline in mental function that is severe enough to disrupt daily life. It can cause problems with people's memory and how well they think and plan. It is caused by different types of disorders or diseases. Alzheimer's disease is the most common cause of dementia. When people say "dementia," *major neurocognitive disorder* is the diagnosis described in DSM-5-TR.
- The neurocognitive disorders are diagnosed as either "major" or "mild" based on the level of decline in mental function. A *major neurocognitive disorder* occurs when someone can no longer do daily mental tasks without help, such as balancing a checkbook or keeping track of medicines. A *mild neurocognitive disorder* occurs when someone can still perform daily mental tasks, but may need extra time, structure, or reminders to complete them.
- Caring for a loved one with dementia is stressful. It's helpful to know what resources are available; seek help from support groups, family, and friends; practice relaxation techniques; and take time for yourself. Giving kindness, patience, respect, and dignity to the person who has dementia is a key aspect of good care.

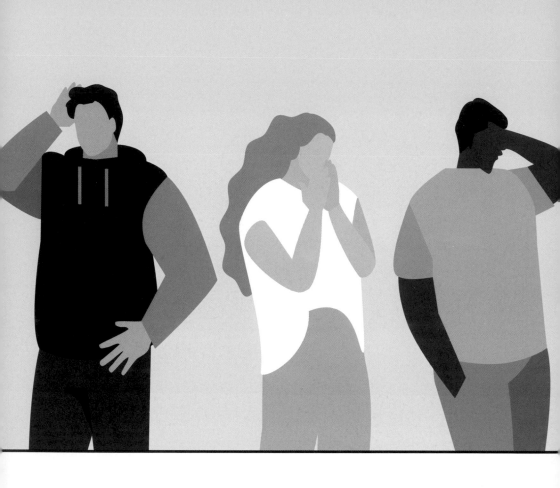

Borderline Personality Disorder

Antisocial Personality Disorder

Schizotypal Personality Disorder

Other Personality Disorders

 Paranoid Personality Disorder

 Schizoid Personality Disorder

 Histrionic Personality Disorder

 Narcissistic Personality Disorder

 Avoidant Personality Disorder

 Dependent Personality Disorder

 Obsessive-Compulsive Personality Disorder

For a complete list of DSM-5-TR disorders, see Appendix A.

CHAPTER 18

Personality Disorders

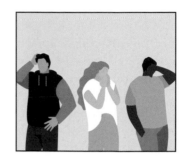

*P*ersonality refers to how people behave, their thoughts and views, and how they relate to others. All people have *personality traits* that make them unique and different from others. These traits are lasting patterns of how people tend to think about and relate to their own world, others, and self. Some people are outgoing; others are shy. Some people are self-assured; others are more humble. Personality traits can sometimes lead the person to have mild problems in relationships, or at school, work, or at home.

A *personality disorder* reflects deeper, more severe problems than the challenges caused by a personality trait. A personality disorder can greatly impair how someone thinks, feels, lives, works, and perceives and loves others every day. These are not sudden changes in the person but have been their way of life. People with a personality disorder tend to be unwilling to change, and often see little reason to change. Many people with these disorders do not realize they are not thinking or acting in a normal or healthy way.

DSM-5-TR describes 10 different personality disorders. All vary in their features. Some people with personality disorders often have trouble trusting others, and some may ignore their own safety, act on impulse, or risk the safety of others. They can behave in harmful ways, sometimes hurting themselves or breaking the law. Others can have shallow relationships and lifestyles. Still others make frequent demands based on their own needs and desires without regard for others. Some may always blame other people for their own behavior or problems. They often are not able to respond in a healthy way to others and to the changes and demands of life. Any of these features can cause distress for the person or for other people with whom they have relationships.

Personality disorders tend to arise in the late teen years or early 20s. It is rare for children to be diagnosed, which should be done with great caution because they are still growing and developing. The symptoms must be present for at least 1 year if so. Children often outgrow personality traits that might appear like a personality disorder by the time they are adults. Unlike other personality disorders, antisocial personality disorder cannot be diagnosed until the person is at least age 18.

A sudden change in personality in middle age or late life is unusual and requires a doctor's thorough review for a medical condition or substance use disorder. A sudden personality change at these ages is likely due to one of these causes rather than a personality disorder.

Features of a Personality Disorder

All types of personality disorders have these **common features**:
- A pattern of disturbed behavior that is different in an extreme way from what is expected in a person's culture, as shown in at least two of the following areas:
  - Ways of thinking about self, others, and events.
  - Ways of having and showing feelings in diverse settings. This includes the range and strength of feelings.
  - Ways of relating to other people.
  - Ways of controlling feelings and conduct.
- The pattern is fairly constant across a range of personal and social settings.
- The pattern causes marked distress or problems in social life, work, and other parts of daily life.
- The pattern started in the teen or early adult years.
- The behavior is not due to another mental disorder or the effects of a substance or another medical condition.

Personality disorders are grouped into three clusters based on their features and symptoms (Table 1). The personality disorders covered in full detail in this chapter are *borderline, antisocial,* and *schizotypal personality disorders;* other personality disorders are reviewed briefly. Most people who have a personality disorder will not have a single "pure" disorder, but will also have features of other personality disorders described in this chapter.

There has been much debate about the concept of personality and how personality disorders are diagnosed. Finding the line between personality traits and personality disorders involves many questions. Personality disorders are complex and the subject of a growing field of research.

Table 1. Personality disorders by DSM-5-TR cluster	
Cluster (or type) and key features	**Personality disorders**
Cluster A—appear odd or eccentric (marked by odd or strange thoughts, feelings, or behavior)	Paranoid personality disorder Schizoid personality disorder Schizotypal personality disorder
Cluster B—appear dramatic, emotional, or erratic (marked by drama, extreme shifts in feelings, and frequent changes in behavior beyond what is normal)	Antisocial personality disorder Borderline personality disorder Histrionic personality disorder Narcissistic personality disorder
Cluster C—appear anxious or fearful (marked by fear or worry)	Avoidant personality disorder Dependent personality disorder Obsessive-compulsive personality disorder

Borderline Personality Disorder

People with *borderline personality disorder* have a pattern of stormy relationships, extreme moods, and impulsive behavior that begins by early adulthood. They have intense fears of being abandoned. Extreme moods may include intense bouts of anger or anxiety that last a few hours, beyond what might be expected. At times, people with the disorder can hurt themselves (often by cutting with a sharp knife or razor) and ignore the safety of others. These extreme emotions and impulsive behaviors are not easy for them to prevent or control.

Bonds with family and friends are also strained and stressful because of their extreme moods. People with borderline personality disorder may profess intense love or esteem for someone that can quickly turn to intense anger or hate.

Borderline personality disorder affects about 2% of people in the United States. The rate of those with the disorder may decrease in older age. Symptoms tend to lessen and become more stable over time, often within 1–8 years of diagnosis.

☑ Borderline Personality Disorder

Borderline personality disorder is diagnosed when a pattern of troubled relationships, extreme changes in self-image, and acting on impulse begins by early adulthood, as shown by at least five of the following:

- Frantic efforts to prevent someone from leaving them.

- Pattern of unstable and intense relationships (may switch between extremes of loving someone one moment and then hating that person the next).

- A self-image marked by extreme and frequent changes (may switch between great self-confidence and very poor self-esteem).

- Risky behavior prone to impulse and self-damage, such as spending sprees, risky sex, substance abuse, reckless driving, and binge eating.

- Pattern of suicidal behavior or self-injury.

- Intense bouts of sadness or being anxious that last a few hours and only rarely more than a few days.

- Often feeling empty (such as feeling bored, sense of having no meaning or purpose).

- Intense anger beyond the scope of the issue, or problems with anger control (such as frequent physical fights or displays of temper, constant anger).

- Fleeting, stress-induced paranoid thoughts or feelings (may suspect others have bad motives or plans against them), or feeling "unreal" or detached from self or the world.

Risk Factors

Physical abuse, sexual abuse, and emotional neglect that occur in childhood are risk factors for the disorder. The disorder is about five times more common among first-degree blood relatives (parent or sibling) of those with the disorder.

Maria's Story

Maria, a single woman without a job, sought therapy at age 33 for treatment of depressed mood, chronic thoughts of killing herself, and having no social contact for many months. She had spent the last 6 months alone in her apartment, lying in bed, eating junk food, watching TV, and doing more online shopping than she could afford.

Maria was the middle of three children in a wealthy immigrant family. The father was said to value work success over all else. He often cursed at and hit all three children, Maria most of all. She felt alone through her school years and had bouts of feeling depressed. Within her family, she was known for angry outbursts. She had done well in high school but dropped out of college because of problems with a roommate and a professor. She had a series of jobs with the hope that she would return to college, but she kept quitting because "bosses are idiots." These "traumas" always left her feeling bad about herself ("I can't even succeed as a clerk!") and angry at her bosses ("I could run the place better than any of them").

She had dated men when she was younger but after a few weeks of "bliss at finding the perfect partner," she would feel hurt and angry when they did not pay enough attention to her or return her calls fast enough. She would end the relationship before they could "hurt me even more."

Maria sometimes cut herself (would make herself bleed using a knife on purpose) when she was feeling empty and depressed. She said that she was often "down and depressed," but that dozens of times for 1–2 days, she would act on impulse with great risk to her safety. This involved drug abuse and reckless driving. Doing these things would often make her feel better.

She had been in psychiatric treatment since age 17 and had stayed in a psychiatric hospital three times after overdoses. During the session, Maria described shame at her lack of job success. She believed she was very able and simply didn't know why she hadn't done better in life. Toward the end of the first session, she became angry with the doctor after he glanced at the clock (asking him, "Are you bored?"). In terms of social contact, she said she knew people who lived in her building, but most of them had become "frauds or losers." There were a few people from school who were "online friends" on social media who were doing "big things all over the world."

Maria was diagnosed with *borderline personality disorder* and *major depressive disorder*. She could not stay at jobs or in school and has problems with anger control, reckless acts, and self-harm (such as cutting). She often feels empty and has paranoid thoughts. Maria refused prescribed medications, stating, "When I take those drugs, I have no feelings. I can't even cry at a sad movie." Instead, she was referred for a form of psychotherapy called *dialectical behavior therapy* or DBT. It helps people know and manage their thoughts and feelings and teaches calming methods. DBT helped Maria learn how to feel more in control of her extreme feelings, as well as when she felt empty or paranoid. She learned skills to stop judging herself and others. After many months, she was able to get and keep a job. She was slowly able to have more healthy friendships with both women and men, but still struggled at times to get along with others.

Antisocial Personality Disorder

People with *antisocial personality disorder* have a widespread pattern of disregard for others. They may often be violent or hostile, break the law, con people, and ignore or infringe on the rights of others. These symptoms have an onset by age 15 years, and symptoms in those younger are diagnosed as conduct disorder. People with antisocial personality disorder often have been abused and neglected in childhood. They have learned to expect the world to be that way. They tend not to have remorse or regret for their actions—which can include fighting, lying, cheating, and stealing.

In relationships, those with antisocial personality disorder often show contempt for others' feelings, hardships, and pain that they may have caused. They may abuse their partners, have many partners, and act without regard for safe sex. They may fail to pay child support and neglect their children, who may not receive enough food, clothing, bathing, or other care and comfort. They can also suffer from tension, boredom, and *depressive, anxiety, substance use,* and *gambling disorders. Attention deficit/hyperactivity disorder* can also occur in people with antisocial personality disorder.

Up to 4% of adults in the United States have antisocial personality disorder, and it is more common in men. The disorder is common among those with severe *alcohol use disorder* and settings such as jails and prisons. People with this disorder tend to show the most extreme behaviors when they are younger and tend to improve as they grow older.

People with antisocial personality disorder often do not believe that they have any problem, nor do they seek mental health care. Their behaviors may be controlled in settings where there is great discipline, structure, and rules that prevent them from making bad choices, such as prison.

 Antisocial Personality Disorder

Since age 15, a person with antisocial personality disorder ignores or violates the rights of others as a common way of life, as shown by at least three of the following antisocial behaviors:

- Fails to follow social norms and laws, as shown by frequent acts that are grounds for arrest.
- Lies, uses fake names, or cons others for profit or pleasure.
- Lacks impulse control and fails to plan ahead.
- Is quickly annoyed, angry, and hostile, as shown by frequent fights or assaults.

- Lacks concern or care for the safety of self or others.
- Often shirks or ignores major duties, as shown by frequent failure to hold a job or pay debts.
- Lacks remorse (doesn't care about hurting, mistreating, or stealing from others).

In addition to the above, the person must meet each of these standards for the disorder:

- Is at least 18 years old.
- Shows signs of *conduct disorder* before age 15 (this involves breaking rules at home and school, or violating the rights of others, such as skipping school, fighting, or stealing).
- Displays antisocial behavior outside an episode of *bipolar disorder* or *schizophrenia*.

Risk Factors

Men with a first-degree blood relative (parent or sibling) with the disorder are at increased risk. Many persons with antisocial personality disorder have a history of emotional, physical, or sexual abuse in childhood.

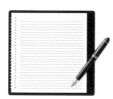

Liam's Story

Liam was a 32-year-old man referred for mental health treatment by the human resources (HR) department of a large construction firm where he had worked for 2 weeks. Before he began working there, Liam appeared very eager and gave proof of two carpentry school degrees that showed a high level of skill and training. Once Liam was employed, his boss noted he was often absent, argued with other workers, did poor work, and made mistakes that might have harmed others. When approached about these problems, Liam was not concerned, blaming the issues on "cheap wood" and "bad management" and said that if someone got hurt, "it's because they're stupid."

When the head of HR tried to fire Liam, he quickly pointed out that he had both attention-deficit/hyperactivity disorder (ADHD) and bipolar disorder. He said that if not granted a waiver under the law, he would sue. He demanded a psychiatric evaluation.

During the interview, Liam focused on how the firm was unfair and on how he was "a better carpenter than anyone else there." Twice divorced, he claimed that his two marriages had ended because of his wives' envy and doubt. He said that they were "always thinking I was with other women," which is why "they both lied to judges and got restraining orders saying I'd hit them." As payback for the jail time because he broke the judges' orders, he refused to pay child support for his two children. He had no desire to see either of his two boys because they were "little liars" like their mothers.

Liam said he "must have been smart" because he made Cs in school despite showing up only half the time. He spent time in a jail for youth at age 14 for stealing "kid stuff, like tennis shoes and wallets that were almost empty." He left school at age 15 after being "framed for stealing a car" by his principal. Liam said he smoked marijuana as a teen and started drinking alcohol on a "regular basis" after he first got married at age 22. He denied that use of either substance was a problem.

Liam ended the exam by asking the doctor to write a note that he had "bipolar" and "ADHD." He said that he was "bipolar" because he had "ups and downs" and got "mad real fast." He learned about ADHD because "both of my boys got it." He ended the exam with a demand for medications, adding that the only ones that worked for him were the "stimulant" medicines that his sons also received for ADHD.

The head of HR did a background check during the psychiatric evaluation, which revealed that Liam had been expelled from two carpentry training programs and that both his degrees were fakes. He had been fired from one local construction firm after a fistfight with his boss and from a second firm after leaving a job site. A quick review of their records showed that he had given them the same false papers. There was also a report that he tried to sell prescribed medicines to his coworkers for cash.

Liam was diagnosed with *antisocial personality disorder*. He has been arrested twice for partner violence—once from each marriage—and has spent time in jail. Liam has faked his carpentry degrees and gives ample proof of frequent fights and quickness to anger, both at work and within his relationships. He has no desire to see either of his young sons and neglects paying any child support. He shows no remorse for how his actions harm or deceive his family, coworkers, or employers. He often quits jobs and fails to plan for his next one. These factors and behaviors meet all seven symptoms for antisocial personality disorder.

Schizotypal Personality Disorder

People with *schizotypal personality disorder* are often seen as odd, strange, or quirky. They tend to distrust others and have bizarre beliefs. For instance, they may believe they have special powers to control others, read other people's minds, or predict events before they happen. They may seem stiff or awkward to others because their feelings are hard for them to manage.

They have few, if any, close ties other than with their parents or siblings. They prefer to keep to themselves. It is hard for them to pick up on social cues, such as eye contact. As they spend more time in a social setting, they tend not to become more relaxed around others (as do many people who are shy). Instead, they grow more tense and have more distrust of those around them. As children or teens, they may be often alone, may attract teasing because they appear odd to others, may be prone to social anxiety, may do poorly in school, and may have strange thoughts, language, and daydreams. They may have unusual interests, such as learning about the paranormal (spirit world) or telepathy (using thoughts to communicate with other people).

About 1% of the population may have this disorder. The disorder can first appear in children or teens and may be slightly more common in males. Between 30% and 50% of people with schizotypal personality disorder also suffer from *major depressive disorder.*

Some cultures or faiths have customs that are normal and accepted within these groups but that might be seen as schizotypal traits by those from outside. These customs might include mind reading or speaking in tongues. In these settings, the disorder is not diagnosed.

Schizotypal Personality Disorder

Schizotypal personality disorder involves a lasting pattern of impaired social contact as shown by extreme unease with—and reduced capacity for—close bonds, and includes odd thoughts and behavior and an altered sense of what is real. The pattern starts by early adulthood and is present in a range of settings, as shown by at least five of the following:

- Thoughts that daily, chance events have special meaning or contain a certain message for the person, when they do not.

- Odd beliefs that the person has special powers (such as sensing events before they happen, reading other people's minds, controlling other people through the person's own thoughts).

- Strange events perceived through the senses (such as sensing another person is in the room who is not there, or hearing a voice saying the person's name).

- Odd thinking and speech (such as speech that is vague or marked by tangents, strange phrasing or ways of linking words).

- Distrust of others or their motives (such as beliefs that others intend to harm the person or damage the person's status at work).

- Flat emotions or responses that do not fit the setting or event.

- Behavior or appearance that is outside social norms (such as not making eye contact, often wearing soiled or stained clothing when clean clothing exists).

- Lack of close friends outside close family.

- Extreme social anxiety that does not go away in known settings and is caused by distrust rather than the person's negative judgments about themself.

The pattern of behavior does not occur during the course of *schizophrenia* or a *bipolar, depressive, other psychotic,* or *autism spectrum disorder*.

Risk Factors

Schizotypal personality disorder runs in families. People with a first-degree blood relative (parent or sibling) who has *schizophrenia* are at a higher risk.

Other Personality Disorders

Other personality disorders in DSM-5-TR include *paranoid, schizoid, histrionic, narcissistic, avoidant, dependent,* and *obsessive-compulsive personality disorders.* These disorders are diagnosed when behaviors linked to the disorder are present in a range of home and social settings. They cause great distress or impair social, work, or other key aspects of function. They often begin in the late teen years or early adulthood.

Paranoid Personality Disorder

People with *paranoid personality disorder* distrust others and suspect others have ill motives toward them. They view the actions of other people as a threat, even those who are close to them or whom they see daily. They want to maintain complete control of close relationships to avoid being betrayed. They may challenge the places, actions, aims, and loyalty of their spouse or partner. They look for clues to support their fears. Because of their distrust, they tend to blame others for their own mistakes or verbally attack them. They can be guarded, hostile, and aloof, keeping their thoughts and feelings to themselves. The disorder is diagnosed when at least four of the following are present:

- Suspects, without good reason, that others exploit, harm, or deceive them.
- Is fixed on unfounded doubts about whether friends or fellow workers are loyal.
- Is slow to confide in others due to baseless fears of spiteful or unjust use of the information.
- Reads hidden insults or threats into harmless remarks or events.

- Holds lasting grudges (does not forgive insults or slights).
- Believes others attack their honor and standing when it is clear to others that this is not the case, and is quick to react with anger or verbal attacks.
- Often suspects, without good reason, that a spouse or sexual partner is cheating on them.

Symptoms do not occur during a time of *schizophrenia, bipolar* or *depressive disorder,* or another *psychotic disorder,* and are not due to another medical condition.

Schizoid Personality Disorder

People with a *schizoid personality disorder* lack a desire for close bonds with other people, are detached, and have a reduced range of feelings. They may be viewed as extreme loners. Praise or insults seem not to affect them. Anger may be hard for them to express, even if provoked. They may seem to drift through life without goals and seem passive to life events. They have few friends, tend not to marry, and yet may work well when left alone. They tend to seek out jobs where they have little contact with people. The disorder is diagnosed when at least four of the following are present:

- Neither desires nor enjoys close bonds with others, even if family.
- Almost always chooses to do things alone.
- Has little, if any, desire for sex with another person.
- Enjoys few, if any, activities.
- Lacks close friends other than first-degree blood relatives (parents, siblings).
- Appears not to care whether others praise, find fault, or insult them.
- Appears cold or detached, without any feelings.

Symptoms do not occur during a time of *schizophrenia, bipolar* or *depressive disorder*, another *psychotic disorder*, or *autism spectrum disorder*, and are not due to another medical condition.

Histrionic Personality Disorder

The word *histrionic* means "dramatic or theatrical." People with *histrionic personality disorder* have frequent, extreme feelings and seek constant attention. They strive to be "the life of the party" wherever they are. Those with this disorder use their looks, flirting, clothing, and other means to draw notice to themselves with others, even when they have no romantic interest in the other person. They may become depressed and upset if they are not the center of attention. The disorder is diagnosed when at least five of the following are present:

- Is not at ease or feels less valued when outside the center of attention.
- Relates to others by flirting or trying to seduce when it is not proper.
- Changes feelings quickly.
- Uses physical appearance to draw attention to themself (such as spending much time and money on grooming, hair, makeup, fancy clothing).
- Has a style of speech that is very vague and lacks detail or facts.
- Acts with extreme feelings and public displays of emotion and drama even with people not known well (such as nonstop sobbing, temper tantrums).
- Is easily swayed by others, current fads, or changes in events.
- Thinks of ties with others as closer and of more value than they actually are (for instance, someone met just once is a "dear, dear friend").

Narcissistic Personality Disorder

People with *narcissistic personality disorder* believe that they are more important and talented than other people and that others should admire them. They tend to have little or no concern for the needs of other people. They expect to be praised and feel they are owed rewards that others may get. They tend to take more credit than they deserve for success, and they don't admit or give credit to those who deserve it. They may not be aware that their remarks can hurt others (such as boasting of good health in front of someone who is sick). Despite high success, their work can suffer because they will not accept critiques to adjust or improve their work. The disorder is diagnosed when at least five of the following are present:

- Inflates talents and success and expects to be noticed as better than others.
- Is absorbed with notions of their own great and endless success, power, genius, beauty, or ideal love.
- Believes they are "special" and unique, and can only be known by or relate to other special or high-status people.
- Requires others to admire them on a constant basis.
- Believes they deserve or are owed special treatment (such as not needing to wait in lines) or that others should comply quickly with their demands.

- Exploits (takes advantage of) others to achieve their goals.
- Lacks concern or does not notice others' feelings or needs.
- Envies others' success or rewards, or believes that others envy them.
- Shows an arrogant (haughty, snobbish) behavior and/or attitude.

Avoidant Personality Disorder

People with *avoidant personality disorder* have extreme shyness, often feel inadequate (not good enough), fear criticism, are quickly hurt by rejection (being unwanted or turned away), and shun closeness or contact with others because of these feelings and fears. When in social settings, a person with avoidant personality disorder may be afraid to speak up for fear of saying the wrong thing or being shamed, teased, or put down. They greatly desire to be liked and to enjoy social contacts, but their extreme fears and shyness keep them from reaching out to others. The disorder is diagnosed when at least four of the following are present:

- Avoids work that requires social contact because of fears that others will criticize (find fault) or reject them.
- Avoids getting involved with people unless certain of being liked.
- Is restrained in close relationships because of the fear of being shamed or mocked.
- Greatly concerned about being criticized or rejected in social settings.
- Shy in new settings because of feelings of inadequacy (not being good enough).
- Feels inept, unpleasing, or inferior to others (low self-esteem).
- Doesn't take risks to engage in new social contacts or other pursuits (such as looking for a new job) for fear of being ashamed.

Dependent Personality Disorder

People with *dependent personality disorder* have a constant and extreme need to be taken care of that leads to meek and clinging behaviors and fears of separation (being parted from another person). They have an extreme need for support and being nurtured. They are passive and have trouble making daily choices (such as what to wear to work) without getting advice from someone else. They believe they cannot function on their own and must depend on someone else. They rely on others to solve their problems and often do not learn skills to live on their own. From early adulthood, they have a profound fear that the person they depend on will leave them. The disorder is diagnosed when at least five of the following are present:

- Has problems making daily choices without getting advice and support from others.
- Needs others to take charge of most major areas of their life.
- Does not express thoughts that differ from others for fear of losing support or approval.
- Has problems starting projects or doing things on their own because of lack of self-confidence.
- Goes to extremes to get support and care from others (may offer to do unpleasant tasks or withstand abuse if doing so seems to secure desired care).
- Feels distressed or helpless when alone because of fears that they cannot care for themself.
- Quickly seeks a new close relationship for care and support when the prior one ends.
- Maintains extreme focus on fears of being left to take care of themself.

Obsessive-Compulsive Personality Disorder

People with *obsessive-compulsive personality disorder* are very focused on order, being perfect, and controlling their own thoughts and the behavior of others who relate to them. As a result, they have trouble accepting unplanned changes and are not open to help from others unless things are done their way. They can become angry when they are not in control. They are often unable to express warm or tender feelings. The disorder is diagnosed when at least four of the following are present:

- Is absorbed with details, rules, lists, order, and schedules to the extent that the major point of the task is lost.
- Hinders or stops a project because their extreme and strict standards are not met (for instance, staying so focused on making each detail perfect that the project is never finished).
- Consumed by work and productivity at the expense of leisure pursuits and friendships (for instance, does not take a day off to go on an outing, does not relax on the weekend).
- Holds extreme, high moral and ethical standards (and may force others to follow these rigid rules).
- Cannot throw away worn-out or worthless objects even when they have no sentimental value.
- Is slow to give tasks or work to others unless their way of doing things is followed.
- Adopts a stingy spending style (frugal with self and others) and lives far below what they can afford in case of future bad events.
- Is rigid and stubborn.

Treatment

Many people with personality disorders get better over time with treatment. Some improve as they grow older. A personality disorder may worsen for a time if the person is under stress, such as with the loss of a loved one or a job. People with certain types of personality disorders are unlikely to seek treatment on their own, but if convinced to seek help, they can often benefit. Treating these disorders mostly involves forms of psychotherapy—often with both the person and group sessions. Many types of psychotherapy work well for people with borderline personality disorder, which can be quite disabling and can involve risky behavior.

There are no medications that are often used to treat any of the personality disorders. However, medications can help in treating some of the symptoms, such as feeling depressed or anxious. Medications can help those who tend to act on impulse, a common problem in people with borderline personality disorder. Types of medications that may help symptoms of personality disorders include the following:

- *Antidepressants* can help with low mood or feeling hopeless, guilty, or worthless.
- *Mood stabilizers* can help reduce extreme moods or mood swings of highs and lows.
- *Antipsychotics* may be used to help improve odd thinking and distrust, such as in schizotypal personality disorder. These medications can help stabilize moods and reduce impulsive behavior in borderline personality disorder.

Tips for Relating to People With Personality Disorders

- People with personality disorders should be treated with respect and kindness, even when their behavior is vexing and hard to deal with.
- It is hard for people with personality disorders to accept or grasp another person's point of view. By nature, people with personality disorders often have an intense and sole focus on themselves.
- People with personality disorders also can have many pleasing traits and major career success or other triumphs.
- Be honest about the person's behavior and its effect on the relationship.
- Set limits on harmful behavior and take steps to avoid repeat abuse.
- The underlying causes of a personality disorder are complex.
- A caring mental health care provider can help you to better know yourself, your choices, and the person with a personality disorder.

Source. Adapted from Yudofsky SC: *Fatal Flaws: Navigating Destructive Relationships With People With Disorders of Personality and Character.* Washington, DC, American Psychiatric Publishing, 2005. Copyright © 2005 American Psychiatric Publishing. Used with permission.

Key Points

- *Personality* refers to how people behave, their thoughts and views, and how they relate to others. All people have *personality traits* that make each person unique. These traits are lasting patterns of how people tend to think about and relate to their own world, others, and self. Personality traits can sometimes cause challenges in relationships or other settings from time to time.
- A *personality disorder* reflects deeper, more serious problems than the challenges sometimes caused by a personality trait. These disorders greatly impair how someone thinks, feels, lives, works, and perceives and loves others every day. Many people with these disorders do not realize they are not thinking or acting in a normal or healthy way.
- Many people with personality disorders get better over time as they grow older. People with certain types of personality disorders seldom seek treatment on their own. When convinced to seek help, they can often benefit.
- Treating these disorders mostly involves forms of psychotherapy—often with both individual and group sessions. No medications are approved as the main or sole treatment of any personality disorder. However, medications can help to treat some of the symptoms that a person with a personality disorder may have, such as feeling depressed, anxious, suspicious, moody, or prone to act on impulse.
- A mental health care provider can also help people in close or frequent contact with someone who has a personality disorder. Therapy can help them to know themselves and the other person better and find healthy ways to cope.

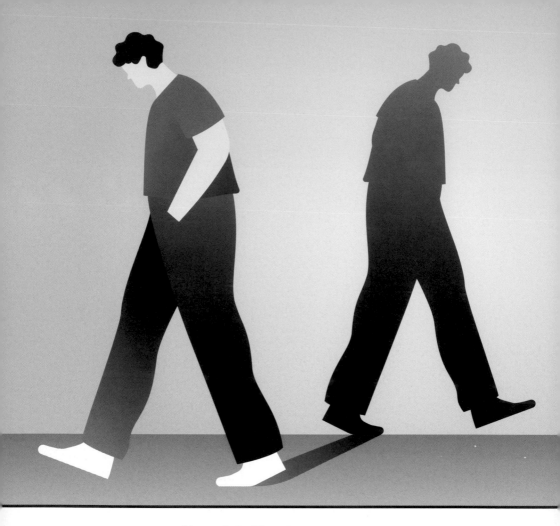

Voyeuristic Disorder

Exhibitionistic Disorder

Frotteuristic Disorder

Sexual Masochism Disorder

Sexual Sadism Disorder

Pedophilic Disorder

Fetishistic Disorder

Transvestic Disorder

For a complete list of DSM-5-TR disorders, see Appendix A.

CHAPTER 19

Paraphilic Disorders

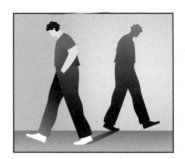

A*paraphilia* is a sexual interest or preference outside the sexual norm. Paraphilias tend to exclude actual sexual intercourse and do not cause harm or distress to self or others. Many types of paraphilias exist, and a person can have more than one type. Having a paraphilia does not by itself lead to a paraphilic disorder.

In contrast, a *paraphilic disorder* involves a paraphilia that causes distress; impaired work, social, or other key functions; or harm or risk of harm to self or others. These disorders often involve repeated, intense sexual fantasies and urges that the person then enacts in real life. Some of the paraphilic disorders are crimes because they risk harm to those who have not given consent for the action. Harm includes physical pain and mental anguish, torment, or distress. People with these disorders devote much time and energy to satisfying their sexual preference, and it may well cause problems in their job, marriage, and other aspects of life.

These disorders are more common in men and tend to be rare in women. Rates of these disorders are unknown. People with a paraphilic disorder may deny that they have the interest and behavior of the disorder. The disorders tend to begin in the teen years or 20s and are often lifelong.

Eight paraphilic disorders in DSM-5-TR are discussed in this chapter:

- *Voyeuristic disorder* (watching others engage in private acts without their consent).

- *Exhibitionistic disorder* (exposing one's genitals to someone who has not given consent).
- *Frotteuristic disorder* (touching or rubbing against a person who has not given consent).
- *Sexual masochism disorder* (seeking one's own pain or humiliation for sexual arousal).
- *Sexual sadism disorder* (causing hurt or humiliation of another person for one's own sexual arousal when the other person has not given consent).
- *Pedophilic disorder* (forcing children to engage in sexual activities because of being sexually aroused by children).
- *Fetishistic disorder* (using nonliving objects for sexual arousal or having a highly specific focus on nongenital body parts).
- *Transvestic disorder* (dressing in the clothes of the opposite gender for sexual arousal).

Voyeuristic Disorder

People with *voyeuristic disorder* are sexually aroused by spying on another person who is naked, undressing, or having sex.

 Voyeuristic Disorder

- For at least 6 months, there has been repeated and intense sexual arousal—as shown in fantasies, urges, or behaviors—from watching an unsuspecting person who is naked, undressing, or engaging in sexual activity.
- The person has acted on these sexual urges without consent of the person watched, or the sexual urges or fantasies cause much distress or impair social, work, or other key aspects of function.
- The person who is aroused or acting on the urges is at least 18 years old.

Exhibitionistic Disorder

People with *exhibitionistic disorder* expose their genitals to strangers (children or adults) who have not given consent for this act. This is often referred to as "flashing."

Exhibitionistic Disorder

- For at least 6 months, there has been repeated and intense sexual arousal—as shown in fantasies, urges, or behaviors—from exposing one's genitals to an unsuspecting (unaware) person.
- The person has acted on these sexual urges without consent of the other person, or the sexual urges or fantasies cause much distress or impair social, work, or other key aspects of function.

Frotteuristic Disorder

People with *frotteuristic disorder* touch or rub against others without their consent. This often happens in crowded places, such as a busy sidewalk or subway car. This may or may not include touching someone's genitals or breasts.

 FrottLeuristic Disorder

- For at least 6 months, there has been repeated and intense sexual arousal—as shown in fantasies, urges, or behaviors—from touching or rubbing against a person who has not given consent.
- The person has acted on these sexual urges without consent of the other person, or the sexual urges or fantasies cause much distress or impair social, work, or other key aspects of function.

Sexual Masochism Disorder

Sexual masochism disorder involves getting sexually aroused when being beaten, bound (tied up), humiliated, or otherwise made to suffer. People with the disorder may also inflict pain on themselves by choking or pricking themselves with sharp objects. Sexual acts may occur with a partner and include being tied up, spanked, or whipped. One dangerous form of sexual masochism involves cutting off oxygen by tying a noose around their neck or putting a plastic bag over their face. There is a risk of accidental death with these acts.

Sexual Masochism Disorder

- For at least 6 months, there has been repeated and intense sexual arousal—as shown in fantasies, urges, or behaviors—from being humiliated, beaten, bound (tied up), or made to suffer in other ways.
- The fantasies, sexual urges, or behaviors cause much distress or impair social, work, or other key aspects of function.

Sexual Sadism Disorder

People with *sexual sadism disorder* get sexually excited by causing pain, suffering, or humiliation in another person without their consent. The other person's distress, physical harm, risk of harm, or mental anguish counts toward the diagnosis. If the sexual sadism urges or fantasies are not acted on, having distress or impaired work or social function meets the standards for the diagnosis.

 Sexual Sadism Disorder

- For at least 6 months, there has been repeated and intense sexual arousal—as shown in fantasies, urges, or behaviors—from the physical or mental suffering of another person.
- The person has acted on these sexual urges without consent of the other person, or the sexual urges or fantasies cause much distress or impair social, work, or other key aspects of function.

Pedophilic Disorder

People with *pedophilic disorder* have a strong sexual interest in or sexual preference for children who have not started puberty and have acted on these urges. Use of pornography that features young children (generally age 13 years and younger) is a strong sign of the disorder, because it reflects sexual interest. When a person acts on this interest or urge and engages in sexual activity with a child, it is a criminal act.

Pedophilic Disorder

- For at least 6 months, repeated, intense sexually arousing fantasies, sexual urges, or behaviors involving sexual activity with a child (generally age 13 years or younger) have been present.
- The person has acted on these sexual urges, or the sexual urges or fantasies cause much distress or relationship problems.
- The person is at least 16 years old and at least 5 years older than the child or children involved in the act.

Fetishistic Disorder

People with *fetishistic disorder* become sexually excited by objects, such as women's underwear, rubber articles, and men's or women's shoes. A fetish (sexual fixation) also may involve a body part, such as feet, toes, and hair. Having contact with these objects (for instance, through holding, tasting, or rubbing) often leads to intense arousal and masturbation. Some people with the disorder may have a large collection of desired objects.

 Fetishistic Disorder

- For at least 6 months, there has been repeated and intense sexual arousal—as shown in fantasies, urges, or behaviors—from either using nonliving objects or a highly specific focus on nongenital body part(s).
- The fantasies, sexual urges, or behaviors cause much distress or impair social, work, or other key aspects of function.
- The fetish objects are not limited to articles of clothing used in cross-dressing or devices designed for genital stimulation (such as a vibrator).

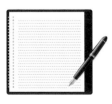 ## Leonard's Story

Leonard is a 65-year-old salesman for a large firm. He sought an evaluation by a psychiatrist after his wife threatened to leave him because of his sexual interest in women's undergarments. Although he said he was embarrassed to discuss this issue with a stranger, he described his sexual interest in a matter-of-fact manner. This interest had begun decades earlier, but he hadn't acted on it until recently.

Leonard's habit began with his wife's severe arthritis and likely depression, both of which reduced her overall activity and interest in sex. His "fetish" was the bright spot during his frequent and otherwise dreary business trips. He masturbated about twice weekly, using bras and panties that he had collected over several years. He also masturbated at home with these undergarments but waited until his wife was out of the house. He said that intercourse with his wife had faded to "every month or two" but was still mutually satisfying.

He was caught masturbating by his wife 6 weeks before the evaluation. Upon seeing him dressed in panties and a bra, she "went nuts." She "shut him out" and hardly spoke to him. When they argued, she called him a "pervert" and made it clear that she was considering divorce unless he "got help."

Leonard had been married for over 30 years, and the couple had two grown children. He had planned to retire comfortably later that year, but not if the two choices were either to "split the assets or to sit around the house and be called a pervert all day." He had made a show of throwing away a half dozen pieces of underwear, which had seemed to reassure his wife, but he had saved his "favorites" and "could always buy more." He did not want to end his marriage, but he saw nothing harmful in his fetish. "I'm not unfaithful or doing anything bad," he says. "It just excites me, and my wife certainly doesn't want to be having sex a few times a week."

Leonard denied any problems with his sexual function, adding that he could maintain erections and achieve orgasm without women's undergarments. He recalled being aroused when he touched women's underwear in his teenage years and had masturbated often to that experience.

Leonard was diagnosed with *fetishistic disorder*. His long history of sexual arousal from women's underwear had not caused problems until he was caught wearing women's underwear by his wife. At that point, Leonard began to feel distress. If his wife accepted or embraced his fetish and his own distress faded, he would likely no longer have a disorder.

Leonard was referred to an expert in sexual disorders. In therapy, Leonard learned that while the fetish harmed no one, it distressed his wife, who felt that he had lost interest in her. Leonard was encouraged to better communicate with his wife, and to focus on satisfying their mutual sexual needs. Leonard was still aroused by women's undergarments, but learned to make these fantasies a part of his sexual relationship with his wife.

Transvestic Disorder

People with *transvestic disorder* become sexually aroused from dressing in the other gender's clothing (cross-dressing). It often involves a man wearing only one or two articles of women's clothing (such as underwear), or it can involve dressing completely in a woman's inner and outer garments, as well as wigs and makeup. Transvestic disorders tend to begin in childhood or early teenage years.

 Transvestic Disorder

- For at least 6 months, there has been repeated and intense sexual arousal—as shown in fantasies, urges, or behaviors—from cross-dressing.
- The fantasies, sexual urges, or behaviors cause much distress or impair social, work, or other key aspects of function.

Treatment

People with paraphilic disorders can receive treatment that helps improve their day-to-day function. Paraphilic disorders are usually treated with psychotherapy to help the person become aware of their paraphilic thoughts and behaviors and to gain control over them. This may involve cognitive-behavior therapy (CBT). CBT helps the person gain control over their interests and acts, and to achieve goals in healthy ways. For some paraphilic disorders, psychotherapy can help to focus on the other partner and satisfying the partner's sexual needs. A paraphilia may still exist, but in some cases it may be used as a healthy part of sexual relationships. Relaxation training is often a part of the therapy to help lower the anxiety and stress that the paraphilic disorder may cause. Relapse prevention techniques help the person avoid falling back into an unhealthy or harmful cycle of inappropriate sexual behavior. These techniques also may help target problems with eating, sleeping, and social function.

There are no medications approved to treat paraphilic disorders, but these disorders are often linked with depression or anxiety that may benefit from treatment. Treatment for these symptoms may include one of the selective serotonin reuptake inhibitor (SSRI) antidepressants. Because *depressive* or *anxiety disorders* may help fuel the paraphilic disorder, treating these disorders may be an important first step in helping the person regain control over their desires and behavior. The SSRIs also may help to reduce the fantasies and urges that can fuel the paraphilic disorder. In some cases, medications that lower testosterone (hormone) levels are sometimes given to men whose sexual behavior is out of control and could cause harm to others, such as those with pedophilic disorder.

Key Points

- A *paraphilia* is a sexual interest or preference outside the sexual norm. Paraphilias tend to exclude actual sexual intercourse and do not cause harm or distress to self or others. Many types of paraphilias exist, and a person can have more than one type. Having a paraphilia does not by itself lead to a paraphilic disorder.

- A *paraphilic disorder* involves a paraphilia that causes distress; impaired work, social, or other key functions; or harm or risk of harm to self or others. These disorders often involve repeated, intense sexual fantasies and urges that the person then enacts in real life. Some of the paraphilic disorders are crimes because they risk harm to those who have not given consent for the action. Harm includes physical pain and mental anguish, torment, or distress.

- People with paraphilic disorders can receive treatment that helps improve their day-to-day function. Paraphilic disorders are usually treated with psychotherapy to help the person be aware of their paraphilic thoughts and behaviors and to gain control over them. This often involves cognitive-behavior therapy.

- For some paraphilic disorders, psychotherapy can help to focus on the other partner and satisfying the partner's sexual needs. A paraphilia may still exist, but in some cases it may be used as a healthy part of sexual relationships.

- There are no medications approved to treat paraphilic disorders, but these disorders are often linked with depression or anxiety that may benefit from treatment. Because *depressive* or *anxiety disorders* may help fuel the paraphilic disorder, treating these disorders is an important first step in helping the person regain control over their desires and behavior.

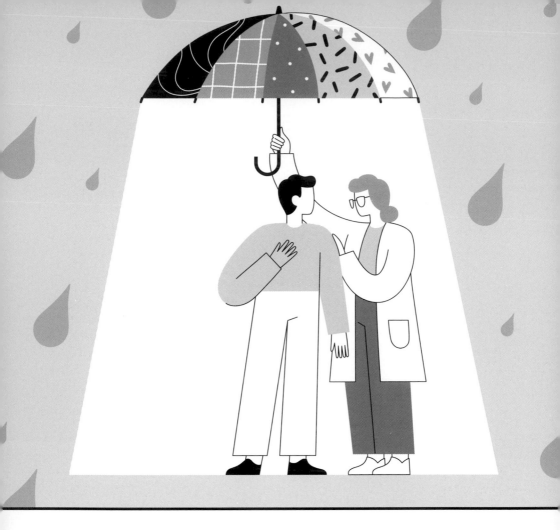

Who Can Help

What Happens Next

    Interview

    Diagnosis

    Treatment

Forms of Treatment

    Psychotherapy

    Psychiatric Medications

    Neuromodulation Techniques

Getting Better and Staying Healthy

    Caring for Your Body

    Caring for Your Mind and Emotions

    Caring for Others

For a complete list of DSM-5-TR disorders, see Appendix A.

CHAPTER 20

Treatment Essentials

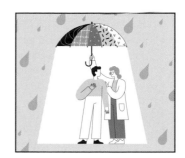

Mental illness, just like other medical disorders, can be treated with success. Treatment can bring relief from distressing symptoms, provide better coping skills, and give hope. All the mental disorders in this book can be treated using one of the methods described in this chapter.

How does someone know when to seek help? A helpful approach is to think about how much a problem has caused trouble or bothered someone, and how long it has lasted. These problems may be hard to admit or say aloud, such as a secret substance habit, a childhood trauma, or frequent fears and worries. When these problems cause great distress or disrupt work, relationships, or other key aspects of life, it is wise to seek help (see box for early warning signs). What makes mental disorders differ from the normal problems of daily life is how serious they are and how long they last. The sooner a person seeks treatment, the sooner they can begin their recovery.

Who Can Help

There are several types of mental health care providers who can help.

- **In case of emergency:** In the United States, anyone can call or text **988** if they are having thoughts of suicide or are concerned about someone who is. The line is open 24 hours a day, 7 days a week for any mental health crisis.

- *Psychiatrists* are licensed medical doctors who have finished medical school, as well as a 4-year psychiatric residency. The residency program gives in-depth training in neurology (study of the human brain), psychopharmacology (how medicines work in the body and brain), psychotherapy ("talk therapy"), and patient care in hospitals and clinics. A psychiatrist can prescribe medication for patients and can provide psychotherapy. If the patient desires, a psychiatrist may suggest a psychologist, licensed clinical social worker, or marriage and family therapist for psychotherapy. Psychiatrists also can admit patients to a hospital for treatment and can provide electroconvulsive therapy (ECT; described later in this chapter in "Forms of Treatment") if that is needed. Psychiatrists have M.D. or D.O. degrees.
- *Psychologists* have finished a graduate program, which includes clinical training, an internship, and postdoctoral clinical experience (client care) in various forms of psychotherapy and psychological testing. They cannot prescribe medications or admit people to hospitals in most states. States require that psychologists be licensed to treat cli-

ents. The degree is either a Ph.D. or Psy.D. Some specialize in treating children or families.

- *Licensed clinical social workers* have finished a 2-year graduate program in specialized training helping people with mental health problems in addition to conventional social work. Some social workers also have doctorate degrees. To practice, they must be licensed by a state. Their credential is L.C.S.W.
- *Marriage and family therapists* are licensed in some, but not all, states and have a graduate or doctoral degree in psychology or a similar field. To practice, they must have at least 2 years of postdegree supervised clinical training with a focus on couples and family treatment. They must also pass a state or national exam. Their credential is L.M.F.T.
- *Psychiatric nurses* have nursing degrees and have passed a state examination. They usually have special training and experience in mental health care, although no special licensing or certification is required. Their credential is R.N.
- *Nurse practitioners* and *physician assistants* can treat patients and prescribe medications under the general supervision of a doctor. Nurse practitioners are identified by the credentials A.P.R.N. or A.R.N.P., and other credentials depending on specialty. Physician assistants are identified by the credential P.A.

To find a mental health care provider, ask for names from your doctor, other mental health care providers you may know, or friends who know of mental health care providers. Some of the support groups found through organizations listed in Appendix C, "Helpful Resources," may be able to suggest names. If you have health insurance, you can ask for a list of mental health care providers who accept your insurance.

People may also seek help from their primary care doctor or a physician assistant when they have health problems. These health problems (such as problems with sleep) might be linked to a mental disorder. Primary care doctors and physician assistants can prescribe medications for mental health care concerns, may team up with mental health care providers to provide care, or may refer their patients to a mental health care provider.

What Happens Next

The usual way of making first contact with a mental health care provider is to call their office to schedule an appointment. Some mental health care providers may want some background information before the visit. Those seeking mental health care who have served in the U.S. military can contact the U.S. Department of Veterans Affairs (VA).

Interview

The first visit involves an evaluation (or "interview") with the mental health care provider. The provider will talk with you to learn about yourself and the problems you are having. Mental health care providers will ask detailed questions to invite you to discuss your problem. Just as a doctor may ask patients about their health problems, a mental health care provider will have the same approach. This information helps the mental health care provider create a unique treatment plan for you. The first visit may last 45–90 minutes. Some common questions during a first visit include the following:

- What brings you here today? (Be ready to talk about a problem you're having or a change you want to make.)
- How have you been feeling?
- What do you think has caused your problem, if anything?
- What symptoms are bothering you?
- What problems have they caused?

Based on your problems and symptoms, mental health care providers also will ask about the following: family history, work history, education, leisure activities or hobbies, relationships, values, cultural background, medical history, past psychiatric history (if any, such as whether other mental health care providers were seen in the past), developmental history, and sexual history.

The mental health care provider may ask permission to obtain more information (such as from medical records) and suggest psychological or lab tests. You may be asked to schedule a physical exam with your primary care doctor if prescribed medications for a mental disorder are needed—or if a medical disorder needs to be ruled out that may be causing the psychiatric symptoms. In some cases, a diagnosis or an initial assessment will require another one or two sessions, and sometimes the mental health care provider will request permission to interview a partner or family member.

Diagnosis

The mental health care provider will diagnose the problem using DSM-5-TR guidelines. (DSM does not provide treatment guidelines, only guidelines for diagnosis.) The mental health care professional can then form a treatment plan. The mental health care professional and the person seeking care make decisions together about treatment.

More than one disorder may be diagnosed, such as *panic disorder* and *agoraphobia*. Many people with mental disorders also have a *substance use disorder*. People may turn to alcohol or drugs to ease the symptoms or emotional pain they feel. In some cases, the alcohol or drugs may cause a mental disorder, worsen its symptoms, hinder progress and efforts to get better, and disrupt effects of other medications taken for the disorder.

Treatment

Treatment for mental disorders is offered in a range of settings. The most common setting is an outpatient clinic (that is, a mental health care provider's office or a clinic).

People who pose an urgent risk for harming themselves or others, or who are gravely disabled, may need to be hospitalized. Most seriously ill people want to get help, but sometimes they refuse hospital treatment and the doctor may seek a court order to hospitalize them involuntarily (against their will). The amount of time the court grants for involuntary hospital care depends on state law, and these laws differ widely in the United States. Usually, a hearing is held to determine if the person should remain in the hospital (this process may vary by state). If they remain gravely ill, or still are a threat to themselves or others, they may stay in the hospital involuntarily for a longer period of care.

After hospital care, patients often return to the outpatient clinic for needed continued care, but sometimes they are referred to a partial hospitalization service connected with an inpatient psychiatric unit. These programs provide daily treatment on a one-on-one basis with a psychiatrist and other mental health care providers, as well as group therapy. This type of care lasts until patients improve enough to be referred to a psychiatric outpatient clinic—often for about 2–4 weeks.

Left untreated, a mental disorder can increase the risk for suicide. For this reason, those who have suicidal thoughts and feelings, their family members, and their loved ones should learn about warning signs. Thoughts and feelings about suicide should never be ignored. The following tips can help (see box).

Recovery-Focused Care

Recovery from mental illness is a process of change in which people improve their health and wellness and are helped to regain control over their lives. The goal is to have a full life even with mental health symptoms. Recovery-focused care centers on what the person can control; their strengths, abilities, and interests; and ways to maintain hope. Recovery-focused care is not a type of treatment but is an approach to care that can be used with any type of treatment, including medication and psychotherapy. It can also be used in support groups after treatment. This type of care focuses on the person and not on the diagnosis, yet takes into account the person's symptoms. Talking with mental health care providers about this approach at any point of treatment can offer help and guidance. Recovery-focused care can help people with any type of mental illness, including substance use disorders, schizophrenia and other psychotic disorders, and trauma-based disorders.

Forms of Treatment

There are many treatment options for mental disorders (Table 1). Treatment aims to help people cope with their symptoms and lead a full life. The main types of treatment include medication and psychotherapy. Medications and psychotherapy may be used alone or together. Often combining psychotherapy with medication provides a more powerful response. Psychotherapy can also help loved ones know how to better care for those with a disorder and to better cope with the impact of the disorder.

For many disorders, medication can ease symptoms. As people start to improve with use of psychiatric medications, other problems may surface that may have been hidden or were not the main cause of concern in seeking treatment (such as how they relate to others). People may be able to give more focus to other behaviors they see that have added to their problems and need to change. Psychotherapy can help people learn how to better cope and think about their problems. In the process of treatment, even those who have endured trauma or years of suffering often discover within themselves strengths they may have never known. As they work toward recovery, they can learn more gratifying ways of living and acting and rebuild self-esteem.

When medications and psychotherapy have not worked well, some people have found help from *neuromodulation techniques*. These techniques stimulate the nerves to create a natural response. Electroconvulsive therapy (ECT) and transcranial magnetic stimulation are safe and helpful treatments when medications have not worked for severe symptoms of certain disorders, such as *major depression*.

Psychotherapy

Psychotherapy ("talk therapy") refers to any type of counseling based on the exchange of words in the context of the unique relationship that develops between a mental health care provider and a person seeking help. The process of talking and listening can lead to new insights, relief from symptoms that cause distress, changes in unhealthy or maladaptive behaviors, and more effective ways of dealing with the world.

There are many different types of psychotherapy, and some are more effective for certain problems, or for certain people, than others. Most mental health care providers today are trained in a variety of techniques and tailor their approach to the problem, personality, and needs of the person seeking help. Because mental health care providers may combine different techniques during therapy, the lines between the various approaches are often blurred.

Conversations with a mental health care provider are the foundation of mental health treatment. The relationship that grows between the person and the mental health care provider is called the *therapeutic alliance*. This working relationship allows them to work together in a trusting, cooperative manner. The mental health care provider works with the per-

Table 1. Treatments for mental disorders	
Psychotherapy	**Psychiatric medications**
Psychodynamic psychotherapy	Antidepressants
Interpersonal therapy	Antipsychotics
Supportive psychotherapy	Sedatives, hypnotics, and
Cognitive-behavior therapy	anxiolytics
Dialectical behavior therapy	Mood stabilizers
Behavior therapy	Stimulants
Couples, marital, and family therapy	**Neuromodulation techniques**
Group therapy	Electroconvulsive therapy
	Transcranial magnetic
	stimulation

son to develop mental health goals for the person's mental well-being. There will be tasks and activities to move toward these goals. In psychotherapy, the mental health care provider focuses on the needs of the person. Anything shared in a session with a mental health care provider is kept private. Mental health care providers are bound by ethics and the law not to divulge any information without the person's consent. The exception is if there is likely harm to the person or others.

Psychodynamic Psychotherapy

Psychodynamic psychotherapy aims to help people gain insight into their problems and bring about change. This approach involves face-to-face meetings with a mental health care provider, building a therapeutic alliance, and interpretation and clarification of what the person says. This therapy often focuses on conflicts that arose in childhood that have had lingering effects in adulthood. People most likely to benefit from this treatment are those who have enough knowledge and insight to have, express, and explore intense emotions. The therapy may be brief, with fewer than 25 sessions, or longer term, lasting for several years.

Interpersonal Therapy

Interpersonal therapy is intended to enhance relationships and social interactions and improve interpersonal skills. It uses techniques such as reassurance and support, clarification of feelings, and improving interpersonal communication. People most likely to benefit are those with *major depression,* marital problems, or problems building relationships and interacting with others. The therapy often consists of 12–16 sessions, but may be longer for maintenance treatment (after problems are under control, therapy may go on to prevent relapse). This approach, first used for research into the treatment of depression, focuses on relationships to help deal with unrecognized feelings and needs and improve interpersonal and communication skills. Unlike other psychodynamic treatments, it does not deal with the psychological root of symptoms but focuses on current problems.

Supportive Psychotherapy

Supportive psychotherapy is the most common type of psychotherapy. It seeks to maintain or restore a person's highest possible level of function. It involves the therapist's concern, advice, reassurance, suggestion, reinforcement (a technique that encourages desired response through a system of rewards and/or punishment), discussion of alternative behaviors, teaching of social/interpersonal skills, and help in problem solving. People most likely to benefit from this approach are those in highly stressful situations, those with severe medical illness, and those with mental disorders who do not benefit from other approaches. The therapy may be brief (a single session or several sessions over a period of days or weeks) to long term (over many years), based on the nature of the problem.

Any form of psychotherapy or counseling that offers reassurance, empathy, and education is supportive. The goal of supportive psychotherapy is to help people to adapt and to return to their normal or prior best level of function to the extent possible given personality, life events, ability, or illness.

Cognitive-Behavior Therapy

The goal of *cognitive-behavior therapy* (CBT) is to identify and change distortions in thinking, as well as problem behaviors. It uses such techniques as identifying beliefs and attitudes; spotting negative thought patterns and unhelpful behaviors; education in other ways of thinking and responding; cognitive rehearsal (reviewing in one's mind how to respond differently than in the past); and homework assignments. CBT addresses negative views of oneself, negative understandings of experience, and negative views of the future. Sometimes people are not aware that they hold these automatic negative views of themselves or their experiences. CBT helps people learn that they can achieve small successes that make a meaningful and positive difference in their lives. People most likely to benefit are those with *major depression, anxiety disorders, obsessive-compulsive disorder, eating disorders, insomnia, substance use disorder,* and *trauma-related disorders.* The length of treatment often is brief, about 15–25 sessions.

Dialectical Behavior Therapy

Dialectical behavior therapy (DBT) helps people know and manage their thoughts and feelings and teaches calming methods. It can teach people to learn how to feel more in control of extreme feelings. At the same time, the mental health care provider coaches people to understand their own duty to change behavior that is risky and causes upset or problems.

DBT builds a strong and equal relationship between the person in treatment and the mental health care provider. The mental health care provider often reminds the person when behavior is not healthy or causes problems, such as when limits are broken. Needed skills are taught to better deal with future events. DBT involves both one-on-one and group therapy. One-on-one sessions are used to teach new skills, while group sessions provide the chance to practice these skills.

DBT has been helpful in the treatment of those who have *borderline personality disorder* and thoughts of suicide. It is also used for those with *major depression, posttraumatic stress disorder, eating disorders, substance use disorders,* and traumatic brain injury.

Behavior Therapy

Behavior therapy aims to replace unhealthy patterns of behavior with more healthy ways of behaving and coping with stress, fear, or worry. It uses a range of techniques to help people who want to change their behavior. People most likely to benefit are those who want to change habits and those with *anxiety disorders* (such as *phobias*), panic attacks, and *substance use* or *eating disorders.* The length of treatment often is brief and consists of less than 25 sessions.

The basic methods of behavior therapy include:

- *Behavior modification*, which focuses on a negative habit or behavior.
- *Systematic desensitization*, which teaches how to reduce or control fear triggered by certain things (such as animals or elevators) or settings (such as being out in public).
- *Relaxation training,* which helps individuals to control their physical and mental state.
- *Exposure therapy,* which involves gradual stages of direct exposure to a feared object or situation to control anxiety without the use of relaxation techniques. *Exposure and response prevention therapy* can be helpful for people with *obsessive-compulsive disorder*. This teaches them to stop doing a compulsion (a repeated act, such as hand washing) when exposed to the feared or unpleasant object.
- *Flooding,* which exposes people to what they fear most and keeps them exposed to the feared item or setting with the aid of the mental health care provider until their fear lessens.
- *Assertiveness training,* which teaches people to express their feelings and thoughts honestly and directly.

Couples, Marital, and Family Therapy

Couples, marital, and family therapy seeks to change relationships, improve communications and interactions, and teach better ways to resolve conflicts. Those most likely to benefit are couples or families who want to change their basic ways of interacting, and children or teenagers with mental disorders or troubling behaviors. The treatment can last for weeks or months. In one-on-one psychotherapy, the focus is on the person within a couple or family. In couples, marital, and family therapy, the focus is on the two persons in a relationship, or on the entire family. The way they relate to one another or feel about the other is the focus. Depending on the nature of the problem, mental health care providers may suggest a mix of one-on-one and couples or family therapy.

Although some mental health care providers work with individuals as well as with couples and families, many specialize in marital and family therapy. It can be hard for couples or families to know when they should seek help for their problems. Their concerns may seem minor or petty, but even small things sometimes can be a sign of a greater underlying problem. As with individual symptoms, the key issue is to find out how severe or how long the problem has endured.

Couples or marital therapy tends to be brief, lasting for weeks or months. Common issues include communication difficulties, sexual problems, and differing views of what partners expect from the relationship. The goal is to identify and resolve the issues as quickly as possible. Therapy begins with the partners identifying problems or areas in which they would like to see some change. A husband may report that his wife complains that he neglects his share of child care, while the wife may feel overwhelmed by the demands of their young children. The mental health care provider may help them pinpoint target behaviors that need to be changed and contract with each other to modify these behaviors in small, specific ways. The techniques are the same for opposite-sex and same-sex couples.

Family therapy involves treatment with one person who is the patient or client and at least one member of their family. Often the entire family is involved. The mental health care provider may meet with various family members separately, as well as with the entire family. The focus is on the *interaction* between people rather than on a single person's way of thinking or the content or nature of a certain problem.

There are two common types of family therapy. *Behavioral family therapy* views problem behaviors as the result of family attention and rewards that support the behavior. *Structural family therapy* stresses the value of family structure for helping the family function, as well as its impact on the well-being of its members.

Group Therapy

Group therapy seeks to change ways of relating with others and relieve distressing psychological symptoms. It provides a helpful way for mental health care providers to follow up with and monitor a group of patients or clients at the same time. It also provides patients or clients with a social environment (and peer group) that will help them learn new and healthier ways to interact with others in a controlled and supportive environment.

It uses basic approaches of supportive, cognitive-behavior, psychodynamic, or interpersonal therapy; self-disclosure and catharsis (the release of feelings through talking and expressing them); sharing of insight and information; and feedback from peers and the mental health care provider. Group therapy most often benefits those who have a similar mental or physical disorder (for instance, an *eating disorder* or *posttraumatic stress disorder*); teens; psychiatric patients in hospital care; and families of people with mental disorders. Group therapy has a brief or long-term time frame.

Groups take place in many settings such as psychiatric hospitals, community mental health centers, health maintenance organizations, teaching hospital clinics, and private offices. Mental health care providers in private practice may organize groups based on similar issues or needs. Psychotherapy groups that usually meet once a week can be a key part of treatment for a wide range of common mental health problems.

Psychiatric Medications

Many kinds of psychiatric medications are labeled by what they work against, with the use of "anti" in their name (for example, *anti*psychotics, *anti*depressants). It's helpful to know that psychiatric medications do not rid a person of a mental illness or cure it, but they can greatly help the person's symptoms.

Psychiatric medications are thought to work by helping the person's body make more or less of the chemical substances called *neurotransmitters* already in their brain and other parts of their body. These chemical substances (such as serotonin and dopamine) are stored in the nerves. They are released throughout the day, traveling from one nerve and into the next. Over time, a medication can change the amount of a neurotransmitter. The effect can help a person with a mental illness make desired changes in their behaviors, moods, and thoughts that are not possible to make through their own effort.

Psychiatric medications can affect every aspect of a person's physical, mental, and emotional function, such as alertness, attention, coordination, energy, mood, judgment, sleep patterns, and interpersonal relationships. Some of these medications take effect at once; others do not have an effect right away. Some continue to exert their effects long after they are no longer being taken. Medications often used to treat mental health problems and shown to be helpful are listed in Appendix B, "Medications."

The doctor will consider each person's needs and symptoms to prescribe the medications that have a good fit. Medications or doses can be adjusted as needed to ensure the person's best response. In prescribing these medications, psychiatrists and other doctors must consider many factors (see box below).

What Doctors Review Before They Prescribe Medications

- **Allergies**—Allergies to certain chemicals in medications will rule out those medicines.
- **Lifestyle**—Some medications must be taken at certain times or have detailed rules for taking them.
- **Age**—This affects how medications are metabolized (or processed) in the body. Older adults may metabolize certain drugs more slowly or may be more prone to certain side effects.
- **Family history**—Presence of mental disorders in family members.
- **General medical health and history of medical problems**—Some illnesses can cause symptoms that mimic or bring on a mental health disorder. If not recently done, a full physical exam is given, along with blood and laboratory tests and, if needed, brain-imaging scans.
- **Other medicines and supplements used**—These may cause side effects or other problems with certain prescribed medications.
- **Medication issues**—Benefits and risks of certain medications for the person seeking care:
  - Although most psychiatric medications are not habit forming, some can be addicting and must be prescribed with care.
  - Many medications can cause side effects that range from mildly irritating (such as dry mouth) to more bothersome (dizziness or constipation) to life threatening (seizures or irregular heart rhythm). In general, side effects tend to be most common and troubling when the drugs are first taken, and most tend to lessen or end after a few weeks.
  - Patients' concerns about side effects—often a different medication can be prescribed if certain side effects do not make the medication a good match for the patient.

Tips to Help Medications Work Best

- Take the medication as the doctor directs.
- Ask if there are any foods, other medications, or supplements to avoid with the prescribed medication.
- Ask if the medication should be taken with food or at certain times of day.
- Know what to expect with side effects. Ask questions and talk about any concerns with the doctor. Ask about how best to cope with side effects.
- Set a helpful routine to make sure the medications are taken every day.
- **Do not stop a medication right away or decrease the dose without checking with the doctor first.** If some medications are stopped right away or the dose is quickly reduced, they may cause harm and unpleasant symptoms—or can make symptoms of the mental disorder worse.
- Pay close attention to how the medicines are working or not working, even as time passes. After a while, the body can adjust to medications, symptoms can improve or worsen, and the doctor may need to adjust the dose or switch medications.
- Even after you feel better and seem to have no symptoms—or if you dislike the side effects—know that medications will help you get and stay better. You may feel better because the medicines are working.
- Seek your doctor's advice for any questions or concerns that you have about your medications.

People who take psychiatric medication should have follow-up visits with their doctor to see whether it is working, or perhaps causing side effects that are unhealthy or unpleasant (see box above on tips to help medications work best). The right medication and dose are needed to help resolve symptoms. This may take time as the dose is adjusted or another medication is tried. Trying different medications or doses may be needed to see what works best. The medication must be taken long enough for them to work. Sometimes weeks or months must pass for the full effects to take hold.

For some mental disorders, people may need to take the medication every day for the rest of their lives, just as a person might take insulin or high blood pressure medicines every day. When this happens, a person is in *maintenance treatment*. This means a person's symptoms are under control or improved enough so that they function better in daily life. The person should keep taking the medication under the doctor's care to maintain its positive effects. The person should see the doctor at scheduled office visits from time to time. The doctor will make sure the medicine is still working, that no side effects are causing problems, and that the person is doing well, with their symptoms well controlled. This will help to prevent *relapse*—a return to harmful symptoms of the disorder and problems that can result.

Antidepressants

Most of today's antidepressants help relieve symptoms and have few side effects. The word "antidepressant" is somewhat misleading because these medications are used to treat many conditions other than depression. They can be effective in treating *panic disorder, posttraumatic stress disorder, generalized anxiety disorder, social phobia, obsessive-compulsive disorder, borderline personality disorder, bulimia nervosa,* irritable bowel syndrome, *attention deficit/hyperactivity disorder, autism spectrum disorder,* smoking cessation, chronic pain, and migraine headaches.

The major types of antidepressants include the selective serotonin reuptake inhibitors (SSRIs), serotonin-norepinephrine reuptake inhibitors (SNRIs), tricyclic antidepressants, tetracyclic antidepressants, and monoamine oxidase inhibitors (MAOIs). About 60%–70% of people who are prescribed a medication will improve. Combined treatment, which involves both drug therapy and psychotherapy, has proved most effective in treating depression and in lowering relapse rates.

Doctors weigh many factors in choosing an antidepressant, such as the person's medical status, history of manic or hypomanic episodes, prior bouts of depression, prior responses to an antidepressant, and the presence of symptoms such as increased sleep, weight gain, or anxiety, or psychotic symptoms, such as delusions or hallucinations.

Antidepressants do not work right away. A good response to these medications takes time. Although a few people may have some improvement, such as increased energy, by the end of the first week, most do not see major benefits for 3–4 weeks. Because doses are increased slowly for some medications, 5–6 weeks may pass from the time a person takes the first pill until the symptoms are relieved, and 8 weeks or longer until the medication has its full impact.

The various types of antidepressants produce different side effects. Many common side effects, such as dry mouth or nausea, subside after several weeks. Although bothersome, these effects do have a positive meaning: the drug is working and levels of the drug in the body are rising. Even when side effects are annoying, it is critical to keep taking the medication long enough for it to be of help and to keep increasing the dose as directed until symptoms improve.

Antipsychotics

Antipsychotics are used to treat psychotic symptoms, such as delusions and hallucinations. These medications can be roughly divided into two groups: 1) older antipsychotics first introduced in the 1950s and 1960s; and 2) newer, or atypical, antipsychotics introduced in the 1990s and later. The atypical antipsychotics account for most antipsychotic prescriptions now.

Antipsychotics are the preferred medications for the treatment of *schizophrenia* and other psychoses, and they have also been a key part in the treatment of manic and depressive symptoms in persons with *bipolar disorder*. Antipsychotic medications are also used to treat psychotic symptoms linked with drug abuse, behavior problems that may occur with *dementia* and *autism spectrum disorder*, and moodiness and impulsivity that occur in patients with *borderline personality disorder*.

The choice of antipsychotic agents is based on their safety and how well side effects are tolerated. Some side effects are extreme but can be treated. One side effect is a symptom called *akathisia*, which is a feeling of restlessness in the lower limbs and inability to sit still. Other side effects are more serious. *Tardive dyskinesia* consists of movements of the mouth and tongue (and sometimes other parts of the body) not done on purpose; the side effect is less common with the newer atypical antipsychotics. A rare but serious side effect is *neuroleptic malignant syndrome.* It causes someone to become rigid and develop fever, rapid heartbeat, abnormal blood pressure, rapid breathing, and changes in mental state ranging from confusion to coma. This condition is a medical emergency.

Antipsychotic medications may cause a drop in blood pressure, dizziness, increased blood lipids, increased blood glucose (sugar levels), high blood pressure, and weight gain. Like most other drugs, antipsychotic agents should be avoided if possible during pregnancy and when mothers are breast-feeding. This is a hard decision since the doctor must balance the low risk of birth defects in the child with the high risk of psychosis in the mother. Use of some antidepressants may increase or decrease the amount of antipsychotic medication to treat the underlying condition. Cigarette smoking can decrease the levels of some antipsychotic medications in the blood, thus making them less effective.

Sedatives, Hypnotics, and Anxiolytics

Sedatives or *anxiolytic medications* are often used to treat anxiety and insomnia. *Hypnotic* agents are medications that are used to cause and maintain sleep.

In some cases, anxiolytics are used to treat *panic disorder* until the effects of the antidepressant medication take hold. *Benzodiazepines* are one class of anxiolytics. They have muscle relaxant and anticonvulsant features (that is, they help control seizures). They need to be used with care because they can be habit forming (addicting). Only a few of the benzodiazepines are approved for the treatment of insomnia, but almost all are used for this purpose. Alcohol should be used in moderation or avoided because its effects are increased with these medications.

All benzodiazepines have similar effects. The choice should be based on how long the medication stays in the blood, how fast it works, how it is processed in the body, and how potent it is. Major side effects of benzodiazepines are sedation, dizziness, and impairment in use of machinery, such as driving a car. Benzodiazepines are sometimes abused; in these cases, patients may be at risk for drug withdrawal if the medication is stopped too quickly. Withdrawal could include symptoms such as nausea, vomiting, tremors, and even seizures. Other common signs of withdrawal are increased blood pressure, rapid heartbeat, panic attacks, memory problems, and worsening of anxiety.

Another anxiolytic is buspirone. It does not interact with alcohol or benzodiazepines, affect the ability to complete tasks or operate machinery, or pose a risk of abuse. It is prescribed for the treatment of *generalized anxiety disorder*, but is not used to treat *panic disorder*. Common side effects are nausea, nervousness, insomnia, and dizziness.

Hypnotic agents, or sleep medications, are prescribed for a brief time to help with sleep. They are short-acting drugs that produce a limited amount of daytime sleepiness. They should only be used in the short term, to decrease the risk of dependence. Another agent that causes sleep is ramelteon, which works on melatonin, a hormone that controls sleep and wake cycles.

Mood Stabilizers

Mood stabilizers help reduce mood swings from highs and lows that occur in patients with *bipolar disorder*. Mood stabilizer medications include lithium, valproate, carbamazepine, lamotrigine, and atypical antipsychotics. Some mood stabilizers are also anticonvulsant medications and are useful in treating seizures. Mood stabilizers each vary in side effects, potential for drug interactions, and the way the body processes them.

- *Lithium* is effective for the acute and preventive treatment of both manic and depressive episodes in patients with *bipolar disorder*. It is also effective in preventing future depressive episodes in patients with recurrent *major depression*. Lithium is the only mood stabilizer for which blood levels of the drug are measured to ensure it is within the needed range to help. As with most medications, lithium is started at a low dose and slowly increased over time. It may produce hypothyroidism, a change in the heartbeat, weight gain, tremors, decreased blood count, and stomach symptoms.
- *Valproate* is used to treat mania and other phases of *bipolar disorder*. Initial side effects of valproate are nausea, sedation, and hand tremor.

Doctors may slowly increase the dose to reduce the side effects. Some people may start at a much higher dose. Valproate should not be used in someone with liver disease. Valproate also may produce changes in blood counts, heartburn, indigestion, weight gain, or drowsiness.

- *Carbamazepine* and *oxcarbazepine* are used to prevent and treat mania. The most serious side effects of carbamazepine are a major decrease in white blood cell count and red blood cells (aplastic anemia) and the ability of the blood to clot. It also may affect the liver, cause a rash, and lower thyroid hormone levels in the blood. It also can produce drowsiness, dizziness, and difficulty walking. Oxcarbazepine does not require blood or liver tests and has fewer side effects than carbamazepine.
- *Lamotrigine* is used to prevent depression in people with *bipolar disorder*. A major side effect is a serious rash that may require treatment in a hospital. To lower the risk of a rash, doctors prescribe lamotrigine at a low dose and slowly increase it over several weeks.

Stimulants

Stimulants are often prescribed for *attention-deficit/hyperactivity disorder* (ADHD), which is more common in boys than girls. These medications are mostly used to treat children but may be used in adults. They are often prescribed by pediatricians and primary care doctors.

There is a major concern in the United States that stimulants are being overused in children and adults with ADHD, and some who do not have the disorder. Most children with ADHD will respond to stimulants, in terms of having improved focus to learn and do schoolwork. Nonstimulant medications are available and can be prescribed to treat ADHD, such as atomoxetine or guanfacine.

Side effects of stimulants are specific to the age group. The principal side effects of stimulants are insomnia, irritable mood, and elevated blood pressure. Side effects such as excitability, increased activity, talkativeness, and irritability may be seen as the last dose of the day wears off or for several days if there is a sudden stop to the stimulant medication. The symptoms would be similar to the original ADHD symptoms. A small number of children being treated with stimulants may develop psychotic symptoms.

Neuromodulation Techniques

Neuromodulation treatments are the least common kind of psychiatric treatment, but they can be very effective when a patient does not respond to other treatments. Neuromodulation treatments actively and safely stimulate nerves, through an electrical or magnetic current, to create a natural response.

Electroconvulsive Therapy

Electroconvulsive therapy (ECT) involves the passage of a controlled electrical current through the brain to induce a brief seizure. ECT is one of the best treatments for *major depression* and some cases of *mania* and *schizophrenia*. As many as 80%–85% of depressed persons who undergo ECT improve.

The mild electrical stimulation affects many of the brain chemicals and receptors involved in depression. Because anesthesia and muscle-relaxing drugs are used before the electrical current is given (through electrodes attached to the scalp), patients do not feel any pain, and their muscles do not shake or jerk. Despite its well-known benefits as a safe, reliable, and effective treatment, ECT is still viewed with distrust by many in the general public. This attitude stems largely from outdated misperceptions of ECT as painful or dangerous.

ECT is the treatment of choice for those with *major depression* who are suicidal, for those who have psychotic symptoms, or for those whose disorder is life threatening, possibly because they refuse to eat and drink. Other people likely to benefit are men and women with depression who:

- Do not improve with other approaches, including psychotherapy and a trial of at least two antidepressant drugs.
- Have psychotic symptoms, such as delusions.
- Need a treatment that produces rapid results because of the danger of suicide or harm to themselves.
- Have had previous depressions that did not improve when treated with antidepressant drugs.
- Have improved with ECT in the past.

Transcranial Magnetic Stimulation

Transcranial magnetic stimulation of the brain is a new form of treatment for *depression* for those whose symptoms have not improved after trying two or three antidepressant medications. The treatment uses a device that creates an electronic pulse that is sent to certain areas of the brain. The pulse is sent through electrodes that are placed on the scalp. Patients report few side effects. In contrast to ECT, a seizure is not induced.

Getting Better and Staying Healthy

Getting help from a mental health care provider is a great start toward getting better. Treatments take time to work and alone will not provide a total cure. Getting better depends on the nature of the problem, the therapy selected, and the skill of the mental health care provider. More than anything else, the hard work of the person seeking help and the support of their loved ones are key. It takes courage to get better. Keep trying each day and don't give up. The following sections list other things to do that can improve your health and treatment.

Caring for Your Body

- Exercise has proven to be good not only for the body, but also for the mind. It is particularly beneficial for depression. It is also an effective means of reducing anxiety. Physical exercise can also relieve tension and enhance the sense of well-being and overall health.
- A healthy, well-balanced diet should be part of every treatment plan. This includes leafy greens, vegetables, fruit, beans, lean meats, fish, and whole grains. Poor eating habits such as skipping meals, eating too quickly, or eating too much junk food (lots of sugar or fast food) can make people physically uncomfortable and psychologically unwell. A healthful balanced diet can improve health and help someone feel better.
- Getting enough sleep each night has great benefits for the mind and body. Aim for 7–8 hours a night and for a set bedtime and wake time. Cut off caffeine, nicotine, alcohol, and exercise a few hours before bedtime, and end screen time (TV, computer, and phone) at least 1 hour before bedtime. Breathing exercises and meditation are helpful to relax and wind down for restful sleep.
- High amounts of caffeine can cause anxiety or panic attacks and worsen these conditions. Alcohol can also make mental health symptoms worse and can interact in sometimes harmful ways with medications.

Caring for Your Mind and Emotions

- Avoid negative self-talk. Focus on things you like about yourself and those things that you do well.
  - Ask others you trust if you cannot think of positive things about yourself.
  - Notice and stop yourself if you often criticize yourself, blame yourself, or feed worries by focusing on the worst outcome over and over. These frequent thoughts can make you feel worse without making anything better. They do not reflect the whole truth and may even be false.

- Create a more positive point of view. See setbacks or losses as one-time events—not as judgments on you or your whole life.
  - The key to change is getting rid of the automatic negative thoughts that may flood your brain.
  - Replace them with positive truths.
  - Keep a list with you of your strengths and what you value in your life to remind yourself of what is important.
- Humor often allows us to express fears and negative feelings without causing distress to ourselves or others. It also may produce enhanced physical well-being. Since we laugh often with others, humor helps in forging supportive relationships.

Caring for Others

- Build friendships to give and receive support. In relationships, people may find that some problems are easier to put into perspective. Reaching out to others is important.
- Doing good things enhances self-esteem and may relieve physical and mental stress. Find ways to help others that you enjoy or are linked to your hobbies.
- Peers or peer-support groups can offer empathy, build morale, and create a new social world for persons dealing with similar life issues. Talking with people who have similar problems is highly useful for those with mental disorders. Hospitals, community health centers, and local mental health organizations often sponsor support groups. By participating, people may develop a sense of connectedness with others who have similar problems.

Key Points

- Seek help for mental health problems when they keep causing distress or problems with work, close relationships, or other key aspects of life. Know the early warning signs for mental illness, such as eating or sleeping too much or too little, pulling away from people and usual activities, having low or no energy, and thinking of harming yourself or others.
- There are many types of qualified mental health care providers available. These include psychiatrists, psychologists, licensed clinical social workers, marriage and family therapists, and psychiatric nurses. These mental health care providers can also work with pri-

mary care doctors, nurse practitioners, and physician assistants who prescribe medicines. Support groups can provide help and improve coping (see Appendix C, "Helpful Resources").

- Many treatments are available for nearly all the psychiatric disorders. Psychotherapy, medication, or a combination of the two can be used. Neuromodulation techniques, such as electroconvulsive therapy (ECT), are also modern, proven, and safe treatments for certain mental disorders when other treatments have not worked.
- Treatment improves health and quality of life. Left untreated, mental disorders often get worse and lead to more problems and distress. Trying to relieve mental health symptoms with drugs or too much alcohol worsens mental disorders and raises the risk of other problems.
- You can improve and maintain your mental health by getting exercise, eating a healthy diet, sleeping well every night, avoiding too much caffeine or alcohol, keeping focused on positive truths, laughing often, building friendships, and helping others.

Complete List of Mental Disorders in DSM-5-TR

These disorders are listed in the order and groupings found in DSM-5-TR.

Neurodevelopmental Disorders

Intellectual Developmental Disorders

Intellectual Developmental Disorder (Intellectual Disability)
Global Developmental Delay
Unspecified Intellectual Developmental Disorder (Intellectual Disability)

Communication Disorders

Language Disorder
Speech Sound Disorder
Childhood-Onset Fluency Disorder (Stuttering)
Social (Pragmatic) Communication Disorder
Unspecified Communication Disorder

Autism Spectrum Disorder

Autism Spectrum Disorder

Attention-Deficit/ Hyperactivity Disorder

Attention-Deficit/Hyperactivity Disorder
Other Specified Attention-Deficit/ Hyperactivity Disorder
Unspecified Attention-Deficit/ Hyperactivity Disorder

Specific Learning Disorder

Specific Learning Disorder

Motor Disorders

Developmental Coordination Disorder
Stereotypic Movement Disorder

Tic Disorders

Tourette's Disorder
Persistent (Chronic) Motor or Vocal Tic Disorder
Provisional Tic Disorder
Other Specified Tic Disorder
Unspecified Tic Disorder

Other Neurodevelopmental Disorders

Other Specified
 Neurodevelopmental Disorder
Unspecified Neurodevelopmental
 Disorder

Schizophrenia Spectrum and Other Psychotic Disorders

Schizotypal (Personality) Disorder
Delusional Disorder
Brief Psychotic Disorder
Schizophreniform Disorder
Schizophrenia
Schizoaffective Disorder
Substance/Medication-Induced
 Psychotic Disorder
Psychotic Disorder Due to
 Another Medical Condition

Catatonia

Catatonia Associated With
 Another Mental Disorder
Catatonic Disorder Due to
 Another Medical Condition
Unspecified Catatonia

Other Specified Schizophrenia
 Spectrum and Other Psychotic
 Disorder
Unspecified Schizophrenia
 Spectrum and Other Psychotic
 Disorder

Bipolar and Related Disorders

Bipolar I Disorder
Bipolar II Disorder
Cyclothymic Disorder
Substance/Medication-Induced
 Bipolar and Related Disorder
Bipolar and Related Disorder Due
 to Another Medical Condition
Other Specified Bipolar and
 Related Disorder
Unspecified Bipolar and Related
 Disorder
Unspecified Mood Disorder

Depressive Disorders

Disruptive Mood Dysregulation
 Disorder
Major Depressive Disorder
Persistent Depressive Disorder
Premenstrual Dysphoric Disorder
Substance/Medication-Induced
 Depressive Disorder
Depressive Disorder Due to
 Another Medical Condition
Other Specified Depressive
 Disorder
Unspecified Depressive Disorder
Unspecified Mood Disorder

Anxiety Disorders

Separation Anxiety Disorder
Selective Mutism
Specific Phobia
Social Anxiety Disorder
Panic Disorder
Agoraphobia
Generalized Anxiety Disorder
Substance/Medication-Induced
 Anxiety Disorder
Anxiety Disorder Due to Another
 Medical Condition
Other Specified Anxiety Disorder
Unspecified Anxiety Disorder

Obsessive-Compulsive and Related Disorders

Obsessive-Compulsive Disorder
Body Dysmorphic Disorder
Hoarding Disorder
Trichotillomania (Hair-Pulling
 Disorder)
Excoriation (Skin-Picking)
 Disorder
Substance/Medication-Induced
 Obsessive-Compulsive and
 Related Disorder
Obsessive-Compulsive and
 Related Disorder Due to Another
 Medical Condition
Other Specified Obsessive-
 Compulsive and Related Disorder

Unspecified Obsessive-
Compulsive and Related
Disorder

Trauma- and Stressor-Related Disorders

Reactive Attachment Disorder
Disinhibited Social Engagement
Disorder
Posttraumatic Stress Disorder
Acute Stress Disorder
Adjustment Disorders
Prolonged Grief Disorder
Other Specified Trauma- and
Stressor-Related Disorder
Unspecified Trauma- and Stressor-
Related Disorder

Dissociative Disorders

Dissociative Identity Disorder
Dissociative Amnesia
Depersonalization/Derealization
Disorder
Other Specified Dissociative
Disorder
Unspecified Dissociative Disorder

Somatic Symptom and Related Disorders

Somatic Symptom Disorder
Illness Anxiety Disorder
Functional Neurological Symptom
Disorder (Conversion Disorder)
Psychological Factors Affecting
Other Medical Conditions
Factitious Disorder
Other Specified Somatic Symptom
and Related Disorder
Unspecified Somatic Symptom
and Related Disorder

Feeding and Eating Disorders

Pica
Rumination Disorder
Avoidant/Restrictive Food Intake
Disorder
Anorexia Nervosa

Bulimia Nervosa
Binge-Eating Disorder
Other Specified Feeding or Eating
Disorder
Unspecified Feeding or Eating
Disorder

Elimination Disorders

Enuresis
Encopresis
Other Specified Elimination
Disorder
Unspecified Elimination Disorder

Sleep-Wake Disorders

Insomnia Disorder
Hypersomnolence Disorder
Narcolepsy

Breathing-Related Sleep Disorders

Obstructive Sleep Apnea Hypopnea
Central Sleep Apnea
Sleep-Related Hypoventilation
Circadian Rhythm Sleep-Wake
Disorders

Parasomnias

Non–Rapid Eye Movement
Sleep Arousal Disorders
Nightmare Disorder
Rapid Eye Movement Sleep
Behavior Disorder

Restless Legs Syndrome
Substance/Medication-Induced
Sleep Disorder
Other Specified Insomnia
Disorder
Unspecified Insomnia Disorder
Other Specified Hypersomnolence
Disorder
Unspecified Hypersomnolence
Disorder
Other Specified Sleep-Wake
Disorder
Unspecified Sleep-Wake Disorder

Sexual Dysfunctions

Delayed Ejaculation
Erectile Disorder
Female Orgasmic Disorder
Female Sexual Interest/Arousal
  Disorder
Genito-Pelvic Pain/Penetration
  Disorder
Male Hypoactive Sexual Desire
  Disorder
Premature (Early) Ejaculation
Substance/Medication-Induced
  Sexual Dysfunction
Other Specified Sexual
  Dysfunction
Unspecified Sexual Dysfunction

Gender Dysphoria

Gender Dysphoria
Other Specified Gender Dysphoria
Unspecified Gender Dysphoria

Disruptive, Impulse-Control, and Conduct Disorders

Oppositional Defiant Disorder
Intermittent Explosive Disorder
Conduct Disorder
Antisocial Personality Disorder
Pyromania
Kleptomania
Other Specified Disruptive,
  Impulse-Control, and Conduct
  Disorder
Unspecified Disruptive, Impulse-
  Control, and Conduct Disorder

Substance-Related and Addictive Disorders

Substance-Related Disorders

Alcohol-Related Disorders

Alcohol Use Disorder
Alcohol Intoxication
Alcohol Withdrawal
Alcohol-Induced Mental Disorders
Unspecified Alcohol-Related
  Disorder

Caffeine-Related Disorders

Caffeine Intoxication
Caffeine Withdrawal
Caffeine-Induced
  Mental Disorders
Unspecified Caffeine-Related
  Disorder

Cannabis-Related Disorders

Cannabis Use Disorder
Cannabis Intoxication
Cannabis Withdrawal
Cannabis-Induced
  Mental Disorders
Unspecified Cannabis-Related
  Disorder

Hallucinogen-Related Disorders

Phencyclidine Use Disorder
Other Hallucinogen Use Disorder
Phencyclidine Intoxication
Other Hallucinogen Intoxication
Hallucinogen Persisting
  Perception Disorder
Phencyclidine-Induced Mental
  Disorders
Hallucinogen-Induced Mental
  Disorders
Unspecified Phencyclidine-
  Related Disorder
Unspecified Hallucinogen-
  Related Disorder

Inhalant-Related Disorders

Inhalant Use Disorder
Inhalant Intoxication
Inhalant-Induced
  Mental Disorders
Unspecified Inhalant-Related
  Disorder

Opioid-Related Disorders

Opioid Use Disorder
Opioid Intoxication
Opioid Withdrawal
Opioid-Induced Mental Disorders
Unspecified Opioid-Related
  Disorder

Sedative-, Hypnotic-, or
Anxiolytic-Related Disorders

Sedative, Hypnotic, or Anxiolytic
Use Disorder

Sedative, Hypnotic, or Anxiolytic
Intoxication

Sedative, Hypnotic, or Anxiolytic
Withdrawal

Sedative-, Hypnotic-, or Anxiolytic-
Induced Mental Disorders

Unspecified Sedative-, Hypnotic-,
or Anxiolytic-Related Disorder

Stimulant-Related Disorders

Stimulant Use Disorder

Stimulant Intoxication

Stimulant Withdrawal

Stimulant-Induced
Mental Disorders

Unspecified Stimulant-Related
Disorder

Tobacco-Related Disorders

Tobacco Use Disorder

Tobacco Withdrawal

Tobacco-Induced Mental Disorders

Unspecified Tobacco-Related
Disorder

Other (or Unknown) Substance–
Related Disorders

Other (or Unknown) Substance
Use Disorder

Other (or Unknown) Substance
Intoxication

Other (or Unknown) Substance
Withdrawal

Other (or Unknown) Substance–
Induced Mental Disorders

Unspecified Other (or Unknown)
Substance–Related Disorder

Non-Substance-Related
Disorders

Gambling Disorder

Neurocognitive Disorders

Delirium

Other Specified Delirium

Unspecified Delirium

Major and Mild
Neurocognitive Disorders

Major or Mild Neurocognitive
Disorder Due to Alzheimer's
Disease

Major or Mild Frontotemporal
Neurocognitive Disorder

Major or Mild Neurocognitive
Disorder With Lewy Bodies

Major or Mild Vascular
Neurocognitive Disorder

Major or Mild Neurocognitive
Disorder Due to Traumatic Brain
Injury

Substance/Medication-Induced
Major or Mild Neurocognitive
Disorder

Major or Mild Neurocognitive
Disorder Due to HIV Infection

Major or Mild Neurocognitive
Disorder Due to Prion Disease

Major or Mild Neurocognitive
Disorder Due to Parkinson's
Disease

Major or Mild Neurocognitive
Disorder Due to Huntington's
Disease

Major or Mild Neurocognitive
Disorder Due to Another
Medical Condition

Major or Mild Neurocognitive
Disorder Due to Multiple
Etiologies

Major or Mild Neurocognitive
Disorder Due to Unknown
Etiology

Unspecified Neurocognitive
Disorder

Personality Disorders

Cluster A Personality Disorders

Paranoid Personality Disorder
Schizoid Personality Disorder
Schizotypal Personality Disorder

Cluster B Personality Disorders

Antisocial Personality Disorder
Borderline Personality Disorder
Histrionic Personality Disorder
Narcissistic Personality Disorder

Cluster C Personality Disorders

Avoidant Personality Disorder
Dependent Personality Disorder
Obsessive-Compulsive
  Personality Disorder

Other Personality Disorders

Personality Change Due to
  Another Medical Condition
Other Specified Personality
  Disorder
Unspecified Personality Disorder

Paraphilic Disorders

Voyeuristic Disorder
Exhibitionistic Disorder
Frotteuristic Disorder
Sexual Masochism Disorder
Sexual Sadism Disorder
Pedophilic Disorder
Fetishistic Disorder
Transvestic Disorder
Other Specified Paraphilic
  Disorder
Unspecified Paraphilic Disorder

Other Mental Disorders

Other Specified Mental Disorder
  Due to Another Medical
  Condition
Unspecified Mental Disorder Due
  to Another Medical Condition
Other Specified Mental Disorder
Unspecified Mental Disorder

Appendix B

Medications

The following medications are commonly used in the treatment of mental disorders. *Note:* Availability of generic and brand name medications can change over time. Where brand names are noted, generic versions are also often available.

Generic name	Common brand name(s)	Medication class/use[a]
acamprosate	generic only	mixed-action agent used to treat chronic alcohol use disorder
alprazolam	Xanax, Xanax XR	benzodiazepine used to treat anxiety
alprostadil injection	Caverject, Caverject Impulse, Edex	prostaglandin inhibitor used to treat erectile disorder
amitriptyline	generic only	tricyclic antidepressant
amoxapine	generic only	tetracyclic antidepressant
amphetamine-dextroamphetamine	Adderall, Adderall XR	combination stimulant used to treat ADHD
amphetamine sulfate	Evekeo, Evekeo ODT, Adzenys XR-ODT	combination stimulant used to treat ADHD
aripiprazole	Abilify, Abilify Mycite	second-generation antipsychotic
aripiprazole (intramuscular injection ER)	Abilify Maintena, Aristada, Aristada Initio	second-generation, long-acting antipsychotic
armodafinil	Nuvigil	stimulant used to treat narcolepsy and sleep apnea

Generic name	Common brand name(s)	Medication class/use[a]
asenapine	Saphris, Secuado	second-generation anti-psychotic
atomoxetine	Strattera	nonstimulant used to treat ADHD
avanafil	Stendra	phosphodiesterase inhibitor used to treat erectile disorder
benztropine	generic only	anticholinergic agent used to treat Parkinson's disease and abnormal movements induced by antipsychotic medications
brexanolone	Zulresso	used to treat postpartum depression
brexpiprazole	Rexulti	used with other therapies to treat major depressive disorder and schizophrenia
buprenorphine	Belbuca, Buprenex, Butrans, Sublocade	partial opioid agonist used to treat chronic opioid use disorder
buprenorphine and naloxone	Zubsolv	partial opioid agonist and an opioid antagonist used to treat chronic opioid use disorder
bupropion	Aplenzin, Forfivo XL, Wellbutrin SR, Wellbutrin XL	mixed-action antidepressant also used to aid smoking cessation and to treat ADHD
buspirone	generic only	anxiolytic used to treat anxiety
carbamazepine	Carbatrol, Epitol, Equetro, Tegretol, Tegretol XR, Teril	anticonvulsant also used to treat bipolar disorder and pain disorders
cariprazine	Vraylar	second-generation antipsychotic also used to treat bipolar disorder

Generic name	Common brand name(s)	Medication class/use[a]
chlordiazepoxide	Librium	benzodiazepine used to treat anxiety and alcohol withdrawal
chlorpromazine	generic only	first-generation antipsychotic
citalopram	Celexa	SSRI antidepressant
clomipramine	Anafranil	tricyclic antidepressant that acts like an SSRI, used primarily to treat OCD
clonazepam	Klonopin	benzodiazepine used to treat anxiety and bipolar disorder
clonidine	Catapres, Duraclon, Kapvay, Nexiclon XR	blood pressure medication also used to treat ADHD and PTSD
clorazepate	Tranxene	benzodiazepine used to treat anxiety and alcohol withdrawal
clozapine	Clozaril, Versacloz	second-generation antipsychotic
cyproheptadine	generic only	antihistamine used to treat movement disorder and insomnia
desipramine	Norpramin	tricyclic antidepressant
desvenlafaxine	Pristiq	mixed-action antidepressant
dexmethylphenidate	Azstarys, Focalin, Focalin XR	stimulant used to treat ADHD
dextroamphetamine	Dyanavel XR, Xelstrym	stimulant used to treat ADHD
dextromethorphan and bupropion	Auvelity	used to treat major depressive disorder
diazepam	Diazepam Intensol, Valium, Valtoco	benzodiazepine used to treat anxiety, seizures, and alcohol withdrawal

Generic name	Common brand name(s)	Medication class/use[a]
diphenhydramine	Benadryl	antihistamine used to treat movement disorder and insomnia
disulfiram	generic only	aldehyde dehydrogenase inhibitor used to treat chronic alcohol use disorder
donepezil	Adlarity, Aricept	cognitive enhancer used to treat dementia
doxepin	Silenor, Zonalon	tricyclic antidepressant also used to treat insomnia
duloxetine	Cymbalta, Drizalma Sprinkle	mixed-action antidepressant also used to treat anxiety and pain disorders
escitalopram	Lexapro	SSRI antidepressant
esketamine	Spravato	used to treat major depressive disorder and treatment-resistant depression
eszopiclone	Lunesta	hypnotic used to treat insomnia
fluoxetine	Prozac	SSRI antidepressant
fluphenazine	generic only	first-generation antipsychotic
flurazepam	generic only	benzodiazepine used to treat insomnia
fluvoxamine	generic only	SSRI antidepressant
gabapentin	Gralise, Neurontin	anticonvulsant used to treat bipolar disorder and pain disorders
gabapentin enacarbil	Horizant	anticonvulsant used to treat restless legs syndrome
galantamine	Razadyne, Razadyne ER	cognitive enhancer used to treat dementia

Generic name	Common brand name(s)	Medication class/use[a]
guanfacine	Intuniv	blood pressure medication also used to treat ADHD
haloperidol	Haldol	first-generation antipsychotic
iloperidone	Fanapt	second-generation antipsychotic
imipramine	Tofranil	tricyclic antidepressant
isocarboxazid	Marplan	MAOI antidepressant
lamotrigine	Lamictal, Lamictal CD, Lamictal ODT, Lamictal XR	anticonvulsant also used to treat bipolar disorder and depression
levomilnacipran	Fetzima	mixed-action antidepressant also used to treat fibromyalgia and neuropathy
lisdexamfetamine	Vyvanse	stimulant used to treat ADHD
lithium	Lithobid	mood stabilizer used to treat bipolar disorder
lorazepam	Ativan, Lorazepam Intensol, Loreev XR	benzodiazepine used to treat anxiety
loxapine	Adasuve	first-generation antipsychotic
lumateperone	Caplyta	atypical antipsychotic used to treat schizophrenia and bipolar disorder
lurasidone	Latuda	second-generation antipsychotic
memantine	Namenda, Namenda XR, Namzaric	cognitive enhancer used to treat dementia
meprobamate	generic only	used to treat anxiety disorders
methylphenidate	Methylin, Ritalin	stimulant used to treat ADHD

Generic name	Common brand name(s)	Medication class/use[a]
methylphenidate (extended release)	Aptensio XR, Concerta, Jornay PM, Ritalin LA, Metadate CD, Methyline ER, Quillivant XR	long-acting stimulants used to treat ADHD
methylphenidate (topical patch)	Daytrana	topical stimulant used to treat ADHD
milnacipran	Savella	mixed-action antidepressant also used to treat fibromyalgia and neuropathy
mirtazapine	Remeron	mixed-action antidepressant also used to treat insomnia
modafinil	Provigil	stimulant used to treat narcolepsy, sleep apnea, and ADHD
naloxone	Suboxone, Zimhi	narcotic antagonist used to reverse opioid effects from overdose
naltrexone (extended release)	Contrave, Vivitrol	narcotic antagonist used to treat chronic opioid and alcohol use disorders
nefazodone	generic only	mixed-action antidepressant
nortriptyline	Pamelor	tricyclic antidepressant
olanzapine	Zyprexa, Zyprexa Zydis	second-generation antipsychotic
olanzapine (intramuscular injection)	Zyprexa Relprevv	long-acting second-generation antipsychotic
olanzapine and fluoxetine	Symbyax	combination antipsychotic-antidepressant used to treat depressive episodes of bipolar disorder and treatment-resistant depression

Generic name	Common brand name(s)	Medication class/use[a]
olanzapine and samidorphan	Lybalvi	atypical antipsychotic and opioid antagonist used to treat schizophrenia and bipolar disorder
oxazepam	generic only	benzodiazepine used to treat anxiety and alcohol withdrawal
oxcarbazepine	Oxtellar XR, Trileptal	anticonvulsant also used to treat bipolar disorder
oxybate	Xyrem, Xywav	used to treat cataplexy due to narcolepsy
paliperidone	Invega, Invega Hafyera, Invega Sustenna, Invega Trinza	second-generation anti-psychotic
paroxetine	Brisdelle, Paxil, Paxil CR, Pexeva	SSRI antidepressant
perphenazine	generic only	first-generation antipsy-chotic
phenelzine	Nardil	MAOI antidepressant
pimozide	generic only	first-generation antipsy-chotic used to treat Tourette syndrome
pramipexole	Mirapex ER	dopamine agonist used to treat Parkinson's disease and restless legs syn-drome
pregabalin	Lyrica, Lyrica CR	anticonvulsant also used to treat fibromyalgia and neuropathy
protriptyline	generic only	tricyclic antidepressant
quetiapine	Seroquel, Seroquel XR	second-generation anti-psychotic
ramelteon	Rozerem	melatonin agonist used to treat insomnia

Generic name	Common brand name(s)	Medication class/use[a]
risperidone	Perseris, Risperdal, Risperdal Consta	second-generation antipsychotic
rivastigmine	Exelon, Exelon Patch	cognitive enhancer used to treat dementia
ropinirole	generic only	dopamine agonist used to treat Parkinson's disease and restless legs syndrome
rotigotine (topical patch)	Neupro	dopamine agonist used to treat Parkinson's disease and restless legs syndrome
selegiline	Zelapar	MAOI antidepressant
selegiline (topical patch)	Emsam	MAOI antidepressant
sertraline	Zoloft	SSRI antidepressant
sildenafil	Revatio, Viagra	phosphodiesterase inhibitor used to treat erectile disorder
tadalafil	Adcirca, Alyq, Cialis, Entadfi, Tadliq	phosphodiesterase inhibitor used to treat erectile disorder
temazepam	Restoril	benzodiazepine used to treat insomnia
thioridazine	generic only	first-generation antipsychotic
topiramate	Eprontia, Qsymia, Qudexy XR, Topamax, Trokendi XR	anticonvulsant also used to treat bipolar disorder
tranylcypromine	Parnate	MAOI antidepressant
trazodone	generic only	mixed-action antidepressant also used to treat insomnia
triazolam	Halcion	benzodiazepine used to treat insomnia

Generic name	Common brand name(s)	Medication class/use[a]
trifluoperazine	generic only	first-generation antipsychotic
trihexyphenidyl	generic only	anticholinergic agent used to treat Parkinson's disease and abnormal movements caused by antipsychotic medications
trimipramine	generic only	tricyclic antidepressant
valproate	generic only	anticonvulsant also used to treat bipolar disorder
vardenafil	generic only	phosphodiesterase inhibitor used to treat erectile disorder
varenicline	Tyrvaya	nicotinic agonist used to aid smoking cessation
venlafaxine	Effexor XR	mixed-action antidepressant also used to treat anxiety, panic disorder, and pain disorders
vortioxetine	Trintellix	mixed-action antidepressant
zaleplon	Sonata	hypnotic used to treat insomnia
ziprasidone	Geodon	second-generation antipsychotic
zolpidem	Ambien, Ambien CR, Edluar, Zolpimist	hypnotic used to treat insomnia

ADHD=attention-deficit/hyperactivity disorder; CD=extended release; CR=controlled release; ER=extended release; LA=long acting; MAOI=monoamine oxidase inhibitor; OCD=obsessive-compulsive disorder; ODT = orally disintegrating tablet; PM=evening dosed; PTSD=posttraumatic stress disorder; SR=sustained release; SSRI=selective serotonin reuptake inhibitor; XL=extended-release tablet; XR=extended release.
[a]General use noted. See product label for product-specific information.

Helpful Resources

General Mental Health

American Academy of Child and Adolescent Psychiatry
aacap.org

This website for child and adolescent psychiatrists provides Facts for Families, medication guides for parents, a search tool to find child and adolescent psychiatrists, and other resources for seeking help and understanding mental illnesses in children and teens.

American Psychiatric Association
psychiatry.org
LaSaludMental.org (en español)

As world's largest psychiatric organization, the American Psychiatric Association provides a wealth of information on its website for the public. This includes online resources about mental health topics, wellness, coping with disasters, and other issues. It includes videos, ways to find help, a blog and treatment locator, warning signs of mental illness, and information for caregivers. A Spanish-language version of the website is also available.

American Psychiatric Association Foundation
apafdn.org

The American Psychiatric Association Foundation is a nonprofit organization that provides high-impact mental health education and programs in communities, schools, and faith-based organizations, and for psychiatrists in training. Its website features information and videos about mental health concerns and disorders, as well as links to crisis helplines and a podcast.

American Psychological Association
apa.org

This website features a wide range of information for the public on its Psychology Topics page, a Psychologist Locator, and other tools and resources for the general public to learn about psychological issues.

Brain & Behavior Research Foundation
bbrfoundation.org

The Brain & Behavior Research Foundation awards grants that will lead to advances and breakthroughs in scientific research. Its website provides information on mental illnesses, cutting-edge research, and stories of recovery featured in free online videos from the Healthy Minds public television series.

Centers for Disease Control and Prevention
cdc.gov

The Centers for Disease Control and Prevention works to protect public health. Its website provides general health information on wellness, safety, and mental disorders, as well as several web pages on mental health topics, including children's mental health, tools and resources, and coping with stress.

Center for Workplace Mental Health
workplacementalhealth.org

The APA Foundation Center for Workplace Mental Health provides employers the tools, resources, and information needed to promote and support the mental health of employees and their families. Mental Health Topics pages on its website offer information and ways to get help for mental health concerns

MedlinePlus
medlineplus.gov

MedlinePlus is the National Institutes of Health website for patients and their families and friends. It contains information about mental disorders and other medical conditions, treatments, drugs and supplements, health and wellness, and definitions of medical terms.

Mental Health America
mhanational.org

This website provides mental health screens, tips for working with a mental health care provider, mental health wellness and illness information, links to crisis lines and support groups, and more.

National Alliance on Mental Illness (NAMI)
nami.org

NAMI is the largest grassroots mental health organization in the United States dedicated to building better lives for the millions of Americans affected by mental illness. NAMI's website offers information on mental illness and treatment, as well as free education, support, and awareness programs.

National Federation of Families
ffcmh.org

The National Federation of Families focuses on advocacy and support for families whose children have mental health needs, including emotional, behavioral, juvenile justice, and substance use challenges. Its website offers crisis resources, courses and trainings for parents and caregivers, family peer support stories, and more.

National Institute of Mental Health—National Institutes of Health
nimh.nih.gov

The National Institute of Mental Health aims to transform the understanding and treatment of mental illnesses through research, and pave the way for prevention, recovery, and cure. On its website, Health Topics, as well as fact sheets and brochures (in English and Spanish), provide information about mental illnesses, their causes, and treatment.

Addictive Disorders

Alcoholics Anonymous (AA)
aa.org

An international support group for people who have a drinking problem, AA helps its members quit drinking through its Twelve Steps recovery program. Its website includes a self-assessment and information on how to locate local AA programs.

Gamblers Anonymous
gamblersanonymous.org/ga/

This international support group for people who have gambling problems is built on the same 12-step recovery program as Alcoholics Anonymous. Its website includes links to hotlines, a self-assessment, questions and answers, and information on meetings, including phone and online meeting options.

Narcotics Anonymous
na.org

This organization offers an ongoing global support network for addicts who wish to pursue a drug-free lifestyle. Its website includes informational pamphlets and resources for connecting to local chapters, including online and phone meetings.

National Council on Problem Gambling
ncpgambling.org

The National Council on Problem Gambling advocates for programs and services that assist people and families affected by problem gambling. Its website features a 24-hour confidential national hotline, resources for help by state, screening tools, and information on selecting a treatment program or facility.

National Institute on Alcohol Abuse and Alcoholism—Rethinking Drinking
rethinkingdrinking.niaaa.nih.gov

This website provides user-friendly tools and information to assess and address drinking habits, including strategies to cut down, support for quitting, questions and answers, and a free downloadable booklet.

National Institute on Drug Abuse—Parents and Educators
nida.nih.gov/research-topics/parents-educators

This website offers the latest science-based information for parents and teachers about drug use, health, and the developing brain. Conversation starters, videos, lesson plans, life skills activities, and other resources are available.

Partnership to End Addiction
drugfree.org

Partnership to End Addiction is dedicated to addiction prevention, treatment, and recovery. Families can find science and research-based information on how to help their child, including effective communication and parenting skills, how to create a treatment and recovery plan, and other support resources on the website.

Substance Abuse and Mental Health Services Administration
samhsa.gov

This website provides links to find alcohol, drug abuse, and mental health treatment in the United States, as well as ways to cope, how to help someone you care about, and low-cost payment options. It also features a wealth of helpful information on substances, substance use, treatment, and recovery.

Anxiety, Bipolar, and Depressive Disorders

Anxiety and Depression Association of America

adaa.org

The Anxiety and Depression Association of America website helps those with anxiety disorders, depression, obsessive-compulsive disorder, and PTSD find treatment and resources. It offers information on disorders and their treatment, types of therapy and choosing a therapist, free webinars, personal stories, and links to free peer support groups.

Depression and Bipolar Support Alliance

dbsalliance.org

The website for the Depression and Bipolar Support Alliance provides crisis information, support networks for those with depression or bipolar disorders and their loved ones, wellness information, online screening tools, a strengths assessment, and many other empowering tools for recovery and wellness.

Families for Depression Awareness

familyaware.org

The website for Families for Depression Awareness provides information to support families and loved ones of adults and teens with depressive disorders. It offers tools for caregivers to learn about self-care, helping their loved one, treatment, coping with depressive disorders, and other helpful information to get people well and prevent suicides.

International Bipolar Foundation

ibpf.org

The International Bipolar Foundation strives to improve the understanding and treatment of bipolar disorders. Its website provides FAQs, information about symptoms, a library of webinars, and other resources for those living with these disorders and their loved ones.

Juvenile Bipolar Research Foundation

bpchildresearch.org

The Juvenile Bipolar Research Foundation website contains information about bipolar disorder in children and questions to help assess a child's symptoms for bipolar disorder.

Attention-Deficit/Hyperactivity Disorder (ADHD)

Attention Deficit Disorder Association

add.org

The website for the Attention Deficit Disorder Association provides ADHD facts, FAQs, virtual online support groups, webinars, and other information and resources to help adults with ADHD.

Children and Adults With Attention-Deficit/Hyperactivity Disorder
chadd.org

The CHADD website offers a host of information about ADHD, such as fact sheets, toolkits, resources for parents, videos to help learning and organization skills, evidence-based ADHD information, and local support groups for the ADHD community.

Autism Spectrum

Academic Autism Spectrum Partnership in Research and Education (AASPIRE)
aaspire.org

AASPIRE brings together autistic and non-autistic scientists and community members to develop and perform research projects with the goal of improving the lives of autistic adults. Its website includes videos, research study topics (such as employment, health care, mental health, and important outcomes), and more information on research.

Autism National Committee
autcom.org

The Autism National Committee aims to protect and advance the human rights and civil rights of all persons with autism and related differences of communication and behavior. Their website includes a newsletter, position papers, and recommended books.

Autism Science Foundation
autismsciencefoundation.org

The Autism Science Foundation website provides a wealth of information about autism to inform and support families, covering early warning signs of autism to questions that emerge as autistic children grow into adulthood. It includes treatment options and ways for parents and siblings to support their autistic loved one.

Autism Society
autismsociety.org

The Autism Society strives to improve the lives of all affected by autism. It advocates for appropriate services across the life span and provides the latest information on treatment, education, research, and advocacy.

Autistic Self Advocacy Network
autisticadvocacy.org

The Autistic Self Advocacy Network website features toolkits, self-advocacy tools, recommended books, and an action center for autistic adults and youth to stay up to date on issues related to access, rights, and opportunities that impact the autism community.

Dementia and Other Memory Problems

Alzheimer's Association
www.alz.org
The Alzheimer's Association website provides a wealth of information about Alzheimer's disease and caregiving, as well as a community resource finder, 24-hour helpline, links to support groups, and more.

Alzheimer's Foundation of America
alzfdn.org
The Alzheimer's Foundation of America website offers a toll-free helpline, telephone support groups, a memory screening test, coping tools, tips for creating a dementia-friendly home, a wealth of practical information, and free video classes (such as art, fitness, and music) to engage those with Alzheimer's disease and their caregivers.

National Institute on Aging (NIA)—Alzheimer's Disease Education and Referral Center
nia.nih.gov/health/alzheimers
The NIA is the main federal agency for Alzheimer's disease research. Its website provides information on Alzheimer's disease and other dementias, as well as practical information for caregivers and health care providers.

Disorders/Differences of Sex Development

Accord Alliance
accordalliance.org
The Accord Alliance strives to enhance the health and well-being of people and families affected by disorders of sex development. Its website provides FAQs about disorders of sex development, a resource guide, links to support groups, viewpoints on care, and more.

Disruptive and Conduct Disorders

Child Mind Institute—Behavior problems
childmind.org/topics/behavior-problems
This Child Mind Institute web page explains causes of behavior problems such as tantrums and teen anger; it also provides strategies for managing behavior problems, ways to help children and teens with big emotions, information on mental disorders in children and teens, and how to get help.

Child Mind Institute—Intermittent explosive disorder
childmind.org/guide/quick-guide-to-intermittent-explosive-disorder

This Child Mind Institute web page describes for parents the symptoms, diagnosis, and treatment of intermittent explosive disorder, as well as risk factors for other mental disorders in children and teens.

Dissociative Disorders

International Society for the Study of Trauma and Dissociation
isst-d.org

The website for the International Society for the Study of Trauma and Dissociation provides webinars, fact sheets, websites of interest, and self-care resources for the public.

Sidran Institute
sidran.org

For help coping with traumatic stress and dissociation, the Sidran Institute website offers a Resources page with information for survivors and loved ones (including children and teens). Treatment resources and links to hotlines for child abuse, crisis, depression, domestic violence, elders, veterans, and more are available.

Eating Disorders

ANAD (National Association of Anorexia Nervosa and Associated Disorders)
anad.org

The ANAD website provides a helpline, links to free online peer support services, a mentorship program, and other resources to support those who struggle with eating disorders and their loved ones.

NEDA (National Eating Disorders Association)
nationaleatingdisorders.org

The NEDA website includes a helpline, eating disorders screening tool, links to support groups and other resources, and information to learn more about eating disorders.

Elimination Disorders

American Academy of Child and Adolescent Psychiatry— Facts for Families
aacap.org

This website provides fact sheets for families about mental health issues for children. A fact sheet on bed-wetting in children provides information for parents, including causes of the behavior and ways to help their child.

FamilyDoctor.org—Stool Soiling and Constipation in Children
familydoctor.org/stool-soiling-and-constipation-in-children/
This web page contains information on the causes of stool soiling, toilet training tips, and questions that parents can ask their child's doctor.

Ethnically and Racially Diverse Communities

General Resources

Mental Health America—Racism and Mental Health
mhanational.org/racism-and-mental-health
This web page addresses the impact of mental health issues in various racial and ethnic groups and provides general information on racism and mental health, including a glossary of terms.

U.S. Department of Health and Human Services— Office of Minority Health
minorityhealth.hhs.gov/default.aspx
In multiple languages, the Office of Minority Health website provides population health profiles by ethnicity (including mental and behavioral health reports), cultural competency tools, and other resources.

Asian American, Native Hawaiian, and Pacific Islander Communities

Asian Mental Health Collective
asianmhc.org
The Asian Mental Health Collective seeks to normalize and de-stigmatize mental health concerns within the Asian community. Its website includes links to support groups, FAQs, information on Asian mental health, and a therapist directory to locate Asian therapists in the United States and Canada, along with additional resources.

The National Asian American Pacific Islander Mental Health Association
naapimha.org
This organization's website provides links to mental health and behavioral services for Asian Americans, Native Hawaiians, and Pacific Islanders. The website includes webinars, trainings in mental health for youth and young adults, links to crisis helplines, and other resources.

Black Communities

Black Emotional and Mental Health Collective
beam.community

The Black Emotional and Mental Health Collective website offers access to virtual and local community mental health programs, trainings, wellness tools, and a Black virtual wellness directory to connect users to local therapists.

The Boris Lawrence Henson Foundation
borislhensonfoundation.org

The Boris Lawrence Henson Foundation website provides links to resources, connections, and support to end the silence and stigma over mental health in the African American community. It offers a local resource guide to culturally competent mental health resources and a blog that focuses on mental health issues of interest.

Therapy for Black Girls
therapyforblackgirls.com

The website for Therapy for Black Girls offers a blog, podcast, therapist search portal, and other resources to support and encourage the mental wellness of Black women and girls.

Therapy for Black Men
therapyforblackmen.org

The website for Therapy for Black Men provides links to multiculturally competent mental health care for Black men. Website visitors can connect with career counseling coaches and local therapists, and find stories, articles, and other resources in the journey toward better mental health.

Hispanic Communities

La Vida es Preciosa/Life Is Precious
comunilifelip.org

This website describes a program that aims to prevents suicide in young Latinas ages 12–17 in the New York City area. Staffed by experienced Latina women, the program and offers bilingual individual and group counseling, arts therapy, academic support, college counseling and career mentoring, family workshops, and nutritional and fitness activities.

SanaMente/Each Mind Matters
sanamente.org (en español)
takeaction4mh.com

The websites for SanaMente/Each Mind Matters offer a wealth of culturally focused information on mental health in Spanish and English languages. Support services are based only in California.

Intellectual Disability (Intellectual Developmental Disorder)

American Association on Intellectual and Developmental Disabilities
aaidd.org

The American Association on Intellectual and Developmental Disabilities promotes a scholarly and clinical understanding of intellectual disability across varied fields, including a focus on progressive policies, sound research, human rights, and effective practices. Its website provides information about intellectual disability, including FAQs.

The Arc
thearc.org

The Arc advocates for and with people with intellectual and developmental disabilities and strives to serve them and their families. Families can find a resource directory, local chapter, blog, and other helpful information on its website.

National Association for the Dually Diagnosed
thenadd.org

The National Association for the Dually Diagnosed website provides information on developing helpful community-based policies, programs, and opportunities to address the mental health needs of persons with intellectual and developmental disabilities.

Learning Disabilities

Learning Disabilities Association of America
ldaamerica.org

The Learning Disabilities Association of America website offers information on support and resources for parents, students, and adults with learning disabilities.

National Center for Learning Disabilities
ncld.org

The National Center for Learning Disabilities website provides guides and information for young adults and parents about K–12 education services, planning for the future after high school, transition to college, the workplace, and other information to improve the lives of all people with learning difficulties and disabilities.

Understood: For Learning and Attention Issues
understood.org

The Understood website provides a user-friendly interface for those with learning disabilities and their families to find a wealth of practical information and resources for help with behavior, learning, and everyday skills.

LGBTQ⁺ Mental Health

Mental Health America
screening.mhanational.org/content/how-do-i-find-lgbtq-friendly-therapy

This web page provides helpful information on how and where to find LGBTQ⁺-friendly therapy. It also includes links to related information and articles of interest.

National Center for Transgender Equality
transequality.org

The National Center for Transgender Equality website provides information to help end discrimination and violence against transgender people. It offers FAQs and videos to understand transgender people, information on transgender issues and rights, and transgender self-help guides.

National Queer and Trans Therapists of Color Network
nqttcn.com/en

The National Queer and Trans Therapists of Color Network website provides links to helplines and online support, a mental health directory, and other resources to support mental health for queer and trans people of color.

Parents, Families, and Friends of Lesbians and Gays
pflag.org

The website for Parents, Families, and Friends of Lesbians and Gays provides educational resources and links to support to advance equality and societal acceptance of LGBTQ⁺ people.

SAGE Advocacy & Services for LGBTQ+ Elders
sageusa.org

The SAGE website offers information and links to supportive services and resources for LGBTQ+ older people and their caregivers. Its Elder Hotline provides confidential support and crisis response for LGBTQ+ older people and caretakers 24 hours a day, 7 days a week.

Trans Lifeline
translifeline.org

The Trans Lifeline website provides confidential crisis intervention by the trans community, for the trans community, through a 24-hour daily hotline 7 days a week. Links to other resources on a variety of topics for transgender people and their loved ones are also available on its website.

The Trevor Project
thetrevorproject.org

The Trevor Project website provides information on crisis intervention and suicide prevention services to LGBTQ+ and questioning young people ages 13–24. It also offers educational resources and a 24-hour daily hotline available by phone or text 7 days a week.

Military Mental Health

DoD Safe Helpline
safehelpline.org
877-995-5247

This website provides sexual assault support for the Department of Defense community and features a 24/7 hotline that is secure, worldwide, and confidential. Answers to common questions and information for survivors and loved ones are also available.

Iraq and Afghanistan Veterans of America
iava.org

The Iraq and Afghanistan Veterans of America website provides a hotline for information and assistance in a variety of areas, such as mental health, peer support, housing, and employment. Services are available for veterans and their families, Afghan allies who have resettled in the United States, and those helping Afghan allies emigrate from Afghanistan.

U.S. Department of Veterans Affairs—National Center for PTSD
ptsd.va.gov

The National Center for PTSD website provides information to understand PTSD and its treatment, as well as links to find a provider and get help. Information is available for veterans and for their families and loved ones.

Vietnam Veterans of America
vva.org

The Vietnam Veterans of America website provides links to resources and information on health care, claims assistance, outreach programs (such as for PTSD and substance use), and more to promote and support the full range of issues important to Vietnam veterans.

Wounded Warrior Project
woundedwarriorproject.org

The Wounded Warrior Project website provides information on direct programs and services for veterans and service members who served in the military on or after September 11, 2001, and incurred a physical or mental injury, illness, or wound during or after service. Links to mental health and wellness information are available for warriors and their families.

Obsessive-Compulsive and Related Disorders

International OCD Foundation
iocdf.org

The International OCD Foundation website provides resources and support for those with OCD and their loved ones. Its website also provides links to its other hosted websites that focus on these topics: OCD in kids, hoarding disorder, body dysmorphic disorder, anxiety in the classroom, and anxiety in athletes.

The TLC Foundation for Body-Focused Repetitive Behaviors
bfrb.org

The website for the TLC Foundation for Body-Focused Repetitive Behaviors provides information on hair-pulling disorder, skin-picking disorder, and related body-focused repetitive behaviors. It includes FAQs, a health education library, links to treatment referrals and support groups, and more.

Personality Disorders

Borderline Personality Disorder Resource Center— New York-Presbyterian
nyp.org/bpdresourcecenter

The Borderline Personality Disorder Resource Center website provides an online repository of information on borderline personality disorder for patients and their loved ones. The center aims to educate those affected by BPD and connect them to treatment and support in their local area throughout the United States.

National Education Alliance for Borderline Personality Disorder
borderlinepersonalitydisorder.org

The National Education Alliance for Borderline Personality Disorder website offers resources for information and support for families and persons in recovery. The organization advocates to enhance the quality of life for those affected by this serious but treatable mental illness.

Treatment and Research Advancements for Borderline Personality Disorder
tara4bpd.org

This website provides resources and information on causes of borderline personality disorder, treatment, help for families, workshops, and guidelines for finding a therapist.

Prolonged Grief Disorder

Center for Prolonged Grief
prolongedgrief.columbia.edu/for-the-public

The Center for Prolonged Grief website provides webinars, podcasts, informational handouts, a therapist search portal, and a self-assessment tool to help recognize symptoms.

Center for Research on End-of-Life Care—Grief Resources
endoflife.weill.cornell.edu/grief-resources

The Center for Research on End-of-Life Care website offers resources to assist bereaved people and their families who may want more information on grief and coping. A grief intensity scale, videos, and other resources are available.

Schizophrenia and Other Psychotic Disorders

Schizophrenia and Psychosis Action Alliance
sczaction.org

The Schizophrenia and Psychosis Action Alliance website provides a variety of resources for people with schizophrenia-related illnesses and their families, including information about schizophrenia and psychosis, treatment, peer support, toolkits for those diagnosed and their loved ones, and a toll-free helpline.

Sexual and Other Violence

Centers for Disease Control and Prevention—Violence Prevention
cdc.gov/violenceprevention

This website contains facts-at-a-glance, prevention tips, and resources on child maltreatment, community violence, elder abuse, firearm violence, intimate partner violence, sexual violence, and youth violence. The domestic violence and sexual violence pages contain links to hotlines for domestic violence, rape, abuse, and incest survivors.

love is respect.
loveisrespect.org

1-866-331-9474 or text "LOVEIS" to 22522

The loveisrespect. website provides information on dating, healthy relationships, relationship violence, warnings signs of abuse, personal safety, and more. Its hotline is available 24 hours a day, 7 days a week by phone and text.

National Domestic Violence Hotline
thehotline.org

1-800-799-SAFE (7233) or text "START" to 88788

The website for the National Domestic Violence Hotline provides information on domestic abuse, including ways to get other help (such as for health and legal concerns), identifying abuse, planning for safety, ways to support those in abusive relationships, and local resources. Its hotline is available 24 hours a day, 7 days a week by phone and text.

RAINN (Rape, Abuse & Incest National Network)
rainn.org

National Sexual Assault Hotline: 1-800-656-HOPE (4673)

The RAINN website provides information on types of sexual violence; consent; sexual assault; warning signs; information for parents, students, and bystanders; and more. Its hotline is available by phone or online (including in Spanish), 24 hours a day, 7 days a week.

Sleep-Wake Disorders

American Academy of Sleep Medicine—Sleep Education
sleepeducation.org

This web page provides a wealth of information about sleep, sleep disorders, and treatment options for those experiencing sleep disorders, as well as resources for parents, educators, and students.

National Heart, Lung, and Blood Institute
nhlbi.nih.gov

This website provides information on sleep disorders, including causes, risk factors, signs and symptoms, treatments, coping tips, research trials, and links to more information in its Health Topics tab.

National Sleep Foundation
sleepfoundation.org

The National Sleep Foundation website provides information on sleep health, sleep problems and disorders, and a library of sleep tools and tips.

Suicide Awareness and Prevention

988 Suicide & Crisis Lifeline
988lifeline.org

In the United States, call, text, or chat **988** to connect to trained counselors available 24 hours a day, every day. The line is available to those in emotional distress or suicidal crisis, or for those concerned about someone they care about. The website also provides information on mental health for different populations, such as youth, veterans, and survivors.

Active Minds
activeminds.org

The Active Minds website provides information for young adults ages 14–25 on depression, anxiety, and bipolar disorders; signs and symptoms of mental health problems; ways to get help in a crisis; tips for self-care; and more.

American Association of Suicidology
suicidology.org

The American Association of Suicidology website features information on warning signs, support groups, and a variety of other resources and literature to promote the understanding and prevention of suicide and support those who have been affected by it.

American Foundation for Suicide Prevention
afsp.org

The American Foundation for Suicide Prevention website provides practical information on ways to get help for thoughts of suicide, surviving a suicide attempt, finding treatment and support, processing the loss of someone who died by suicide, helping someone who is at risk and struggling, and a wealth of other helpful information.

American Indian and Alaska Native National Suicide Prevention Strategic Plan
ihs.gov/suicideprevention

The American Indian and Alaska Native National Suicide Prevention Strategic Plan strives to provide resources across Tribes, Tribal organizations, and Urban Indian organizations to support suicide prevention efforts. Its website features information on how to talk about suicide, warning signs and risk factors, and links to resources.

The Jed Foundation
jedfoundation.org

The Jed Foundation website provides essential information about common emotional health issues, coping skills, and mental health resources to promote emotional health and prevent suicide among teens and young adults. Information is available for teens and young adults, as well as those who want to help.

Suicide Awareness Voices of Education
save.org

The website for Suicide Awareness Voices of Education provides information and resources for those who need help for themselves or for others in suicide crisis. Information on warning signs, prevention, treatment, peer support, bereavement, coping with loss, and for suicide attempt survivors is available.

Tourette's Disorder

National Tourette Syndrome Association
tourette.org

The Tourette Association of America website offers key facts, stories, tools, webinars, and other information to help people and their families cope with the problems that occur with Tourette syndrome and other tic disorders.

Trauma Recovery

Give an Hour
giveanhour.org

The Give an Hour website offers practical information on mental health concerns and questions for those who have experienced trauma as a result of military service, mass violence, the opioid epidemic, and interpersonal violence. For those who have experienced these traumas, an online portal for free mental health services by volunteer mental health professionals is available.

Women's Mental Health

Center for Women's Mental Health—
Reproductive Psychiatry Resource and Information Center
womensmentalhealth.org

The website for the Center for Women's Mental Health at Massachusetts General Hospital provides information about PMS, fertility and mental health, mood disorders and menopause, mental disorders during pregnancy, and breastfeeding and psychiatric medications.

Moms' Mental Health Matters—
National Child & Maternal Health Education Program
nichd.nih.gov/ncmhep/initiatives/moms-mental-health-matters/moms

This website offers resources and reading materials for moms and their partners, families, and friends on depression and anxiety before, during, and after pregnancy.

Postpartum Support International
postpartum.net

The website for Postpartum Support International is available in English and Spanish and features a helpline, information on mental health issues during and after pregnancy, ways to get help, online support groups, information for friends and family, and links to additional resources.

International Mental Health Organizations

These organizations are based outside the United States and promote mental health wellness, support services, and advocacy.

ABRATA (Associação Brasileira de Familiares, Amigos e Portadores de Transtornos Afetivos—Brazilian Association of Family, Friends, and Patients With Affective Disorders)
abrata.org.br

The ABRATA website features links to online support groups, a telephone service, publications, and answers to common questions about mental health to raise awareness about mood disorders and increase psychosocial support for those with depression and bipolar disorder, as well as their families and friends, in Brazil.

Global Alliance of Mental Illness Advocacy Networks (GAMIAN)—Europe
gamian.eu

The GAMIAN website features mental health and advocacy projects (such as online publications on mental health care topics), newsletters, and more for those living in Europe.

World Health Organization (WHO)
who.int

The WHO website features Health Topics and Fact Sheets on a variety of global health issues, including mental health, well-being, and mental disorders.

Australia and New Zealand

The Australian Association for Infant Mental Health
aaimh.org.au

The website for The Australian Association for Infant Mental Health provides position statements to support infant mental health for families and professionals, as well as additional resources for parents about infant care and well-being.

Australian Psychological Society
psychology.org.au

The Australian Psychological Society website provides information for the public about psychology, including web pages about how psychologists can help, types of psychologists, psychology topics, and Find a Psychologist.

BeyondBlue
beyondblue.org.au

The BeyondBlue website offers helpful facts about anxiety, depression, and suicide prevention. Its 24/7 support service of trained mental health professionals listens to concerns and provides information and advice.

Black Dog Institute
blackdoginstitute.org.au

The Black Dog Institute website contains helpful information on depression and bipolar disorder and ways to get help in Australia.

Headspace—National Youth Mental Health Foundation
headspace.org.au

The Headspace website provides links to hotlines and other helpful information to support young people in Australia ages 12–25 regarding their mental health, physical health (including sexual health), alcohol and other drug concerns, as well as work and study support.

Mental Health Foundation of New Zealand
mentalhealth.org.nz

The website for the Mental Health Foundation of New Zealand provides wellness information, suicide prevention and loss resources, support networks, and links to additional information and resources in New Zealand.

New Zealand Psychological Society
psychology.org.nz

The New Zealand Psychological Society website features a Find a Psychologist link and a community resources page that provides parenting, family, and mental health information and helplines.

The Royal Australian and New Zealand College of Psychiatrists
ranzcp.org

The website for The Royal Australian and New Zealand College of Psychiatrists features Find a Psychiatrist and other information for the public on mental illnesses, psychiatry, treatments and medication, and caring for someone with mental illness.

United Kingdom

Carers UK
carersuk.org

The Carers UK website offers practical information, help and advice, and online tools for unpaid carers (such as family, friends, and neighbors) in the United Kingdom.

Centre for Mental Health
centreformentalhealth.org.uk

The Centre for Mental Health website features blogs, publications, and information on mental health topics, with a focus on mental health policies and systems, including the impact of poverty and discrimination on mental health.

Mental Health Foundation
mentalhealth.org.uk

The Mental Health Foundation website contains mental health topics from A to Z for the public, free publications, ways to get help, personal stories, and more.

MIND
mind.org.uk

The website for MIND includes tips for everyday living, personal stories, online peer support, helplines, and other resources to support and empower those with a mental health problem.

SANE
sane.org.uk

The website for SANE provides information to improve the quality of life for those affected by mental illness. It offers a helpline, information on mental disorders and treatment, and an online support forum where people share their experiences.

Together
together-uk.org

The website for Together provides links to crisis support, a service finder, and other information to help people deal with the personal and practical impacts of mental health issues.

Young Minds
youngminds.org.uk

The Young Minds website provides practical mental health information for young people and their parents. It includes information on feelings, coping with life, mental disorders, medications, ways for parents to talk with and seek help for their child, and links to helplines for parents and for young people.

Index

Page numbers printed in **boldface** type refer to tables.

Acute stress disorder, 118–121
Adaptive servo-ventilation (ASV), 179–180
Addictive disorders, 224–241. *See also* Substance use disorders
   about, 225–227
   gambling disorder, 236–238
   intoxication and withdrawal, 228, 231–235, **232–233**, 240, 246–247
   key points, 240–241
   misused substance classes, **226**
   recovery guidelines, 239–240
   tips for relating to people with, 227
   treatment, 238–240
   types of, 228–238. *See also specific disorders*
ADHD. *See* Attention-deficit/hyperactivity disorder
Adjustment disorders, 121–123
   about, 108, 121–122
   diagnosis and symptoms, 122
   co-occurring with, disruptive and conduct disorders, 220
   risk factors, 122
   treatment, 122–123
Aging, vs. Alzheimer's disease, 249
Agoraphobia, 79–80, 88–90
Akathisia, 310

Alcohol use, **226**
   depressive disorder and, 235
   intoxication and withdrawal, **231**, 246–247
   sexual dysfunctions and, 192–193
   statistics on, 234–235
Alcohol use disorder. *See also* Substance use disorders
   about, 228, 234
   co-occurring with,
     bipolar disorder, 52
     eating disorders, 155
     memory loss, 243
     other substance use disorders, 79
     personality disorders, 272
     sleep disorders, 172
   diagnosis and symptoms, 229
   intoxication and withdrawal, **231**, 246–247
   personal story, 230
   tips for relating to people with, 227
   as traumatic brain injury risk factor, 254
   treatment, 238–240
Alprazolam, 89
Alzheimer's disease, 248–252
   about, 244, 248–250
   age-related changes vs., 249

Alzheimer's disease *(continued)*
  caregiver tips, 252
  diagnosis, 250
  personal story, 251
  risk factors, 250
  treatment, 251–252
American Academy of Child and
    Adolescent Psychiatry, 117, 128
American Psychiatric Association
    (APA), xv, xx
Amnesia, types of, 133–134
Amphetamines, 13, 193, **226**, 235
Animal hoarding, 101
Anorexia nervosa
  about, 150–151
  co-occurring with, 151
      depressive disorders, 60
  diagnosis and symptoms, 151
  healthy mind, body, and weight
      for, 150, 151, 156–157
  personal story, 152
  risk factors, 152
  treatment, 155–156
  types of, 151–152
Anti-anxiety medications. *See* Seda-
    tive medications
Anticonvulsant medications, includ-
    ing valproate, 8, 38, 50, 310, 311–
    312
Antidepressant medications
  about, 64, 185, 193, 198, 309
  for adjustment disorders, 123
  for anxiety disorders, 89
  for bipolar disorders, 54
  for dementia, 252
  for depressive disorders, 64–65
  for disruptive and conduct disor-
      ders, 215
  for dissociative disorders, 135
  for eating disorders, 156
  for obsessive-compulsive disor-
      ders, 95, 97, 99, 103
  for paraphilic disorders, 291
  for personality disorder symp-
      toms, 281

for sexual dysfunctions, 197
for sleep-wake disorders, 174, 176
for somatic symptom disorders,
    145–146
for trauma and stress disorders,
    115, 126
Antipsychotic medications
  about, 35, 193, 309–310
  for Alzheimer's disease, 252
  for eating disorders, 156
  for personality disorder symp-
      toms, 281
  for psychotic disorders, 35, 38
Antisocial personality disorder, 272–
    274
  about, 272
  co-occurring with, 272
      addictive disorders, 238
  diagnosis, 218, 272–273
  personal story, 273–274
  risk factors, 273
  treatment, 281
Anxiety disorders, 74–91
  about, 75–76
  co-occurring with,
      autism spectrum disorder, 5
      bipolar disorders, 46, 52
      depressive disorders, 66
      eating disorders, 151, 153, 158–
        159, 172
      obsessive-compulsive disor-
        ders, 95
      paraphilic disorders, 291
      personality disorders, 272
      psychotic disorders, 37
      sexual dysfunctions, 195, 200
      somatic symptom disorders,
        141
  fear vs. anxiety, 75–76
  healthy mind and body for, 90
  key points, 90–91
  as sexual dysfunction risk factor,
      200
  suicide risk with, 83
  treatment, 88–90

types of, 76–88, 235. *See also*
    specific disorders
APA (American Psychiatric
    Association), xv, xx
Appetite changes, 48, 61, 69, **231, 232**
Asperger's disorder, 4, 23
Assertiveness training, 304
ASV (adaptive servo-ventilation),
    179–180
Atomoxetine, 13
Attention-deficit/hyperactivity
    disorder (ADHD), 11–15
  about, 11
  co-occurring with,
      autism spectrum disorder, 5
      bipolar disorders, 46
      depressive disorders, 70
      disruptive and conduct disor-
          ders, 214, 220
      eating disorders, 159
      personality disorders, 272
      trauma and stress disorders, 127
  diagnosis and symptoms, 11–13
  personal story, 14
  risk factors, 13
  suicide risk with, 14
  treatment, 13–14, 312
  ways to cope, 14–15
Atypical (second-generation) anti-
    psychotics, 35, 309. *See also* Anti-
    psychotic medications
Auditory hallucinations, 30
Autism spectrum disorder, 4–10
  about, 4–5
  co-occurring with,
      eating disorders, 157, 158, 159
      motor disorders, 25
      trauma and stress disorders,
          127
  diagnosis and symptoms, 5–8
  parent tips, 10
  personal story, 8–9
  risk factors, 8
  social communication disorder
      comparison, 23

statistics on, 4
treatment, **7**, 9–10
vocational rehabilitation services
    for, 5
Autistic disorder (autism), 4
Avanafil, 196
Avoidant personality disorder, 279,
    281
Avoidant/restrictive food intake
    disorder, 5, 158–159

Bedwetting. *See* Enuresis
Behavioral family therapy, 305
Behavior therapy
  about, 304, 305
  for disruptive and conduct disor-
      ders, 220
  for elimination disorders, 162,
      163
  for sleep-wake disorders, 173–
      174, 175–176
Bell-and-pad method, 163
Benzodiazepines
  about, 180, 310–311
  for addictive disorders, 240
  as addictive substance, **226**, 311
  for anxiety disorders, 89
  for sleep-wake disorders, 174,
      181, 186
  for trauma and stress disorders,
      121
Bilevel positive airway pressure
    (BiPAP), 179–180
Binge-eating disorder, 154–157
  about, 155–156
  co-occurring with,
      bipolar disorders 52
      depressive disorders, 155
  diagnosis, 155
  healthy mind and body for, 156–
      157
  risk factors, 155
  treatment, 155–156
Binge-eating episodes, 151, 153–154
Biofeedback, 135

Bipolar disorders
    about, 45
    co-occurring with,
        anxiety disorders, 87
        disruptive and conduct disor-
            ders, 214, 220
        eating disorders, 151, 153
        gambling disorder, 238
        overview, 46, 52
        sexual dysfunctions, 200
        sleep disorders, 172, 174
    differential diagnosis, 35
    key points, 55–56
    as sexual dysfunction risk factor,
        200
    suicide risk with, 46–47, 48, 52
    treatment essentials, 311–312
    types of, 46–55, 235. *See also spe-
        cific disorders*
Bipolar I disorder, 46–51
    about, 46–47
    co-occurring disorders, 46
    diagnosis, 46–48
    healthy mind and body, 51
    personal story, 49
    risk factors, 49
    suicide risk, 46–47, 48
    treatment, 49–51
Bipolar II disorder, 51–54
    about, 51–52
    co-occurring disorders, 52
    diagnosis, 52–53
    personal story, 53–54
    risk factors, 52, 53
    suicide risk, 52
    treatment, 54
Bizarre delusions, 30, 38–39
Bladder retraining exercises, 163. *See
    also* Kegel exercises
Blindness, 142–143
BMI (body mass index), 150, 151
"Body clock," 185–186
Body dysmorphic disorder, 98–100
    about, 98–99
    diagnosis and symptoms, 99

healthy mind and body for, 94
risk factors, 99
treatment, 99–100
Body mass index (BMI), 150, 151
Body movement disorders. *See*
    Motor disorders
Borderline personality disorder, 269–
    271
    about, 269
    diagnosis, 270
    personal story, 270–271
    risk factors, 270
    treatment, 281
Brain function domains, **245–246**
Brain injury. *See* Traumatic brain
    injury
Breathing-related sleep disorders,
    170, 174, 176–180
Brief psychotherapy, 123
Brief psychotic disorder, 40
Bulimia nervosa
    about, 153
    co-occurring with, 153
        depressive disorders, 60
    diagnosis, 153–154
    healthy mind and body for, 156–
        157
    risk factors, 154
    treatment, 155–156
Bupropion, 193
Buspirone, 194, 311

Caffeine
    about, 228
    as addictive substance, **226**
    alcohol and, 173, 234
    avoidance for healthy mind and
        body, 70, 90, 314
    for good sleep hygiene, 172, 173,
        187
    intoxication and withdrawal, 228,
        231
Cannabis. *See also* Substance use
    disorders
    about, 234

as addictive substance, **226**
bipolar disorders and, 49, 52
intoxication and withdrawal, **231**
schizophrenia and, 32
statistics on, 234
tips for relating to people with, 227
Carbamazepine, 50, 312
Cataplexy, 174, 175, 176
Catatonia, 40, 41–42
Catatonic behavior, 31, 32, 38, 40, 41
CBT. *See* Cognitive-behavior therapy
Centers for Disease Control and Prevention (CDC)
on healthy weight, 150
on screening for autism, 7
Central sleep apnea, 179–180
Cerebrovascular disease, 261–262
"Chasing losses," 236, 237
Cheyne-Stokes breathing, 179
Childbirth, bipolar II disorder and, 53
Childhood disintegrative disorder, 4
Childhood disorders
about, 3–4
autism spectrum disorder, 4–10, 23, 25, 127, 157, 158, 159
communication disorders, 21–23
conduct disorder, 70, 164, 217–220, 273
disinhibited social engagement disorder, 108, 126–128
disruptive mood dysregulation disorder, 70–72, 214
eating disorders, 149, 150–151, 157–159
elimination disorders, 160–166
gender dysphoria, 206, 207–208
intermittent explosive disorder, 215–217, 220
key points and special services, 26–27
motor disorders, 24–26
narcolepsy, 174

obsessive-compulsive disorders, 95
obstructive sleep apnea hypopnea, 176–177
oppositional defiant disorder, 164, 214–215, 220
posttraumatic stress disorder, 109–113, 117
prolonged grief disorder, 123
reactive attachment disorder, 126–127
separation anxiety disorder, 86–89
sleep-wake disorders, 182, 183
specific learning disorder, 23–24
Childhood neglect and trauma, 126–128, 154, 270
Cholinesterase inhibitors, 251–252, 260
Chronic (recurrent) insomnia, 171
Cigarette smoking
as addictive substance, **226, 232**
as ADHD risk factor, 13
as erectile disorder risk factor, 195
medication interactions, 310
schizophrenia and, 32
as specific learning disorder risk factor, 23–24
statistics on, 234–235
as substance use disorders risk factor, 235
Circadian rhythm sleep-wake disorders, 185–186
Clomipramine, 97, 194
Clutter vs. hoarding, 100
Cocaine, 193, **226**, 235
Cognitive-behavior therapy (CBT)
about, 115, 303
for anxiety disorders, 89
for bipolar disorders, 50
for depressive disorders, 63
for disruptive and conduct disorders, 215, 221, 222
for dissociative disorders, 135
for eating disorders, 156

Cognitive-behavior therapy (CBT)
(*continued*)
for obsessive-compulsive disorders, 97–98, 99, 103
for paraphilic disorders, 291
for sexual dysfunctions, 199, 201
for somatic symptom disorders, 145
for trauma and stress disorders, 115, 126
Cognitive processing therapy (CPT), 115
Communication disorders, 21–23
Compulsions, 94–95. *See also* Obsessive-compulsive disorders
Conduct disorder
about, 217–218
antisocial personality disorder and, 273
co-occurring with, 70
disruptive and conduct disorders, 220
elimination disorders, 164
diagnosis, 218–219
personal story, 219–220
treatment, 218, 220
Constipation. *See* Encopresis
Continuous amnesia, 133
Continuous positive airway pressure (CPAP) machine, 178, 179, 180
Counseling. *See* Psychotherapy
Couples (marital) therapy
about, 297, 305
for bipolar disorders, 51
for depressive disorders, 63
for sexual dysfunctions, 196, 201
Covert sensitization, 222
CPAP (continuous positive airway pressure) machine, 178, 179, 180
CPT (cognitive processing therapy), 115
Cravings, in addictive disorders, 225, 228, 229, 236, 240
Cyclothymic disorder, 54–55

DBT (dialectical behavior therapy), 303–304
Decluttering, professional help for, 103
Deep brain stimulation, 257
Defecating issues. *See* Encopresis
Delayed ejaculation, 199
Delirium, 244, 246–248
Delusional disorder, 38–40
Delusions
about, 30, 31
delusional disorder and, 38–40
pyromania and, 221
schizoaffective disorder and, 37–38
schizophrenia and, 31, 32–33
schizophreniform disorder and, 41
treatment, 34, 35, 309–310, 313
Dementia and other memory problems, 242–264
about, 243–245, **245–246**
brain injuries and, 252–255
delirium and, 246–248
dementia defined, 264
key points, 264
medical conditions as cause of, 259–264
types of, 248–264. *See also specific disorders*
Dependent personality disorder, 279–280, 281
Depersonalization, defined, 135, 136
Depersonalization/derealization disorder, 134–136
Depression episodes (major depressive episodes), 46, 48, 51, 52–53, 54
Depressive disorders, 58–73
about, 59–60
anxiety disorders as risk factor for, 83
co-occurring with,
alcohol-induced depressive disorder, 235
anxiety disorders, 79, 83, 87

autism spectrum disorder, 5
catatonia, 41
dementia and memory disorders, 248
disruptive and conduct disorders, 214, 220
eating disorders, 149, 151, 153
gambling disorder, 238
paraphilic disorders, 291
personality disorders, 272
sexual dysfunctions, 195, 196, 200
sleep disorders, 172, 174
somatic symptom disorders, 141
substance-induced depressive disorder, 235
as delirium risk factor, 247
key points, 72–73
as sexual dysfunction risk factor, 196, 200
types of, 60–72, 235. *See also specific disorders*
Depressive mood swings, 55
Derealization, defined, 135, 136
Developmental coordination disorder, 5, 24–25
Developmental disorders. *See* Neurodevelopmental disorders
Diagnosis process, viii–ix, xvii–xviii, xix, xx, 298–299
Diagnostic and Statistical Manual of Mental Disorders (DSM), xv, xix–xx
Dialectical behavior therapy (DBT), 303–304
Diazepam, 89
Diet and exercise recommendations, 314
for anxiety disorders, 90
for bipolar disorders, 51
for depressive disorders, 65–66
for eating disorders, 156–157
healthy weight, defined, 150, 151, 156–157

for obsessive-compulsive disorders, 94
for premenstrual dysphoric disorder, 70
for sexual dysfunctions, 202
for trauma and stress disorders, 117
Discomfort and pain. *See* Somatic (physical) symptom disorders
Disinhibited social engagement disorder, 108, 126–128
Disorganized (abnormal) motor behavior, 30, 31, 32, 38, 40, 41
Disorganized thinking and speech, 30, 32, 38, 40, 41
Disruptive and conduct disorders, 212–223
about, 213–214
key points, 222–223
parent tips, 221
types of, 214–222. *See also specific disorders*
Disruptive mood dysregulation disorder, 70–72
about, 70–71
co-occurring disorders, 70
diagnosis and symptoms, 71
treatment, 71–72
ways to cope, 72
Dissociative amnesia, 133–134
Dissociative disorders, 131–136
about, 132
definitions, 131
key points, 136
suicide risk with, 131, 132, 134
trauma and stress disorders with dissociative symptoms, 111, 112–113, 118, 119
types of, 132–136. *See also specific disorders*
Dissociative identity disorder, 132–133
Dopamine, 256, 306
Dopamine agonists, 186, 257, 260
Dopamine-norepinephrine reuptake inhibitors, 64

Doxylamine, 174
Drugs. *See* Psychiatric medications
Drug use. *See* Substance use disorders
DSM *(Diagnostic and Statistical Manual of Mental Disorders)*, xv, xix–xx

Early (premature) ejaculation, 195, 196–197
Eating disorders, 148–159
  about, 149–150
  co-occurring with, 149
    bipolar disorders, 52
  healthy mind, body, and weight for, 150, 151, 156–157
  key points, 159
  risk factors, 149
  suicide risk with, 151
  types of, 150–159. *See also specific disorders*
Ejaculation. *See* Sexual dysfunctions
Electroconvulsive therapy (ECT), 42, 50, 54, 301, **302,** 313
Elimination disorders, 160–166
  about, 161–162
  key points, 165–166
  parent tips, 162, 165
  types of, 162–165
Emergency suicide hotline, 295–296, 300
Encopresis (fecal incontinence), 162–165
  about, 161, 162–163
  diagnosis, 164
  parent tips, 165
  risk factors, 163–164
  treatment, 164–165, 166
Enuresis (urine incontinence)
  about, 161, 162
  diagnosis, 162–163
  parent tips, 165
  treatment, 162–163, 166
Episodic insomnia, 171

Erectile disorder (impotence), 195–196
Erotomanic delusions, 30
Exercise, 314. *See also* Diet and exercise recommendations
Exhibitionistic disorder, 286–287, 291
Exposure and response prevention therapy, 98, 115, 222, 304
Externalizing disorders, 213
Eye movement desensitization and reprocessing (EMDR), 115

Factitious disorder, 140, 144–146
Family therapy
  about, 297, 305–306
  for bipolar disorders, 50, 51
  for disruptive and conduct disorders, 218
  for eating disorders, 156
  for major depressive disorder, 63
  parent management training, 214, 218, 220, 221
  for trauma and stress disorders, 127
Fears (specific). *See* specific phobia
Fear vs. anxiety disorders, 75–76. *See also* Anxiety disorders
Fecal incontinence. *See* Encopresis
Female orgasmic disorder, 197–198
Female sexual interest/arousal disorder, 200–201
Fentanyl, 234
Fetishistic disorder, 286, 289–290, 291
FFT (functional family therapy), 218
Fire-setting, 220–221
First-generation (typical) antipsychotics, 35, 309. *See also* Antipsychotic medications
Flooding (exposure therapy), 304
Fluoxetine, 89, 194, 197. *See also* Selective serotonin reuptake inhibitors

Frontotemporal neurocognitive disorder, 257–258
Frotteuristic disorder, 286, 287, 291
Functional family therapy (FFT), 218
Functional neurological symptom disorder, 140, 142–143, 145

Gambling disorder, 236–238
    about, 236–237
    co-occurring with, personality disorders, 272
    diagnosis, 237–238
    risk factors, 238
    tips for relating to people with, 227
    treatment, 238
Gender diverse people, 192, 205
Gender dysphoria, 204–211
    about, 205–207
    in children, 206, 207–208
    key points, 211
    personal story, 208–209
    risk factors, 208
    sex characteristics, 206, 207
    suicide risk with, 207
    in teens and adults, 206–207, 208
    treatment, 209–211
Gender nonconforming behavior, 206
Generalized anxiety disorder
    about, 81
    co-occurring with,
        anxiety disorders, 86
        bipolar disorders, 52
        obsessive-compulsive disorders, 101
    diagnosis and symptoms, 81–82
    as eating disorder risk factor, 154
    healthy mind and body for, 90
    risk factors, 82
    treatment, 88–89, 311
Generalized dissociative amnesia, 133

Genito-pelvic pain/penetration disorder, 199–200
Grandiose delusions, 30
Grief, 59–60, 62, 108, 123–126
Grossly disorganized behavior, 31, 32, 38, 40, 41
Group therapy
    about, 306
    for adjustment disorders, 123
    for eating disorders, 156
    for major depressive disorder, 63
    for prolonged grief disorder, 126
Guanfacine, 13

Habit reversal techniques, 103
Hair-pulling disorder, 103–104
Hallucinations, 30, 32, 38, 40, 41, 174
Hallucinogens, **226**
    intoxication and withdrawal, **232**
Health problems. *See* Somatic (physical) symptom disorders
Healthy weight, 150, 151, 156–157
Hearing loss, 142–143
Histrionic personality disorder, 277–278, 281
HIV infection, 262–263
Hoarding disorder, 100–103
    about, 100–101
    co-occurring disorders, 101
    diagnosis and symptoms, 101
    healthy mind and body for, 94
    personal story, 102
    risk factors, 101
    treatment, 103
Hormones
    for gender dysphoria, 209–211
    for paraphilic disorders, 291
    for premenstrual dysphoric disorder, 70
    of sleep-wake cycle (melatonin), 174, 311
Hospitalizations, 299

Hotline for suicide prevention, 295–296, 300
Huntington's disease, 263–264
Hypersomnolence disorder, 185
Hypnotic agents ("sleeping pills"), 174, 193, **226**, **302**, 310, 311
Hypochondriasis, 143. *See also* Illness anxiety disorder
Hypomanic episodes, 46, 48, 51–53
Hypopnea, 176–179
Hypothalamic mood swings, 55

IDEA (Individuals with Disabilities Education Act), 10, 15, 20, 27
Illness anxiety disorder, 140, 143–144, 145
Impotence (erectile disorder), 195–196
Individuals with Disabilities Education Act (IDEA), 10, 15, 20, 27
Inflammatory bowel disease, 79
Inhalants, **226**
    intoxication and withdrawal, **232**
Inpatient psychiatric units, 299
Insight, levels of, 35, 42, 94
Insomnia disorder, 171–174
    about, 171–172
    diagnosis, 172
    personal story, 173
    risk factors, 172
    treatment, 173–174
Intellectual disability, 15–20
    about, 15–16, **16–18**
    co-occurring with, 5
        autism spectrum disorder, 5
        eating disorders, 157, 158, 159
        movement disorders, 25
    diagnosing, 19
    risk factors, 20
    treatment, 20
Intermittent explosive disorder
    about, 215
    diagnosis, 216
    personal story, 216–217
    treatment, 220
Internalizing disorders, 213

Interpersonal therapy, 50, 63, 302–303, 306
Interventions, for addictive disorders, 226–227
Intoxication. *See* Substance intoxication and withdrawal
Involuntary hospital care, 299
Iron deficiency, 104, 157, 186

Kegel exercises, 163, 198, 200
Kleptomania, 221–222

Lamotrigine, 50, 311, 312
Language disorder, 5, 21
Language skills, autism spectrum disorder and, **7**
Language type, of frontotemporal neurocognitive disorder, 257–258
Levels, of intellectual disability function, **16–18**
Levodopa, 257
Lewy body disease, 259–261
Licensed clinical social workers, 297
Life changes. *See* Adjustment disorders; Prolonged grief disorder
Lithium, 38, 50, 311
Localized amnesia, 133
Lorazepam, 89

Major depressive disorder, 60–66. *See also* Persistent depressive disorder
    about, 60
    co-occurring with, 60
        anxiety disorders, 77
        bipolar disorders, 52
        depressive disorders, 70
        eating disorders, 155
        obsessive-compulsive disorders, 95, 99, 100, 103
        overview, 60
        personality disorders, 275
        trauma and stress disorders, 124

diagnosis and symptoms, 61
differential diagnosis, 35
grief vs., 59–60, 62
healthy mind and body for, 65–66
maintenance treatment, 65
personal story, 62–63
risk factors, 61, 85, 122
suicide risk with, 60, 61, 313
treatment, 63–65, 301, 313
Major depressive episodes, 46, 48, 51, 52–53, 54
Major neurocognitive disorder, 134, 244, **245–246**, 247, 264
Male hypoactive sexual desire disorder, 201
Manic-depressive disorder, 46. *See also* Bipolar I disorder
Manic episodes, 46, 47–48, 51
Manic mood, 38
MAOIs (monoamine oxidase inhibitors), 64, 309
Marijuana. *See* Cannabis
Marriage therapy. *See* Couples therapy
Meaning-centered therapy, 126
Medical transition, for gender dysphoria, 210–211
Medications. *See also* Psychiatric medications; Side effects
tips for using, 36, 308
Melatonin, 174, 311
Memantine, 252
Memory problems. *See* Amnesia, types of; Dementia and other memory problems
Menstruation disorders, 52, 68–70
Mental disorder, defined, xvi
Methylphenidate, 13, 14, 176, 234
Mild neurocognitive disorder, 134, 244–245, **245–246**, 247
Military (service members), xi, 114, 116, 134, 298
Mirtazapine, 193
Modafinil, 176

Monoamine oxidase inhibitors (MAOIs), 64, 309
Mood stabilizers
about, 50, 311–312
autism spectrum disorder and valproate, 8
for bipolar disorders, 50, 54
for disruptive and conduct disorders, 215
for eating disorders, 156
for personality disorder symptoms, 281
for psychotic disorders, 38
Mood swings (dramatic). *See* Bipolar disorders
Motor disorders
developmental coordination disorder, 5, 24–25
functional neurological symptom disorder, 140, 142–143
Parkinson's disease, 79, 256–257
stereotypic movement disorder, 25–26
tic disorders, 26, 95
"Multiple personality disorder." *See* Dissociative identity disorder

Naltrexone, 25, 222, 240
Narcissistic personality disorder, 278–279, 281
Narcolepsy, 174–176
about, 174
co-occurring disorders, 174, 184
diagnosis, 170, 175
risk factors, 175
treatment, 175–176
Negative symptoms, 31, 32, 38, 41
Neurocognitive disorders. *See also* Dementia and other memory problems
about, 244–245, **245–246**, 264
as amnesia cause, 134
as delirium risk factor, 247
medical conditions causing, 259–264

Neurodevelopmental disorders, 2–27
about, 3–4
key points, 26–27
types of, 4–26. *See also specific disorders*
Neuroleptic malignant syndrome, 310
Neuromodulation techniques
about, 301, **302**, 312–313
electroconvulsive therapy, 50, 54, 301, 313
transcranial magnetic stimulation, 301, 313
Neurotransmitters, 306
Nicotine, 234. *See also* Cigarette smoking
Nightmare disorder, 183
Nihilistic delusions, 30
Nonbizarre delusions, 38–39
NREM (non–rapid eye movement) sleep arousal disorders, 181–182
NREM (non-REM) sleep, 170–171
Nurse practitioners, 297
Nutrition and diet. *See also* Diet and exercise recommendations
counseling, for eating disorders, 159

Obsessive-compulsive disorder (OCD), 94–98
about, 94–95
co-occurring with, 95
anxiety disorders, 87
depressive disorders, 60
eating disorders, 149, 159
other obsessive-compulsive disorders, 99, 101
psychotic disorders, 32
diagnosis and symptoms, 95
personal story, 96–97
risk factors, 96
treatment, 97–98
Obsessive-compulsive disorders, 92–105
about, 93–94, 103
diagnosis, 99

healthy mind and body for, 94
key points, 104
suicide risk with, 99
treatment, 304
types of, 94–104. *See also specific disorders*
Obsessive-compulsive personality disorder, 280–281
Obstructive sleep apnea hypopnea
about, 176–177
co-occurring with, 177
narcolepsy, 174
diagnosis, 177
personal story, 177–178
risk factors, 178
treatment, 178–179
OCD. *See* Obsessive-compulsive disorder
Opioid use, sexual dysfunction and, 192–193
Opioid use disorder
about, 231
intoxication and withdrawal, **232**, 234
tips for relating to people with, 227
Oppositional defiant disorder, 164, 214–215, 220
Organizers (professional), 103
Orgasm issues. *See* Sexual dysfunctions
Outpatient clinics, 296–297, 299
Oxcarbazepine, 312

Pain and discomfort. *See* Somatic (physical) symptom disorders
Panic attacks, 76, 77, 78–79
Panic disorder
about, 76–77
co-occurring with, 77
bipolar disorders, 46
depressive disorders, 60
eating disorders, 149
psychotic disorders, 32
diagnosis and symptoms, 77

healthy mind and body for, 90
personal story, 78–79
risk factors, 78
treatment, 88–89
Paralysis
functional neurological symptom
disorder and, 140, 142–143
sleep paralysis, 174, 176
Paranoid personality disorder, 276–
277, 281
Paranoid thoughts
in borderline personality disorder, 270, 271
with delusions, 30
Paraphilic disorders, 284–292
about, 285–286
key points, 292
treatment, 291
types of, 286–291
Parasomnias, 181–185
Parent management training, 214,
218, 220, 221
Parkinson's disease, 79, 256–257
Paroxetine, 89, 115, 197
Pedophilic disorder, 286, 288–289,
291
Pee. *See* Enuresis
Peer-support groups, 315
Persecutory delusions, 30
Persistent (chronic) motor or vocal
tic disorder, 26
Persistent depressive disorder
about, 66
diagnosis and symptoms, 66–67
personal story, 67–68
risk factors, 67, 68
treatment, 68
Persistent insomnia, 171
Personality disorders, 266–282
about, 267–269
clusters of, **269**
co-occurring with,
anxiety disorders, 87
depressive disorders, 66
features of, 268–269, **269**

"multiple personality disorder,"
132–133
suicide risk with, 270, 304
tips for relating to people with,
281
treatment, 281, 304
types of, 269–280. *See also specific
disorders*
Personality traits, 267–269
Pervasive developmental disorder
not otherwise specified, 4, 23
Phobias. *See also* specific phobia
Physical problems. *See* Somatic
(physical) symptom disorders
Physician assistants, 297
Pica, 157
PMDD. *See* Premenstrual dysphoric
disorder
Polysomnography, 170
Poop. *See* Encopresis
"Poor insight," 35, 42, 94
Posttraumatic stress disorder
(PTSD), 108–117
about, 107, 108–109
co-occurring with,
anxiety disorders, 79, 87
dissociative disorders, 134
trauma and stress disorders,
124
coping with, 116, 117
diagnosis and symptoms, 109–
111, 112–113
in children under 6, 111–113
healthy mind and body for,
117
personal story, 114
risk factors, 113
as sexual dysfunction risk factor,
196
symptoms, 109–111
treatment, 115–116
for children, 117
Pragmatic (social) communication
disorder, 22–23
Pramipexole, 186, 257

Premature (early) ejaculation, 195, 196–197
Premenstrual dysphoric disorder (PMDD), 68–70
   about, 68–69
   co-occurring with, bipolar disorders, 52
   diagnosis and symptoms, 69
   healthy mind and body for, 70
   risk factors, 69–70
   treatment, 70
Premenstrual syndrome, 52, 68–69
Primary enuresis, 162
Prion disease, 263
Professional organizers, 103
Prolonged exposure therapy, 115
Prolonged grief disorder, 123–126. *See also* Grief
   about, 108, 123–124
   diagnosis and symptoms, 124–125
   major depressive disorder vs., 62
   personal story, 125–126
   risk factors, 125
   treatment, 126
Provisional tic disorder, 26
Psychiatric medications. *See also* Side effects
   about, **302**, 306–308
   anticonvulsant medications, including valproate, 8, 38, 50, 310, 311–312
   antidepressants (overview), 64, 185, 193, 309. *See also* Antidepressant medications
   antipsychotics, 35, 36, 38, 156, 193, 252, 281, 309–310
   hypnotic agents ("sleeping pills"), 174, 193, **226**, **302**, 310, 311
   mood stabilizers (overview), 50, 311–312. *See also* Mood stabilizers
   overview, **302**, 309–312
   sedatives medications (overview), 180, **226**, **232**, 310–311. *See also* Sedative medications

stimulants, 13, 175–176, **232**, 235, 312
Psychiatric nurses, 297
Psychiatrists, vii–x, 296. *See also* Psychiatric medications; Psychotherapy
Psychodynamic psychotherapy, 302
Psychologists, 296–297
Psychotherapy
   about, 301–302, **302**
   for adjustment disorders, 123
   for bipolar I disorder, 50
   for depersonalization/derealization disorder, 135–136
   for disruptive and conduct disorders, 220
   for elimination disorders, 161–162
   for gender dysphoria, 209–210
   for hoarding disorder, 103
   for major depressive disorder, 63, 64–65
   mental health care providers for, 296–297
   for obsessive-compulsive disorder, 95
   for paraphilic disorders, 291
   for somatic symptom disorders, 145–146
   therapeutic alliance in, 145
   types of, 63, 302–306. *See also* Behavior therapy; Cognitive-behavior therapy; Couples therapy; Family therapy; Group therapy
Psychotic disorders, 28–43
   about, 28–31
   features of, 30–31
   key points, 42–43
   suicide risk with, 32, 37, 40
   types of, 31–42, 235. *See also specific disorders*
PTSD. *See* Posttraumatic stress disorder
Purging episodes, 151, 153–154
Pyromania, 220–221

Ramelteon, 311
Rapid cycling, of manic, depressive, or hypomanic episodes, 46
Rapid eye movement. *See* REM behavior disorder; REM sleep behavior disorder
Reactive attachment disorder, 108, 126–127
Recovery-focused care, 32, 63, 299–300
Recovery tips, for addictive disorders, 227, 239–240
Recurrent (chronic) insomnia, 171
Referential delusions, 30
Regurgitation, 157–158
Relapse, 151, 238
   prevention, 302, 308, 309
     addictive disorders, 239–240, 241
     bipolar disorders, 49, 54
     conduct disorder, 218
     depression, 65
     enuresis, 163
     paraphilic disorders, 291
     schizophrenia, 36, 37, 43
Relaxation training, 135, 174, 291, 304
REM (rapid eye movement) sleep, 170–171
REM (rapid eye movement) sleep behavior disorder, 170, 174, 184–185, 256
Restless legs syndrome, 174, 186
Retrospective memory loss, 133
Rett's disorder, 4
Reward system, 225
Ropinirole, 257
Rumination disorder, 157–158

Schizoaffective disorder, 37–38
Schizoid personality disorder, 277, 281
Schizophrenia, 31–37
   about, 31–32
   co-occurring disorders, 32
   diagnosis and symptoms, 32–33, 34–35

differential diagnosis, 34–35
personal story, 33–34
"poor insight" and, 35, 42
treatment, 34–36
Schizophreniform disorder, 41
Schizotypal personality disorder
   about, 274–275
   diagnosis, 275–276
   risk factors, 275–276
   treatment, 281
Secondary enuresis, 162
Second-generation (atypical) antipsychotics, 35, 309. *See also* Antipsychotic medications
Sedative (anxiolytic or anti-anxiety) medications, including benzodiazepines
   about, 180, 310–311
   for addictive disorders, 240
   as addictive substance, **226**, 311
   for anxiety disorders, 89, 311
   intoxication and withdrawal, **232**
   sexual dysfunction and, 193, 194
   for sleep-wake disorders, 174, 181, 186
   for trauma and stress disorders, 121, 123
Seizures
   delirium and, 248
   functional neurological symptom disorder and, 140, 142–143
   as intellectual disability risk factor, 20
   neuromodulation techniques and, 313
   sedative withdrawal and, **232**
   traumatic brain injury and, 253, 254
   treatment of, 8, 50, 310, 311
Selective amnesia, 133
Selective serotonin reuptake inhibitor (SSRI) antidepressants
   about, 193, 198, 309
   for disruptive and conduct disorders, 215

Selective serotonin reuptake inhibitor (SSRI) antidepressants *(continued)*
  for dissociative disorders, 135
  for obsessive-compulsive disorders, 97, 99, 103
  for paraphilic disorders, 291
  for sexual dysfunctions, 197
  for trauma and stress disorders, 115
Sensate focus method, 198
Senses, loss of, 142–143
Separation anxiety disorder, 86–89
  about, 86–87
  diagnosis and symptoms, 87
  healthy mind and body for, 90
  personal story, 87–88
  risk factors, 87–88
  treatment, 88–89
Serotonin-norepinephrine reuptake inhibitors (SNRIs), 64, 309
Sertraline, 115, 194, 197
Service members (military), xi, 114, 116, 134, 298
Sex characteristics, 206, 207. *See also* Gender dysphoria
Sexual dysfunctions, 190–202
  about, 191–192
  healthy mind and body for, 202
  key points, 202
  substance/medication-induced, 192–195, 235
  types of, 192–201. *See also specific disorders*
Sexual masochism disorder, 286, 287–288, 291
Sexual response stages, 192
Sexual sadism disorder, 286, 288, 291
Side effects, of medication, 36, 307, 308
  antidepressants, 64, 309
  antipsychotics, 310
  benzodiazepines, 89, 311
  clomipramine, 97
  dopamine agonists, 257
  Lewy body disease and, 259–260

  memory problems as, 243
  mood stabilizers, 311–312
  selective serotonin reuptake inhibitors, 136
  sexual problems as, 193
  stimulants, 312
Sildenafil, 196
Situational insomnia, 171
Skin-picking disorder, 103, 104
Sleep apnea, 174, 176–180
Sleep cycle, 170–171
Sleep hygiene, 169, 187, 314
"Sleeping pills" (hypnotic agents), 174, 193, **226**, **302**, 310, 311
Sleep log, 170
Sleep paralysis, 174, 176
Sleep-related hypoventilation, 180
Sleep terrors, 181–182
Sleep-wake disorders, 168–188
  about, 169–171
  diagnosis, 170
  key points, 187–188
  treatment, 187
  types of, 171–186, 235. *See also specific disorders*
Sleepwalking, 174, 181–182
Smoking. *See* Cannabis; Cigarette smoking
SNRIs (serotonin-norepinephrine reuptake inhibitors), 64, 309
Social (pragmatic) communication disorder, 22–23
Social anxiety disorder, 84–86
  about, 84–85
  co-occurring with,
    bipolar disorders, 46, 52
    obsessive-compulsive disorders, 99, 100–101
  diagnosis and symptoms, 85
  as eating disorder risk factor, 154
  healthy mind and body for, 90
  personality disorders and, 276
  risk factors, 86
  treatment, 88–89
Social workers, 297

Somatic (physical) symptom
disorders, 138–146
about, 139–140
key points, 146
treatment, 145–146
types of, 140–145. *See also specific
disorders*
Somatic delusions, 30
Somatic symptom disorder
about, 140–141
diagnosis and symptoms, 141
risk factors, 141–142
treatment, 145
Specific learning disorder, 23–24
Specific phobia
about, 82–83
co-occurring with,
anxiety disorders, 86
bipolar disorders, 52
diagnosis and symptoms, 83–84
healthy mind and body for, 90
risk factors, 84
treatment, 88–89
Speech, loss of, 142
Speech sound disorder, 21–22
SSRI. *See* Selective serotonin
reuptake inhibitor antidepressants
Stereotypic movement disorder, 25–
26
Stimulants
about, 13, 312
for ADHD, 13
intoxication and withdrawal, **232**,
235
side effects, 312
for sleep-wake disorders, 175–176
Stool issues. *See* Encopresis
Stress
of caring for loved ones with
dementia, 252
defined, 75, 107, 128. *See also* Anxiety disorders; Obsessive-
compulsive disorders;
Trauma and stress disorders

depressive disorders and, 61, 67,
69
dissociative disorders and, 132,
134–135
eating disorders and, 151, 154,
157–158
elimination disorders and, 161–
162, 163
gambling disorder and, 237
psychotherapy for dealing with,
301–306
sexual dysfunctions and, 191, 196,
197, 201–202
sleep-wake disorders and, 171,
172, 175, 182, 187
somatic symptom disorders and,
141–143
stereotypic movement disorder
and, 25
stuttering and, 22
tic disorders and, 26
Strokes, 177, 179, 244, 261
Structural family therapy, 305–306
Stuttering, 22
Substance intoxication and withdrawal
about, 228, 231–235
delirium and, 246–247
diagnosis and symptoms, **231–
232**, 233
treatment, 240
Substance/medication-induced
mental disorders, 235–236
Substance/medication-induced sexual dysfunction, 192–195
about, 192–193
diagnosis, 193–194
personal story, 194
treatment, 194–195
Substance use disorders
about, 226, 228
co-occurring with,
anxiety disorders, 79, 85
bipolar disorders, 46, 52
depressive disorders, 60, 66, 70

Substance use disorders *(continued)*
  co-occurring with *(continued)*,
    disruptive and conduct disorders, 214, 220
    eating disorders, 149
    gambling disorder, 238
    obsessive-compulsive disorders, 99
    personality disorders, 272
    psychotic disorders, 32, 35, 37
    sleep disorders, 172, 180
    trauma and stress disorders, 124
  diagnosis, 229
  differential diagnosis, 35
  maintenance treatment, 308
  personal stories, 230–231
  recovery guidelines, 239–240
  risk factors, 83
  tips for relating to people with, 227
  as traumatic brain injury risk factor, 254
  treatment, 238–240, 308
Suicide prevention and hotline, 295–296, 299, 300, 304, 313
Suicide risk
  ADHD and, 14
  anxiety disorders and, 83
  bipolar disorders and, 46–47, 48, 52
  depressive disorders and, 60, 61, 313
  with dissociative disorders, 131, 132, 134
  eating disorders and, 151
  gender dysphoria and, 207
  obsessive-compulsive disorders and, 99
  personality disorders and, 270, 304
  psychotic disorders and, 32, 37, 40
  trauma and stress disorders and, 109, 122, 124, 125

Supportive psychotherapy, 63, 303
Support levels, for autism spectrum disorder, **7**
Systematic desensitization, 304
Systematized amnesia, 133

Tadalafil, 196
"Talk therapy." *See* Psychotherapy
Tardive dyskinesia, 310
TBI. *See* Traumatic brain injury
Tetracyclic antidepressants, 309
Therapeutic alliance, 145
Tic disorders, 26, 95
Tobacco, 202, **226**. *See also* Cigarette smoking
  intoxication and withdrawal, **232**
Toilet training, 161
Tolerance for substances, 228
Tourette's disorder, 26
Transcranial magnetic stimulation, 301, 313
Transient ischemic attacks (ministrokes), 261
Transvestic disorder, 286, 290–291
Trauma and stress disorders, 106–128
  about, 107–108
  key points, 128
  suicide risk with, 109, 122, 124, 125
  types of, 108–128. *See also specific disorders*
Traumatic brain injury (TBI), 252–255
  about, 252–253
  diagnosis, 253–254
  personal story, 254–255
  risk factors, 254
  treatment, 255
Traumatic events
  childhood neglect and trauma, 126–128, 154, 270
  defined, 107, 128
  reactions to, 107–108
Treatment essentials, 295–316
  about, vii–viii, ix–x, xi–xiii, xviii–xix, xx, 295
  caring for others, 315

diagnosis process, viii–ix, xvii–xviii, xix, xx, 298–299
early warning signs of mental health problems, 296
first visit with health care provider, 297–300
health care provider options, 295–297
interview portion of first visit, 298
key points, 315–316
recovery-focused care, 299–300
self-care of body and mind, 313–315
for suicide prevention, 295–296, 299, 300, 304, 313
treatment settings, 299
types of treatments, 300–313. *See also* Neuromodulation techniques; Psychiatric medications; Psychotherapy
Tricyclic antidepressants, 176, 309
12-step groups, 240
Typical (first-generation) antipsychotics, 35, 309. *See also* Antipsychotic medications

Urinary incontinence, 163. *See also* Enuresis
U.S. Department of Veterans Affairs (VA), 298

Valproate, 8, 38, 50, 311–312
Vaping, in teens, 234
Vardenafil, 196
Vascular neurocognitive disorder (dementia), 244, 261–262
Veterans, xi, 114, 116, 134, 298
Vitamin B, 243
Voyeuristic disorder, 285, 286, 291

Warning signs, for mental health problems, 296
Weight. *See also* Eating disorders.
    changes in, xvi
        major depression, 48, 61
        narcolepsy, 174
        premenstrual dysphoric disorder, 69
    healthy, 150, 151, 156–157
    low birthweight, 13, 23, 24, 96
    medication side effects and, 36, 64, 309, 310, 311, 312
    sleep apnea and, 176, 178
Withdrawal. *See* Substance intoxication and withdrawal
World Health Organization, on healthy weight and BMI, 150, 151
Worrying. *See also* Anxiety disorders; Obsessive-compulsive disorders
    and sleep hygiene tips, 187